www.wadsworth.com

wadsworth.com is the World Wide Web site for Wadsworth and is your direct source to dozens of online resources.

At *wadsworth.com* you can find out about supplements, demonstration software, and student resources. You can also send email to many of our authors and preview new publications and exciting new technologies.

wadsworth.com
Changing the way the world learns®

ENVIRONMENTAL HEALTH

THIRD EDITION

Monroe T. Morgan, B.A., M.S.P.H., Dr.P.H.
East Tennessee State University

Contributing Authors:

Darryl B. Barnett, Dr.P.H.
Eastern Kentucky University

Joe E. Beck, M.P.A.
Eastern Kentucky University

Franklin B. Carver, Ph.D.
North Carolina Central University

Trenton G. Davis, Dr.P.H.
East Carolina University

L. Fleming Fallon, Jr., M.D., Dr.P.H.
Bowling Green State University

Frank C. Gomez, Dr. P.H.
Touro University International

Larry Gordon, M.S., M.P.H.
University of New Mexico

Carolyn Hester Harvey, Ph.D.
Eastern Kentucky University

Albert F. Iglar, Ph.D.
East Tennessee State University

Maurice Knuckles, Ph.D.
Meharry Medical College

R. Steven Konkel, Ph.D.
Eastern Kentucky University

David McSwane, H.S.D.
Indiana University-Purdue University of Indianapolis

Burton R. Ogle., Ph.D.
Western Carolina University

Welford C. Roberts, Ph.D.
The Uniformed Services University of the Health Sciences

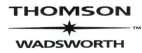

THOMSON
™
WADSWORTH

Australia • Canada • Mexico • Singapore • Spain • United Kingdom • United States

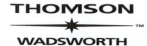

Publisher: Peter Marshall
Acquisitions Editor: April Lemons
Assistant Editor: Andrea Kesterke
Technology Project Manager: Star MacKenzie
Marketing Manager: Jennifer Somerville
Marketing Assistant: Mona Weltmer
Advertising Project Manager: Shemika Britt
Project Manager, Editorial Production: Karen Haga
Print/Media Buyer: Rebecca Cross
Permissions Editor: Bob Kauser

Production Service and Compositor: UG / GGS
  Information Production Services, Inc.
Text Designer: Sue Hart
Photo Researcher: Jane Sanders
Copy Editor: Julie Kennedy
Illustrator: UG / GGS Information Services, Inc.
Cover Designer: Belinda Fernandez
Cover Images: Maurer Photo and Photonica
Text and Cover Printer: Transcontinental Printing, Inc.

Printed in Canada
3 4 5 6 7 06 05

For more information about our products, contact us at:
Thomson Learning Academic Resource Center
1-800-423-0563
For permission to use material from this text,
contact us by: **Phone:** 1-800-730-2214
Fax: 1-800-730-2215
Web: http://www.thomsonrights.com

Library of Congress Control Number: 2002110784

ISBN 0-534-51717-X

Wadsworth/Thomson Learning
10 Davis Drive
Belmont, CA 94002-3098
USA

Asia
Thomson Learning
5 Shenton Way #01-01
UIC Building
Singapore 068808

Australia
Nelson Thomson Learning
102 Dodds Street
South Melbourne, Victoria 3205
Australia

Canada
Nelson Thomson Learning
1120 Birchmount Road
Toronto, Ontario M1K 5G4
Canada

Europe/Middle East/Africa
Thomson Learning
High Holborn House
50/51 Bedford Row
London WC1R 4LR
United Kingdom

Latin America
Thomson Learning
Seneca, 53
Colonia Polanco
11560 Mexico D.F.
Mexico

Spain
Paraninfo Thomson Learning
Calle/Magallanes, 25
28015 Madrid, Spain

Dedication

This book is dedicated to Monroe T. Morgan Jr., Marcus T. Morgan, Katrien and Natasha, Shirley L. Morgan, Marie Morgan Rice, and all of my former students.

This generation's contributions to society will not be determined by the height of our buildings, by how far we have traveled into space, by the depth of ocean explorations, by how many atomic bombs we have, or by how advanced our technology, but, rather, by how fast we learn to live together as human beings and how well we manage our fragile environment.

We environmentalists are partially responsible for overpopulation by controlling the vectors of and the causative agents of death. Therefore, it is incumbent upon us to be the advocators of family planning (preventing unwanted pregnancies) lest humanity become a hungry mass of people living in poverty with a pitiable quality of life.

Brief Contents

Contents

Preface

I wrote this text in an attempt to place the more important principles of environmental health in one convenient volume. This book does not concentrate on practices because practices change. The principles, however, seldom do. The third edition of *Environmental Health* is aimed at the human population rather than just the environmental sciences. Illustrating the requirements for human life with emphasis on the means for supporting human existence, *Environmental Health* also focuses on the need to control factors that are harmful to human life. Therefore, the chapters outline the requisites of life, water, air, food, space, and shelter. Furthermore, they address methods of controlling agents that cause disease (in other words, communicable disease control, wastewater treatment, swimming pool guidelines, solid waste management, insect and rodent control, radiation control, and environmental management). Chapter 16, "Environmental Planning," covers planning methods as they apply to environmental management. The goal of environmental management is to improve the quality of life for all people by creating a sustainable society.

The third edition of *Environmental Health* discusses such topics as national and international health politics, environmental ethics, global diseases, and global pollution. Comprehensive and expanded coverage of diseases, ecosystems and communities of species, environmental politics, Healthy People 2010, and environmental health topics—including new world population charts and statistics and global air pollution control—are included in this edition. Additionally, new end-of-chapter key terms with page references help to facilitate study, and Web site URL listings provide links to key environmental organizations. *Environmental Health* is accompanied by a comprehensive test bank featuring at least 20 multiple choice questions per chapter (available to qualified adopters; please consult your local sales representative for details).

Community health educators, public health officers, nurses, engineers, physicians, epidemiologists, veterinarians, physical education majors, environmentalists, and many other health professionals will benefit from this knowledge of the role of environmental health in public health and the health care system.

Acknowledgments

I hope this book serves as a medium for the transfer of knowledge to the keen minds of our future much needed environmental and public health professionals. In preparing this book, I received much encouragement from professionals throughout the United States. Friends, environmentalists, engineers, health educators, professors of public health, and other health professionals made valuable, logical, and well-founded suggestions. Without their input, this text would be of far less value. I am grateful to many friends for their suggestions and contributions.

The major contributors to the book are Dr. Albert F. Iglar, professor of environmental health, East Tennessee State University; my son Monroe T. (Monte) Morgan, Jr.; and my wife, Dr. Shirley L. Morgan, M.P.H., M.S.E.H., professor of public health at East Tennessee State University. Without their help, this text would not have become a reality. The assistance provided by Gordon Cox, M.S.E.H., superintendent of water and wastewater treatment for Johnson City, Tennessee, and Alex Broyles, M.P.H., is much appreciated. I am grateful to the graduate students and graduate assistants who helped with the preparation of this book, particularly Rhonda Cook and Hollie Williamson. Also, I give special thanks to East Tennessee State University for providing photos used in the text.

I wrote the first edition of *Environmental Health* after having taught and learned from students from the 50 states and 56 other countries. During the thirty-six years of teaching, I have found that environmental and public health needs are very similar around the world.

For the second edition, realizing there was value in numbers and in a variety of experiences, I asked several friends and former students to contribute by writing a chapter in their area of expertise. That change was so successful that for this edition, I again asked other friends and former students to contribute by writing a chapter. When people read this book, they will agree that the contributing authors have added greatly to the book.

For a job well done by the contributing authors (who are some of the top environmentalists in the world), I say thank you very much. To my many, many former students around the world, I say thanks for your success, because you have been instrumental in giving me the drive to do this book and you make me proud.

1

WORLD POPULATION

OBJECTIVES

☐ Explore the historical aspects of population growth.

☐ Define doubling time and explain its meaning.

☐ Discuss why the population explosion occurred.

■ Explain the effects of urbanization.

☐ Express the need for family planning and describe planning programs.

☐ Describe ideal population levels.

☐ Discuss how to manage human environments.

The world is approximately 4 billion years old. It has taken that many years to form the earth, develop its resources, store energy in various forms, and enable living organisms to adapt to the planet. More human-caused environmental degradation has taken place in the last 2,000 years than in all the previous years combined. Hence, we have a need for courses in planet management, ecosystems management, and human environment management. Humans should become the environment's protecting manager rather than its self-serving destroyer.

For almost 300,000 years, human overpopulation was not a problem. Drought, floods, famine, plagues, pestilence, and war kept early populations in check, as did the lack of heating for homes, the inability to preserve food, and the harsh wilderness. Couples had large families to be certain that some children survived these hazards.

When the Europeans discovered America, approximately 250 million people lived on the earth. By 1650, about 150 years later, the population had increased to about 500 million. In 1850, approximately 1.2 billion people lived on the earth. The population increased 70 years later (1920) to just under 2 billion people. In 1950, another one-half billion inhabitants were added to the earth. By 1980, the earth's population had reached approximately 4.5 billion. That is a more than fivefold increase in 300 years.

As the world population base became larger, the chance of a population increase became much greater. Today, the world population is approximately 6.2 billion and is increasing at a rate of 11.5 new children every second, which equates to 227,000 per day or 83 million people per year. This means future population increases will be even greater than from 1950 to 1980, when the increase amounted to only three times the population of the world in 1650. As of 2000, there were 21 cities in the world with more than 10 million people, 14 of these in developing countries. There are 24 more with over 5 million people. By 2030, global urban populations will be twice the size of rural populations. Over this period, developing countries will grow by 160%.

■ TABLE 1.1 ■

WORLD POPULATION DOUBLING TIME

Year	Estimated World Population	Years to Double
800 B.C.	5 million	1,500
A.D. 1650	500 million	200
A.D. 1850	1 billion	80
A.D. 1930	2 billion	45
A.D. 1975	4 billion	36
A.D. ??	8 billion	??

···············

DOUBLING TIME

The world population increased more rapidly about 200 years ago with the "Great Awakening," followed quickly by the industrial-medical-scientific revolution. At this time, sanitation, immunization, and other measures of environmental and public health greatly reduced the incidence of childhood and other communicable diseases. As three cases in point:

- In 1796 Edward Jenner demonstrated that immunizations could prevent smallpox.

- Walter Reed discovered that the *Aedes* mosquito spread yellow fever.

- Alexander Fleming later discovered penicillin.

Scientists refined flood control, improved agricultural and food technology, and developed public and environmental health practices. All of this activity served to control plagues and epidemics, which led to fewer children dying and a longer life expectancy. As a result, the world population grew rapidly. At the same time, a culture characterized by large families continued, with few of the children dying. Instead of two of twelve children surviving, now eight, nine, and ten, or more survived.

The **doubling time** for the world population is decreasing. Table 1.1 highlights this concept. To find the doubling time, we have to know the **growth rate**. The relationship between growth rate and doubling time is shown in Table 1.2.

■ TABLE 1.2 ■

RELATIONSHIP BETWEEN GROWTH RATE AND DOUBLING TIME

Growth Rate	Years to Double
0.5%	140
0.8%	87
1.0%	70
2.0%	35
3.0%	24
4.0%	18
5.0%	14
7.0%	10
10.0%	7

As the graphs in Figure 1.1 and Figure 1.2 reveal, developing nations tend to have greater potential than developed countries for population increase. This is because the potential for population increase becomes greater as more females enter childbearing ages. The women have babies, and the population base and growth potential increase even further. Many developing countries have a "stair-step" or "Christmas tree" graph. In contrast, when the population of developed nations is plotted, it gives a "stovepipe" effect. More babies are born in countries that are less able to provide food and the other requirements of life.

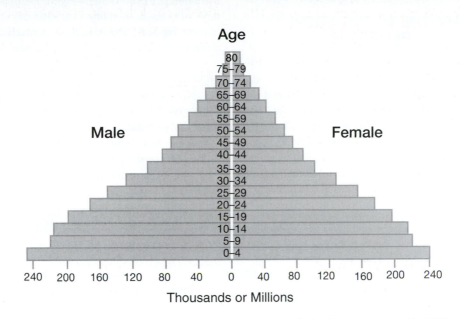

Source: United Nations, Demographic Indicators of Countries: Estimates and Projections, as assessed in 1980

FIGURE 1.1 Age structure pyramid for developing countries.

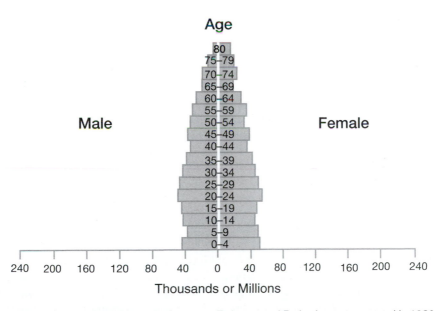

Source: United Nations, Demographic Indicators of Countries: Estimates and Projections, as assessed in 1980

FIGURE 1.2 Age structure pyramid for developed countries.

WHY THE POPULATION EXPLOSION?

Most microorganisms multiply by simple division. One organism divides into two. Each of the two divides into four, four into eight, and so on. Let's assume that these organisms are being grown in a test tube that will hold only a certain number of organisms. Also assume that the organisms divide every 24 hours. If the test tube were inoculated with one organism on day one and the test tube, because of available life requirements, would support only 365 days of growth, then one year (365 days) after inoculation the test tube would have reached its maximum carrying capacity. If asked when the test tube would be one-half full, the answer would be on the 364th day.

Now let's assume that on the 200th day one-fourth of the microorganisms were to die. In that case the population on day 365 would not have filled the test tube. A longer incubation period would be required to fill the test tube. If, then, on day 240 another one-fourth of the population were

■ TABLE 1.3 ■

POPULATION DATA FOR SELECTED COUNTRIES, 2001

Country/Region	Population (millions)	Births per 1,000 pop.	Deaths per 1,000 pop.	Growth Rate (%)	Life Expectancy Male	Life Expectancy Female	Population (sq. mi.)
WORLD	6.137	22	9	1.3	65	69	118
Africa	818	38	14	2.4	52	55	70
Egypt	69.8	28	7	2.1	65	68	181
Ethopia	65.4	14	15	2.4	51	53	153
Ghana	19.9	32	10	2.2	56	59	216
Kenya	29.8	34	14	2.0	48	49	133
Nigeria	126.6	41	14	2.8	52	53	355
South Africa	43.6	25	14	1.2	52	54	99
Tanzania	36.2	41	13	2.8	52	54	99
Zaire	56.6	47	16	3.1	45	50	59
ASIA	3,720	22	8	1.4	65	68	303
Bangladesh	133.5	28	8	2.0	59	59	2,401
China	1,273.3	15	6	0.9	69	73	344
India	10,330	26	9	1.7	60	61	814
Iran	66.1	18	6	1.2	69	71	108
Japan	127.1	9	8	0.2	67	73	872
Philippines	77.2	29	6	2.2	64	70	666
Saudi Arabia	21.1	35	6	2.9	66	69	25
Thailand	62.4	14	6	0.8	70	75	315
Turkey	66.3	22	7	1.5	67	71	221
Vietnam	78.7	20	6	1.4	63	69	623
LATIN AMERICA	525	24	6	1.7	81	76	144
Argentina	37.5	19	8	1.1	70	77	35
Brazil	171.8	22	7	1.5	65	72	52
Chile	15.4	18	5	1.3	72	78	53
Colombia	43.1	24	6	1.8	68	74	98

(continued)

POPULATION DATA FOR SELECTED COUNTRIES, 2001

Country/Region	Population (millions)	Births per 1,000 pop.	Deaths per 1,000 pop.	Growth Rate (%)	Life Expectancy Male	Life Expectancy Female	Population (sq. mi.)
Cuba	11.3	14	7	0.6	73	77	264
Mexico	99.6	24	5	1.9	73	78	132
Nicaragua	5.2	35	6	3.0	66	70	104
Peru	5.2	35	6	1.8	66	71	53
Venezuela	24.6	25	5	2.0	70	76	70
NORTH AMERICA	316	14	9	0.5	76	81	41
Canada	31.0	11	8	0.3	76	81	8
United States	284.5	15	9	0.6	74	80	77
EUROPE	727	10	11	−0.1	74	80	82
Denmark	5.4	13	11	0.2	74	74	322
France	59.2	13	9	0.4	75	83	278
Germany	82.2	9	10	−0.1	74	81	597
Hungary	10.0	10	14	−0.4	66	75	278
Italy	57.8	9	10	−0.0	76	82	497
Poland	38.6	10	10	0.0	68	78	310
Spain	39.8	10	9	0.0	74	82	204
Sweden	8.9	10	11	−0.0	77	82	51
United Kingdom	600	12	11	0.1	75	80	635
CARIBBEAN	37	21	8	1.3	66	71	410
Bahamas	0.3	21	5	1.5	70	75	58
Barbados	0.3	14	9	0.5	70	75	1,620
Grenada	0.1	21	8	1.3	63	66	678
Jamaica	2.6	20	5	1.5	70	73	624
Puerto Rico	3.9	15	7	0.8	71	80	1,139

Source: Population Reference Bureau, Inc.

to die, it would take an even longer period of time to fill the test tube. The death rate slows population growth. Expressed simply, more deaths equate to a smaller population base.

The preceding analogy can be related to the history of the earth's human population. Floods, droughts, famine, war, and disease have all decreased the population. A prime example of population reduction is the pandemic of bubonic plague, which occurred in 430 B.C., and again in the A.D. 1340s, destroying approximately one-fourth of the world's population each time. Now think of the epi-

demics and pandemics of smallpox, cholera, typhoid fever, malaria, yellow fever, typhus, tuberculosis, rabies, and others that have occurred. Imagine how these diseases have kept the world population in check until recent years.

Modern knowledge in medicine, public and environmental health, and agriculture have started to control epidemics. More and more people are living, and living longer. This includes more unwanted, unplanned babies living, and living longer than ever before. Thus, the world is experiencing a human population explosion. Table 1.3 gives

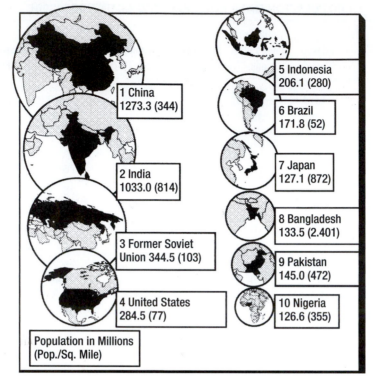

Source: World Population Data Sheet, Population Reference Bureau, Inc., 2001

FIGURE 1.3 Most populous nations.

population data for selected countries. In 1996, one-third of humanity was under 15 years of age. The most populous nations are shown in Figure 1.3. The four most populous nations provide a study in contrasts. First-rated China has an average of 344 people per square mile, and India has a crowded 814. By comparison, Russia and the United States have only 22 and 77 people per square mile, respectively.

In some cultures having large families is socially desirable. The reasons vary. Some want children for working in agriculture, some for military advantage, and some for political influence. Some religions advocate large families and teach that the higher being will provide for the children.

EFFECTS OF OVERPOPULATION

In 1791, Thomas Malthus predicted that the population would grow faster than the ability to feed it. This was before automation of farm life, tractors, synthetic fertilizer, mass transport, freeze-drying, and so forth. He suggested that populations grow geometrically (2–4–8) while food production increases arithmetically (1–2–3–4). Malthus's claim may have an unsettling amount of truth.

Despite several decades of agricultural research aimed at increasing the worldwide food supply, one of every three persons living in poor, underdeveloped countries is unable to find enough to eat. These people suffer from starvation and from diseases such as kwashiorkor, which results from a lack of protein. In many cases large families cannot provide for the children properly and do not receive much-needed health, social, and agriculture services from their government.

Approximately 12 million people die of starvation each year. Thirty million more people each year suffer from diseases made worse by hunger. More disturbing perhaps is that in the areas hit hardest by hunger, the population doubles every 17 to 30 years.

EFFORTS TO CONTROL OVERPOPULATION

Over the years some effort has been made to address the problem of the large family. Slogans such as "zero population growth" (**ZPG**), "Stop at two," "How dense can we get?" and others have brought attention to the need for controlling family size.

Until about 1984, the United States encouraged worldwide population planning and control activities. It gave financial support for family planning programs and research groups such as the International Planned Parenthood Federation and the United Nations Fund for Population Activities (UNFPA). In 1985, however, the U.S. government, as a result of pressure from anti-abortion groups, cut off its contributions to UNFPA.

To combat the problem of overpopulation, some countries have legalized abortion and others have offered free sterilization. Many countries have offered educational programs explaining the need for family planning and discussing the undesirable effect of having too many children. These programs, along with other factors, have been somewhat effective in stabilizing the population in developed countries, but not in less-developed countries (LDCs) where parents are less able to support the children.

Overpopulation causes the majority of undesirable environmental, social, economic, educational, and political problems. Many of the problems discussed in this book are the result, either directly or indirectly, of overpopulation. Improved technology

and a desire for affluence, linked with an ever-increasing population, are factors in causing environmental degradation. The denser the population, the more severe are the potential environmental problems. Many of these have occurred because of refusal to manage the effluent from the affluent society, resulting in noise pollution, hazardous waste, air pollution, water pollution, land pollution, ozone depletion, and crowded, dirty cities.

URBANIZATION

In 1800, approximately 6% of the U.S. population lived in urban areas. By 1900, 45% resided in cities. Presently, over 73% of the U.S. population lives in urban areas. Worldwide, approximately 28% of the population lived in cities in 1950. By A.D. 2020, more than 66% is expected to live in cities, as shown in Figure 1.4. Around the world, as families continue to produce more children than they can support, the children flock to the cities in search of work, where they find that computer-operated machinery and other modern technology reduce the need for manpower. This leads to unemployment, and unemployment leads to problems such as drug addiction, alcoholism, crime, and homelessness. In some cities in developing countries, babies are born in the streets, live there, and die there, with little potential for advancement.

Much of the population growth is the result of unplanned and unwanted pregnancies. Many cities do not provide shanty towns and slums with adequate drinking water, sanitation, food, health care, housing, schools, and jobs because of a lack of money and the fear that improvements will attract even more of the rural poor. In 1994, a report indicated the world's biggest cities were growing by one million a week. Figure 1.4 shows the largest urban agglomerations in the world.

THE NEED FOR FAMILY PLANNING

If we could determine what percentage of the babies born in the world each year are not wanted by the parents, the result no doubt would be embar-

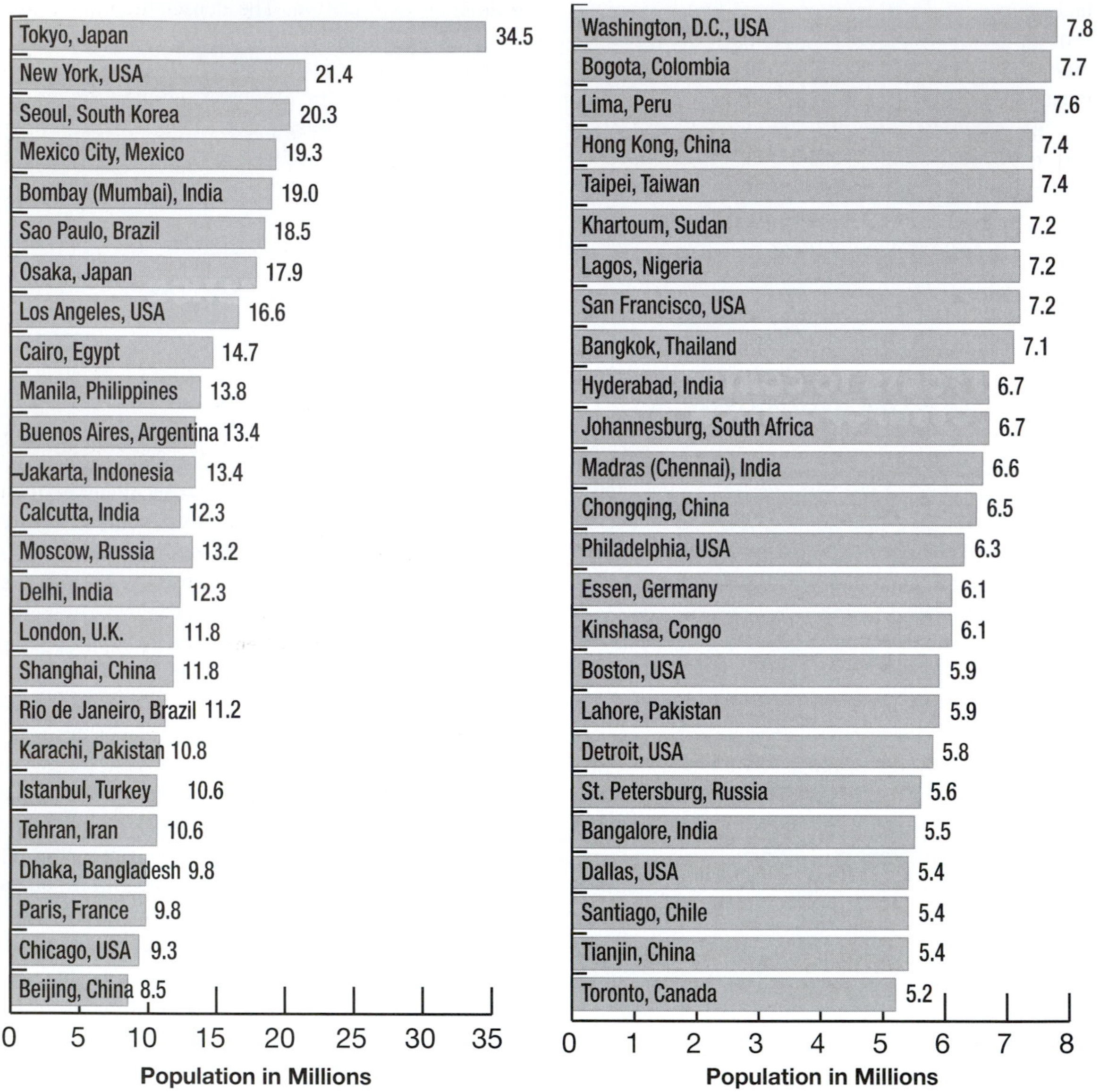

City	Population in Millions
Tokyo, Japan	34.5
New York, USA	21.4
Seoul, South Korea	20.3
Mexico City, Mexico	19.3
Bombay (Mumbai), India	19.0
Sao Paulo, Brazil	18.5
Osaka, Japan	17.9
Los Angeles, USA	16.6
Cairo, Egypt	14.7
Manila, Philippines	13.8
Buenos Aires, Argentina	13.4
Jakarta, Indonesia	13.4
Calcutta, India	12.3
Moscow, Russia	13.2
Delhi, India	12.3
London, U.K.	11.8
Shanghai, China	11.8
Rio de Janeiro, Brazil	11.2
Karachi, Pakistan	10.8
Istanbul, Turkey	10.6
Tehran, Iran	10.6
Dhaka, Bangladesh	9.8
Paris, France	9.8
Chicago, USA	9.3
Beijing, China	8.5

Population in Millions

City	Population in Millions
Washington, D.C., USA	7.8
Bogota, Colombia	7.7
Lima, Peru	7.6
Hong Kong, China	7.4
Taipei, Taiwan	7.4
Khartoum, Sudan	7.2
Lagos, Nigeria	7.2
San Francisco, USA	7.2
Bangkok, Thailand	7.1
Hyderabad, India	6.7
Johannesburg, South Africa	6.7
Madras (Chennai), India	6.6
Chongqing, China	6.5
Philadelphia, USA	6.3
Essen, Germany	6.1
Kinshasa, Congo	6.1
Boston, USA	5.9
Lahore, Pakistan	5.9
Detroit, USA	5.8
St. Petersburg, Russia	5.6
Bangalore, India	5.5
Dallas, USA	5.4
Santiago, Chile	5.4
Tianjin, China	5.4
Toronto, Canada	5.2

Population in Millions

Source: Thomas Brinkhoff, *Principal Agglomerations and Cities of the World*

FIGURE 1.4 World's 50 most populous cities, 2001.

rassingly high. Further, if we could determine how many of the children are not wanted in large families that cannot provide a good quality of life for the children, we probably would be shocked at the high percentage. The point is that each day many of the children born throughout the world in developed and undeveloped countries alike are not planned and are unwanted. In many of these families each new baby adds to the misery of the family. Unwanted babies are a fundamental problem because overpopulation is the underlying cause of so many of the economic, social, and environmental problems.

John D. Rockefeller, III, an authority on population and family planning, remarked in a speech to the U.S. House of Representatives that in the long run no substantial benefits will result from further growth of the nation's population. Rather, population growth is an intensifier and multiplier of many problems: environmental, social, political, economic. The nation has nothing to fear, he said, from a gradual approach to population stabilization.

He further explained that a strong moral consensus is fundamental to any consideration of the population problem. The realization is increasingly widespread that the motivation behind population control is not negative and restrictive but, rather, positive and constructive. The concern is not merely about numbers and fertility; it is about human values and the quality of human life.

Thus, one real need is to prevent unwanted pregnancies around the world. The developed nations need to help their own people and those in less-developed countries to prevent unwanted babies by providing parent education programs. If the number of unwanted babies could be reduced around the world, overcrowding no longer would be a problem and many of the ensuing environmental, political, social, and economic problems would be greatly reduced. A family planning program should be available worldwide to everyone who wants it. Parents should be able to have only the number of children they want.

In Planned Parenthood programs, the two general approaches to decreasing birthrates are family planning and economic growth. Planned Parenthood programs are offered in many developed nations and in some developing countries. Throughout the world, lowering the birthrate is the focus of most of these efforts to control population growth. By 1986, programs to reduce birthrate were available to 91% of the population of less-developed countries. The effectiveness and sources of funding for these programs vary from country to country.

President Lyndon B. Johnson once said: "Let's act on the fact that five dollars spent on population control is equivalent to one hundred dollars in economic growth." Economic development may reduce the number of children parents want by enhancing education, providing economic security, and reducing the need to consider children a substitute for old-age social security. In developed parts of the world such as in North America, Europe, and Japan, family planning services help to reduce the population growth rate by providing guidance to parents in regulating family size and health.

Family planning clinics vary as to the method of preventing pregnancies (progestational agents). However, the methods listed and described in Table 1.4 are the most common methods.

....

IDEAL POPULATION LEVELS

Dr. Theodore Morgan and other ecologists believe that the world population will continue to grow until the quality of life has been degraded for all. Some ecologists believe the growth will continue until it becomes necessary to create a "super" world agency to set and enforce ideal population for the various countries. Some believe that the ideal population level will be determined by factors such as each country's per-capita income, quality of life, length of growing season, topography, quality of waste disposal facilities, size, technology level, and quality of air and water. Even if optimum population levels are determined, though, the difficulty will be in enforcing the population levels.

Something will keep the population in check. What will it be? Will it be the aforementioned "super agency"? Will it be that the air becomes so polluted as to cause population control? Will the 1% of fresh water become so polluted that it spreads diseases and keeps the population in check? Or will the population control agent be toxic materials? Will it be the lack of food? Will it be the lack of sufficient space? Will it be that the lack of space and resources causes war? Or will it be that nations share and support family planning programs and prevent unwanted pregnancies? Let us hope that the population is controlled by family planning rather than by starvation.

SUMMARY OF BIRTH CONTROL/CONTRACEPTIVES

Type	Male Condom	Female Condom	Spermicides Used Alone	Diaphragm with Spermicide	Cervical Cap with Spermicide
Estimated Effectiveness	About 85%	An estimated 74%–79%	70%–80%	82%–94%	At least 82%
Risks	Rarely, irritation and allergic reactions	Rarely, irritation and allergic reactions	Rarely, irritation and allergic reactions	Rarely, irritation and allergic reactions; bladder infection; very rarely, toxic shock syndrome	Abnormal Pap test; vaginal or cervical infections; very rarely, toxic shock syndrome
Protection Against Sexually Transmitted Diseases	Latex condoms help protect against sexually transmitted diseases including herpes and AIDS	May give some protection against sexually transmitted diseases including herpes and AIDS; not as effective as male latex condom	Unknown	None	None
Convenience	Applied immediately before intercourse; used only once and discarded	Applied immediately before intercourse; used only once and discarded	Applied no more than 1 hour before intercourse	Inserted before intercourse; can be left in place 24 hours, but additional spermicide must be used if intercourse is repeated	Can remain in place 48 hours; not necessary to reapply spermicide upon repeated intercourse; may be difficult to insert
Availability	Non-prescription	Non-prescription	Non-prescription	Prescription	Prescription

Oral Contraceptive Pill	Implant Norplant	Injection (Depro-Provera)	IUD	Periodic Abstinence (NFP)	Surgical Sterilization
97%–99%	99%	99%	95%–96%	Highly variable, perhaps 53%–85%	Over 99%
Blood clots, heart attacks, strokes, gallbladder disease, liver tumors, water retention, hypertension, mood changes, dizziness, and nausea; not for smokers	Menstrual cycle irregularity; headaches, nervousness, depression, nausea dizziness, change of appetite, breast tenderness, weight gain, enlargement of ovaries and/or fallopian tubes, excessive growth of body and facial hair; may subside after first year	Amenorrhea, weight gain, and other side effects similar to those with Norplant	Cramps, bleeding, pelvic inflammatory disease, infertility; rarely, perforation of the uterus	None	Pain, infection, and, for female tubal ligation, possible surgical complications
None	None	None	None	None	None
Pill must be taken on daily schedule, regardless of frequency of intercourse	Effective 24 hours after implantation for approximately 5 years; can be removed by physician at any time	One injection every 3 months	After insertion, stays in place until physician removes it	Requires frequent monitoring of body functions and periods of abstinence	Vasectomy is a one-time procedure usually performed in a doctor's office. Tubal ligation is a one-time procedure performed in an operating room
Prescription	Prescription; minor outpatient surgical procedure	Prescription	Prescription	Instructions from physician or clinic	Surgery

MANAGING HUMAN ENVIRONMENTS

The **biosphere** (atmosphere, hydrosphere, and lithosphere) is the same size it was thousands of years ago. The population and its desire for affluence, however, have greatly increased over those thousands of years. With more people living longer and demanding more resources, and consequently producing more effluent, a greater demand is being placed on the environment each year. That demand is divided into two primary areas:

1. The environment must provide food, water, air, fuel, building materials, and other resources for a rapidly expanding population.
2. The environment also must dispose of the effluent (sewage, refuse, hazardous waste, industrial waste, etc.) from the population.

Thus, the solutions might be found in two approaches:

1. Family planning services around the world may prevent unwanted babies.
2. Worldwide environmental management may enable humans and other animals to enjoy a good quality of life—thus a sustainable society.

The remainder of the book will explore the problems and their solutions.

SUMMARY

The earth's population is approximately 6.2 billion and increasing at a rate of about 83 million per year. This necessitates careful planning and management to ensure a healthy environment for the future. The developing countries have a greater potential for population growth coupled with more current health problems. For example, they are still dealing with epidemics of infectious diseases such as dengue, cholera, typhoid fever, malaria, yellow fever, typhus, and tuberculosis—diseases that have been largely eradicated in developed countries through proven sanitation and other environmental measures.

The two broad approaches to managing human environments are (a) family planning and (b) environmental management. The later encompasses means of controlling agents that cause disease, including, among others, water and wastewater treatment, insect and rodent control, and radiation control.

KEY TERMS

Biosphere, p. 12	Growth rate, p. 2
Doubling time, p. 2	ZPG, p. 7

REFERENCES

Brown, Lester R., et al. 1997. *State of the World.* Norton & Company, New York.

Chiras, Daniel D. 1994. *Environmental Science—A Framework for Decision Making.* 4th ed. The Benjamin/Cummings Publishing Company.

"50% of Population to Live in Cities." *World Population News Service Popline.* 1995, Nov.–Dec. Vol. 17.

James, Ian. 1999. *Planet Earth.* Dempsey Paris, Bath, England.

Morgan, Monroe T. "A World Fit To Live In." *World Health.* May 1989.

"World Population Data Sheet." *Population Reference Bureau, Inc.* 2001. Washington, DC.

2

FUNDAMENTALS OF ENVIRONMENTAL HEALTH

OBJECTIVES

■ Identify and discuss what determines our health.

■ Enumerate the requirements for the growth of microorganisms.

■ Name the causative agents of disease.

■ Define environmental health and give a brief history of its evolution.

■ Discuss the portals of entry for microorganisms.

■ Determine the methods of spreading disease.

What determines the health of the over 6 billion people in the world? What determines the health of the 284.5 plus million individuals who currently inhabit the United States of America? The pressure of rising health care costs increases the need to understand the determinants of health and the role of environmental health in the health care system.

. . . .

DETERMINANTS OF HEALTH

The four basic determinants of health are hereditary or biological factors, medical care, lifestyle, and environment.

Hereditary or Biological Factors

Major aspects of human biology are controlled by genetics. A person may be healthy in every other way but may have inherited conditions such as hemophilia, diabetes, mental retardation, various eye problems, lack of **resistance to disease**, or any number of other problems. Research now provides evidence that traits inherited from the mother and father can influence whether a person becomes addicted to alcohol or another drug.

Medical Care

The medical care we receive during our lifetime can determine our health. For example, if a child develops streptococcal infection and does not get medical care, he or she might develop a rheumatic heart condition. Or if a youngster breaks a limb and does not receive proper medical care, he or she might end up with a deformed arm or leg.

Two main aspects of health care affect everyone. One is *technology*, which has been in the limelight for several decades. Ever-increasing technological advances have added productive years to thousands of lives. An example is the computerized axial tomograph or CAT scanner. Other technological devices include sophisticated equipment for kidney patients, artificial organs, monitoring instruments for the human fetus, and electrocardiograph devices worn by patients to detect an oncoming heart attack. These amazing instruments have captured the fancy of society and added to the cost of health care. The second trend in health care is a heightened interest in medical self-help. This trend is illustrated by self-examination of the skin, breasts, mouth, eyes, and nails, for example.

Lifestyle

Lifestyle has a lot to do with one's health. Lack of sleep and rest reduces our resistance to infections and leads to bodily degeneration. A person who has an excellent body but eats poorly, does not exercise enough, and smokes and drinks heavily may develop health problems rather quickly. Many Americans indulge in high-fat, high-sugar, high-salt, low-fiber diets. Moving sidewalks, escalators, elevators, cars, buses, and other means of transportation may be leading people to an early demise. Like all muscles, the heart muscle will waste away if it is not used vigorously. Considering these factors, it is rather easy to understand why heart disease is the number-one killer in the United States.

In contrast to the overindulgence and sedentariness that characterize modern American life, the lifestyle in underdeveloped countries has its own health problems. People in some areas of the world suffer malnutrition and other diseases caused by the lack of proper nutrition. Overall, infectious diseases dominate the health problems of underdeveloped countries.

Of all the health determinants, lifestyle may be the easiest to control. Even so, it will require much effort.

Environment

Considering the world's population as a whole, the environment affects people's health more strongly than any of the other determinants. The environment encompasses the water we drink, the food we eat, the air we breathe. In the past, because of poor environmental management, many people died from environmentally related diseases such as typhoid fever. Some estimates, based on morbidity and mortality statistics, indicate that the impact of the environment on health status is as high as 80%.

Human evolution has been selective. People have adapted to the environment in which they found themselves by, for example, producing biological defenses against disease. People also have acquired intelligence, knowledge, and expertise that have allowed them to make significant changes in the environment, thereby creating conditions that lessen the likelihood of disease. This is accomplished mainly by controlling the causative agents of disease while they are still in the environment, before they reach people, so the body does not have to produce defenses and therapeutic measures are not required.

Environmental health practice, as the name suggests, refers to the relationship between environment and health. Some important elements of environmental health practice—the first line of defense against disease—include:

- Water quality management—ensuring that potable water is available through treatment of water supplies

- Human waste disposal—disposing of human wastes in septic tank systems and sewage treatment plants

- Solid and hazardous waste management—treating and disposing of solid and hazardous wastes

- Rodent control—removing potential harborage and sources of food

- Insect control—utilizing natural, biological, and other methods to reduce insect populations

- Milk sanitation—ensuring that all milk for human consumption is produced under sanitary conditions and is pasteurized

- Food quality management—maintaining surveillance over food from the farm to the consumer so as to prevent contamination

- Occupational health practice—assuring a healthy and safe work environment

- Interstate and international travel sanitation—preventing the spread of communicable diseases between states and nations

- Air pollution control—reducing the emissions of pollutants into the atmosphere

- Water pollution control—reducing the effects of industrial and other waste on water supplies and recreational areas by the pretreatment of industrial and domestic waste

- Environmental safety and accident prevention—designing into the environment features, such as pedestrian ramps, that promote safety or compensate for people's inadequacies

- Noise control—abating high noise levels in industrial settings and in the community to avoid health degradation

- Housing hygiene—promoting housing conditions necessary for the physiological and psychological well-being of inhabitants

- Radiological health control—controlling radiation sources such as X ray equipment, nuclear fission plants, and radioactive waste

- Recreational sanitation—monitoring the environment to prevent unsafe conditions at swimming pools and other recreational facilities

- Institutional environmental management—preventing the spread of nosocomial infections

- Land use management—zoning to direct land use to desirable purposes

- Product safety and consumer protection—ensuring that drugs, toys, appliances, and the like are safe for human use

- Environmental planning—applying environmental design to minimize human stress and accidents

Throughout history, reduction of disease and discomfort has been accomplished largely by altering the environment. Therapeutic programs are glamorous and tend to be successful in obtaining funding and publicity. Prevention programs—the preferable approach—many times are taken for granted and are not funded properly.

················

REQUIREMENTS FOR THE GROWTH OF MICROORGANISMS

We live in a world that harbors countless microorganisms that are both beneficial and detrimental to humans. The disease-causing, or pathogenic, microbes are of particular concern. By better understanding what specific elements are necessary for these biological causative agents of disease to live and reproduce, one also learns ways of controlling their populations. The following eight elements are required for the growth of microorganisms:

1. Favorable oxygen supply
2. Favorable temperatures
3. Food
4. Moisture
5. Favorable pH
6. Favorable osmotic pressure
7. Absence of toxic materials
8. Space

Many microorganisms need free *oxygen* from the atmosphere to survive. These organisms are termed **aerobic**. Other microorganisms live in environments void of free oxygen. These are **anaerobic** organisms. You may have been in a swampy area where a sulfur or "rotten egg" odor was prevalent. Often these odors can be attributed partly to the presence of anaerobic bacteria degrading organic matter. Some bacteria are **facultative**. They have the ability to exist either aerobically or anaerobically, depending on their surrounding environment. For instance, if we were to place an aerobic microbe in an environment without free oxygen, it would not survive. A facultative organism, however, would tolerate a range of oxygen levels.

Growth of microorganisms can be controlled by manipulating their oxygen requirements. For example, because aerobes may hasten the spoilage of perishable products, many foods are vacuum-packed to prevent the growth of aerobic organisms. This oxygen-free environment, however, is desirable for anaerobic organisms such as *Clostridium botulinum*, which produces a toxin that causes botulism.

Microorganisms also have specific *temperature* requirements for growth. At optimal temperature, a cell multiplies most rapidly. At temperature extremes—both very hot and very cold—the cell may stop growing and reproducing or simply die.

Three groups of microorganisms—thermophilic, mesophilic, and psychrophilic—grow in various temperature ranges:

1. **Thermophilic**, or "heat-loving" **microbes**, grow from roughly 113°F to 167°F.

2. **Mesophilic** organisms prefer a medium range roughly from 69°F to 113°F.

3. **Psychrophilic**, or "cold-loving" organisms, grow in a range of roughly 19°F to 68°F.

The psychrophilic organism spoils foods under refrigeration. The bacteria most important from a public health standpoint are the mesophilic because they thrive and reproduce at approximately 98.6°F and thereby are able to exist within the human body.

Temperature affects all of us. At room temperature (68°F to 70°F) we feel comfortable and active. If we lower the temperature to 38°F or below, however, our bodies are stressed and we shiver in an attempt to raise the body's temperature. Because the body is exothermic (must emit heat), we also feel stressed when the surrounding temperature is 98°F or above and the body perspires to cool itself. If the temperature is sufficiently hot or cold for an extended time, the human body becomes overstressed, possibly leading to death.

The same principle applies to bacterial microbial populations, although they are less adaptive to temperature changes than humans are because they lack control of their own cell temperature. By controlling the temperature around the organisms, we can control their activity or induce their death. Through refrigeration or heating of foods, we control many of the pathogens responsible for food-borne illness. This can be accomplished by adjusting the temperature out of the mesophilic range—preferably colder than 45°F or hotter than 140°F. An adage concerning food is "Keep it hot, keep it cold, or don't keep it long."

Food is another growth requirement for microorganisms. Microbes consume many of the foods we eat. Just as with humans, limiting the amount of food available to a microbial population limits growth. By thoroughly cleaning and sanitizing eating utensils and equipment, we can greatly control the growth of many disease-causing microorganisms in restaurants, institutions, and homes.

Just as humans require water, microorganisms require some degree of *moisture*. Removing moisture from an environment inhibits the growth of microorganisms. Freeze-drying, or desiccating, is a good example of such a measure used to protect food. Commercially, the process involves removing moisture from a food product and then sealing the product in a moisture-proof container. The waxed paper surrounding the dried corn flakes you may have eaten for breakfast is a product of this principle. Once you open a package of dried food, the moisture in the air may spark the growth of microorganisms that can spoil the product.

Microorganisms also require a *favorable pH* in order to reproduce. Pathogenic organisms generally prefer a neutral pH, around 7.0. A sudden change in pH, either above or below 7.0, will kill the organisms. Many foods are potentially hazardous to humans because their neutral pH readily supports the growth of pathogens. We can reduce the potential hazard of foods such as cream-filled pastries and mayonnaise by adding vinegar or an acid to reduce the pH. But who likes vinegar in cream-filled pies? Therefore one refrigerates them to create an unfavorable environment for pathogens.

Favorable osmotic pressure is a requirement for growth of microorganisms. Living microbes have a certain saline, or salt, concentration within their cells. Placing these organisms in a surrounding environment that contains either more or less salt than in the organism (cell) itself inhibits their growth. A saline solution surrounding a cell that has a salt concentration equal to that within the cell is **isotonic**, and provides optimum growth potential. The condition in which the saline content within the cell is greater than that of the surrounding environment is called **hypo-**

tonic. A hypotonic environment allows moisture to enter the cell by the process of osmosis. This results in the cell expanding to the extent that it may rupture in a process called **plasmoptysis**. In a third condition, termed **hypertonic**, the environment surrounding the organism contains a greater saline concentration than that within the organism. When a food is surrounded by a high concentration of salt, the moisture within the cells escapes, by the process of an attempt to dilute the surrounding salt solution. This loss of water is called **plasmolysis**. Removing the moisture from food by creating a hypertonic environment produces conditions unfavorable for microbial growth within a food, such as with salt-cured ham.

Another requirement for microbial growth is the *absence of toxic materials*. Many commonly used household products limit the growth of microorganisms because they introduce some form of toxin to the organisms' surrounding environment. Common bleach, spray disinfectants, and various phenol-based compounds are examples. Most municipal water treatment facilities use chlorine as a disinfectant. Chlorine, or a "bleach solution," also is used in food service establishments to sanitize equipment and utensils that may harbor pathogens. Further examples of materials used to kill microorganisms are antibiotics, Mercurochrome, and iodine.

Finally, *space* is a requirement for growth of microorganisms. Microbes multiply exponentially and will heavily populate an area within a short time (several hours for some species if all requirements for growth are favorable). Imagine what would happen if the entire population of a small city of 30,000 people were forced to live in an area no larger than a football field! They would have no means of human waste disposal and only a limited food supply. Within a short time, starvation would occur and disease would spread, causing the population to die out. A similar condition exists within a colony of microorganisms. Without enough space, concentrations toxic enough to kill the vast majority of the colony occur.

Optimal Growth Curve

Altering any of the above growth requirements can result in effectively controlling the growth of microorganisms detrimental to humans. If all requirements for microbial growth exist, the individual organisms will multiply as shown in Figure 2.1. As this figure shows, a phase of acclimation first occurs when a small group of organisms is introduced to a new environment. The stresses of new surroundings may induce death of a few organisms.

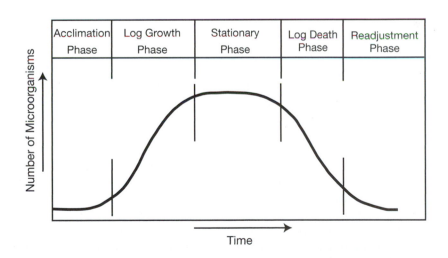

FIGURE 2.1 Optimal growth curve.

The remaining microbes, however, adjust and reproduce. This brings the microbes to the next phase, the logarithmic growth phase.

In the logarithmic, or log, growth phase the organisms reproduce exponentially. One cell divides and becomes two, two then divide and become four, four cells divide and become eight, and so on until the numbers reach the billions. As the numbers of organisms increase, the amount of their toxic waste products also increases. This, coupled with a reduced amount of nutrients available, slowly kills the organisms. The stage in the cycle when the death of the organisms (death rate) equals that of new organisms being produced (birthrate) is called the stationary phase. In this phase the number of organisms reaches equilibrium and remains stationary until onset of the logarithmic death phase.

When the microbes have consumed most or all nutrients and the microbial waste products reach a concentration high enough to destroy the majority of the population, they find themselves in the logarithmic death phase. The overcrowded environment is unfavorable for growth because of lack of food, changes in pH, waste buildup, crowding, and other factors. A few organisms may remain after the log death phase. These organisms proceed into the readjustment phase, as the few surviving organisms of the log death phase attempt to reproduce. Enough nutrients may be available to allow some cell division; however, the death rate will equal or slightly surpass the reproduction rate for a time. Eventually new nutrients may be introduced into the environment and the existing toxins may be diluted. Upon creation of new, favorable environmental conditions, the organisms enter once more into the phase of acclimation. This optimal growth curve cycle can continue time and time again if favorable growth conditions allow.

Controlling Microbial Growth

Communicable diseases pose major public health problems around the world. If a society is to control communicable disease, people must know what is necessary for microbial growth so it can be limited or stopped by creating an unfavorable environment. Much of environmental health practice involves creating an unfavorable environment for the causative agents of disease and thereby creating a favorable environment for humans. In other areas of public and environmental health, such as wastewater treatment, cheese processing, and others, we need to create a favorable environment for microorganisms so they will degrade the waste or produce the food.

....
CAUSATIVE AGENTS OF DISEASE

Now let's take a look at the etiology or causative agents of disease. Specifically, what can make humans sick? The major **causative agents** of disease may be classified as:

1. Biological agents
2. Chemical agents
3. Physical agents
4. Too little of something
5. Too much of something
6. Hereditary disease
7. Stress
8. Diseases of unknown cause

Biological agents of disease are living things that cause disease because of their effect on characteristics associated with life. These agents are living cells that induce a wide range of illnesses. Nearly every year an individual is overcome by some type of *virus*, of which the common cold is an example. Pathogenic *bacteria* can cause diseases such as salmonellosis, typhoid, and strep throat. Other biological disease-causing classifications are fungi (yeasts and molds) and protozoa, such as those that produce some sexually transmitted diseases. Metazoa, such as tapeworms, form the final class. These are illustrated in Figure 2.2.

Chemical agents of disease are substances that cause disease because of their mass or ability to engage in chemical reactions with molecules in the body. Most living quarters contain chemicals that can cause disease. Commonly found items include cleansing agents, pesticides, petroleum products, and chemical drain openers. On crowded interstate highways, too, we view hazardous chemicals in transport. Consequently, the proper treatment, storage, and disposal of these chemicals is of critical concern to human health.

Viruses

Poliovirus
0.03 micrometers
in diameter

Bacteria

Tuberculosis bacilli:
3 micrometers long

Syphilis spirochetes:
10 micrometers long

Fungi

Yeast: causes vaginal infections; 5–30 micrometers long

Mold: causes athlete's foot, ringworm, and jock itch

Protozoa

Trichomonas: causes genital tract infections; 50–100 micrometers long

Amoeba: causes amoebic dysentery

Metazoa (Helminths or parasitic worms)

Tapeworm:
up to several meters long

FIGURE 2.2 Classes of pathogens.

Physical agents of disease do their damage by transferring energy to the body, damaging body cells. For example, ionizing radiation, at high doses, can endanger life, whether its source is X ray equipment or a nuclear power plant. Noise-producing physical agents also may harm health. Excessive noise can lead to hearing loss, hypertension, heart disease, strokes, and other problems. The sun's ultraviolet radiation is another disease-causing physical agent. In America, a dark tan often is associated with physical beauty. The skin tans as a defense against the sun's rays. Overexposure to these rays can damage the skin and cause severe illness or death.

Too little of, or a lack of, certain life-supporting materials can cause disease. For example, if a person takes no food or water into the body, the body weakens and eventually dies. The body requires specific nutrients, without which illness occurs. For example, a lack of Vitamin D will cause rickets, and a lack of niacin in the diet (protein-calorie deficiency) causes kwashiorkor.

Just as too little of certain substances can cause disease, so can *too much of* something. For instance, an individual who eats improperly and excessively may become obese. Even over-consumption of a life-supporting chemical such as water can be fatal. Likewise, a high concentration of carbon dioxide, a natural respiratory waste product, can cause illness.

Heredity can be a disease agent. Poor eyesight, hemophilia, and baldness are examples of inherited genetic traits.

Stress may cause ill health. From time to time, everyone comes under stress. Demands and expectations placed upon a person sometimes are so great that the body becomes overstressed. This may result in emotional disorders, hypertension, stroke, and even heart attack, all of which may lead to death. Stress also can contribute to alcoholism and other drug abuses when individuals prefer to intoxicate their system to "cope" with stressful situations. We would do well to consider the effects of stress upon us and learn to manage it so that we can live healthier lives.

A final causative agent of disease is the *unknown*. Many people die each year because of environmental pollutants working synergistically with other factors. Cancer is a serious problem in today's society. Because it is caused by exposure or a series of exposures to carcinogens in the environment years before the onset of disease, in many cases the exact cause of illness may never be known.

The main three causative agents of disease—biological, chemical, and physical agents—can be spread in several ways—by air, water, food, insects, fomites (inanimate objects such as forks and door knobs) and animals. In environmental health, many programs address the need to control the causative agent while it is in the environment before it gets to the public and causes disease.

HUMAN DEFENSE AGAINST DISEASE

Throughout recorded history, people have tried to reduce suffering and disease. The first attempts consisted of treating the symptoms of disease. Common practice to treat a fever was to put on more quilts and blankets (*after* the causative agent had entered the body) and raise the temperature until the fever "broke." (We now know that the microorganism causing the fever was killed by the high temperature.) In the next era, we administered a medicine such as penicillin to kill the organism *after* it had entered the body. The third era is characterized by immunization. Doctors give people an antigen to cause the body to produce antibodies against specific biological agents. This provides **immunity** so *after* that agent enters the body, the antibodies will kill it. In each of the cases mentioned above, except immunization, the treatment is administered *after* the causative agent had entered the body.

In the mid-19th century, Edwin Chadwick of England and Lemmuel Shattuck of Boston, Massachusetts, wrote reports on the sanitary condition of the environment. They emphasized the environment's role in spreading germs and other causative agents of disease. Thus, they recommended sanitation programs to control the causative agents of disease while they are in the environment, *before* they get inside humans. They also in essence recommended the basis for the fourth era and the first line of defense—environmental health practice. Figure 2.3 lists the four lines of defense through the health care system.

I. Humans' First Line of Defense Against Disease (Environmental Management)

  A. Water quality management
  B. Proper human waste disposal
  C. Solid and hazardous waste management
  D. Rodent control
  E. Insect control
  F. Milk sanitation
  G. Food quality management
  H. Occupational health practice
  I. Interstate and international travel sanitation
  J. Air pollution control
  K. Water pollution control
  L. Environmental safety and accident prevention
  M. Noise control
  N. Housing hygiene
  O. Radiation control
  P. Recreational sanitation
  Q. Institutional environmental management
  R. Land use management
  S. Product safety and consumer protection
  T. Environmental planning

II. Humans' Second Line of Defense Against Disease (Public Health and Preventive Medicine)

  A. Proper nutrition
  B. Good personal health practice
  C. The body's reflexes, chemicals, and barriers
  D. Routine health and dental check-up
  E. Application of health education
  F. Other

III. Humans' Third Line of Defense Against Disease (Public Health and Preventive Medicine)

  A. Phagocytosis (a natural process)
  B. Immunity (active and passive)

IV. Humans' Fourth Line of Defense Against Disease (Curative Medicine)

  A. Surgery
  B. Administering of medication and radiation
  C. Diagnosing by means of various lab methods
  D. Corrective dentistry
  E. Corrective therapy (i.e., speech, hearing, respiratory)

FIGURE 2.3 The role of environmental health in the health care system.

First Line of Defense

Humans have adapted to the environment in which they live by producing biological defenses against disease. As a direct result of this evolution, humans also have acquired knowledge that allows them to make significant changes in the environment. Some changes, such as pollution, may make conditions less suitable to humans. Controlling both man-made and naturally occurring environmental conditions through environmental health practices provides people's first line of defense against disease— *prevention*. Thus, environmental health practice is people's first line of defense against disease, by applying environmental technology and the arts and sciences to control the causative agents of disease in the environment before they reach humans.

Second Line of Defense

Humans' second line of defense against disease is the body's adaptation to prevent the agents of disease from becoming established within it. The human body possesses mechanisms that deter disease-causing agents from entering. The first of these is the *skin* covering the body. Because the skin is relatively impermeable, it provides a barrier to many pathogenic agents. Another protective mechanism consists of the *mucous membranes*, which secrete a protective fluid that traps undesirable particles, microorganisms, and so forth. In addition, *cilia*—tiny, hairlike projections—sweep mucus and other debris from the respiratory tract. The body also has *secretions of various fluids*, such as saliva, gastric juice, and perspiration, containing protective substances. For eye protection, tears contain lysozyme, a chemical that dissolves the cell walls of certain bacteria. Ears secrete wax that keeps out undesirable particles. Reflexes (involuntary movements in response to stimuli) also play a role in protecting the body from disease.

Nutrition is an important defense because an adequately nourished body is able to better resist disease. An individual's *condition of health* also plays a major role in preventing disease. Individuals who are ill are more susceptible to infection by other disease-inducing agents than are persons who are in a good state of health.

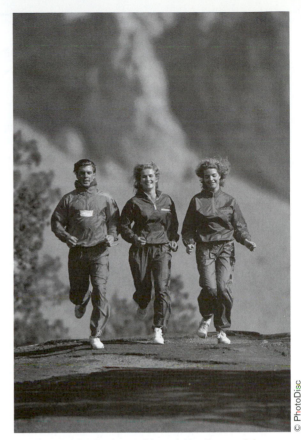

© PhotoDisc

Lifetime participation in aerobic activities is one of the most important factors in preventing cardiovascular disease.

Third Line of Defense

If the aforementioned defense mechanisms are insufficient and do not destroy or prevent the entrance of the causative agent, humans have a third line of defense consisting of phagocytosis and immunity.

Phagocytosis is the primary *cellular* defense against disease. In this defense, cells show an adaptive response to the presence of pathogenic agents. Shortly after pathogens invade host cells, the *inflammation response* occurs. This is characterized by reddening of the affected area because of capillary dilation; swelling from the leakage of plasma through the capillary walls, which increases the fluid content of the tissue; heat/fever, which aids the destruction of some pathogens by increasing the action of white blood cells; and pain, indicating to the body that a problem is present.

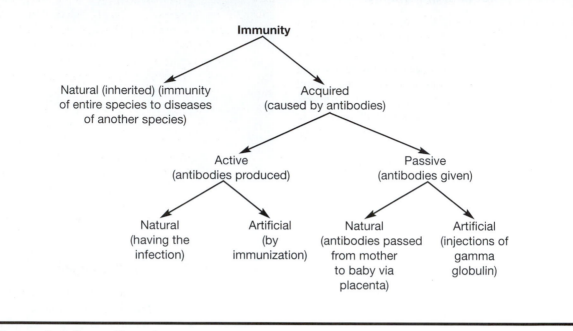

FIGURE 2.4 Types of immunity.

During inflammation, phagocytes destroy the pathogens. In the blood system these phagocytes are leukocytes, or white blood cells. In the lymphatic system microphages and macrophages carry out the process. If phagocytosis fails to destroy the pathogens—possibly because of the number and character of the invading organism—the body has to depend on its own immunity. There are many diseases for which one cannot be immune. Immunity results from the presence of an antibody that attacks the specific microorganism (causative agent). The substance that stimulates the production of antibodies in the body is known as the antigen.

Immunity is divided into categories according to how the body acquires it.

1. *Active immunity*, in which the body of the user produces the antibodies. Active immunity can be acquired either naturally or artificially. To possess naturally acquired active immunity, the individual first must have an infection for which the body produces antibodies, with or without symptoms. To pos-sess artificially acquired active immunity, the body must be vaccinated with weak or attenuated germs, which stimulate antibody production without causing observable signs of disease, or be vaccinated with toxoids. Treatment of the body with a toxoid stimulates the production of antibodies without producing the signs and symptoms of the disease.

2. *Passive immunity*, in which the required antibodies are not produced within the body that needs them but are produced within some other body. Passive immunity can be either naturally or artificially acquired also. Naturally acquired passive immunity results from the transfer of antibodies across the placenta from the immune mother to the fetus or via the mother's colostrum to her breast-fed infant. Artificially acquired passive immunity is acquired from antibodies or antitoxin received from the blood serum of immune human beings or animals. Figure 2.4 depicts the forms of immunity.

Fourth Line of Defense

Admittedly, when one is in pain, sick, or needs surgery, the curative medicine professionals—doctor, dentist, nurse—are the professionals one wants to see. Whenever possible, however, people would rather the pain or sickness be prevented by the environmental health, public health, or preventive medicine specialist. Thus, because of high cost of curative medicine, there is greater need for environmental health practice, public health, and preventive medicine than ever before. The public would rather pay for prevention than the fourth line of defense—curative medicine. *To help the public better understand the role of environmental heath practice in the health maintenance system, this book emphasizes the need to prevent disease rather than have to utilize curative medicine.*

....

PORTALS OF ENTRY

If microorganisms are to have an optimum chance to establish themselves, they must enter a host through an appropriate portal. They must enter the body where they can obtain nutrients, reproduce, and ultimately cause disease. As examples, organisms such as salmonella enter the body through the host's digestive tract, whereas the virus of yellow fever enters via an insect (mosquito) bite. The major portals of entry to the human body are the skin, the reproductive organs, the respiratory tract, and the digestive tract.

The Skin

About two square meters of skin, on average, insulate the human body—obviously providing a large surface area for the potential ingress of chemicals and microorganisms. The outermost layer of skin, the **epidermis**, provides the defense against the entry of causative agents of disease. The epidermis is essentially a layer of dead skin in the process of being shed, much like an insect molts or sheds its outer protective layer—although with humans the process is much more gradual. Cuts or breaks in the epidermis weaken this protective layer, allowing microorganisms to enter. This can occur, for example, when a blood-sucking insect feeds by puncturing the epidermis and, in the process of taking blood, introduces contaminated materials or pathogens into the body.

Hair follicles originate in the dermis. They are spread throughout the epidermis, concentrating on the arms, legs, and head. Oils and sweat are secreted through pores of the epidermis. When the ducts becomes clogged, as with acne, the sweat and oils are retained and the area becomes swollen or festered. Bacteria and other microorganisms colonize the affected area, resulting in increased blood flow to the area, elevated body temperature, and more white blood cells to fight the infection. The infection may become widespread, causing severe and possibly permanent damage to the affected areas.

The Reproductive Organs

Human reproductive organs—in males, the penis and testicles; in females, the uterus and ovaries—require direct bodily contact to transmit disease. Sexually transmitted diseases—syphilis, gonorrhea, AIDS, and others—rely on intimate contact because the infecting organisms are incapable of survival outside the body. Preventive measures include prophylactics or abstention from sex.

The Respiratory Tract

The human respiratory tract consists of the nose, trachea, left and right bronchi, bronchioles, alveolar ducts, and alveoli. Microbes such as *Mycobacterium tuberculosis*, which causes tuberculosis, enter the body through the nose (or mouth) during breathing and progress into the lung tissues. Eventually they reach the bloodstream, where infection may spread throughout the body. Often, foreign materials (smoke, dust) precipitate lung diseases as they, too, irritate sensitive lung tissue. Black lung disease, common to coal miners and others who inhale large quantities of dust or dirt, is a good example.

The human respiratory tract is not totally defenseless against disease. The nose and lungs have a number of protective devices. Nose hair filters inhaled air, removing large particulate matter that otherwise might become imbedded in the lungs. The mucus of the nose and throughout the respiratory tract traps various other foreign matter, both macroscopic (visible to the naked eye) and microscopic. The cough reflex is yet another protective device, triggered when the nasal sinus passages are irritated. Cilia—short, fingerlike projections that line the inner wall of the lungs and have a constant and coordinated motion—trap fine particles that escape the nasal filter.

The Digestive Tract

The human digestive tract consists of the mouth, esophagus, stomach, small intestine, and large intestine. Harmful microorganisms can enter the digestive tract in food or liquids. Many food-borne and liquid-borne diseases such as botulism and salmonellosis, respectively, are quite severe.

The digestive tract has two basic protective mechanisms. The mucous membrane that lines the digestive tract is hard for pathogens to penetrate and entraps many particles. Also, the digestive tract secretes chemicals, the most important of which are:

- HCl, secreted by the stomach, which kills some germs and incapacitates others;
- bile, secreted by the liver into the intestinal tract, which has an antiseptic power because of its high pH.

If the built-in defenses against disease fail, modern medicine has developed to such an extent that the disease can be treated successfully in many cases. The body, however, is not people's first line of defense. Environmental health practice—controlling the causative agent before it can reach a person—precludes a challenge to the body's defenses and renders the advances of modern medicine unnecessary. Environmental health practice, therefore, arguably is the most important consideration in preventing disease in the future.

The offering of environmental health courses and public health education (particularly family planning) were not part of the education systems until recent years. Hence, there is a critical need for environmental and public health education if mankind is to avert disaster.

"In the spring of 1992, the National Academy of Sciences and the Royal Society of London, in a first ever joint statement, warned that 'if current predictions of population growth prove accurate and patterns of human activity on the planet remain unchanged, science and technology may not be able to prevent either irreversible degradation of the environment or continued poverty for much of the world.'" When we consider the above statement, we realize such problems as crime that are precipitated by crowdedness, poverty, and hunger; the need for environmental and public health education become apparent.

The author developed the first BSEH environmental health curriculum to be accredited in 1969. At that time, it was felt and hoped that by now an environmental health course would be a core class in high school and college. That has not come to be, but if we are to have a healthy, sustainable society, the material presented in this book must become part of educational systems and the news media.

> There is a midrashic story: A man is on a boat. He is not alone, but acts as if he were. One night, he begins to cut a hole under his seat. His neighbors shriek: "Have you gone mad? Do you want to sink us all?" Calmly, he answered them, "What I'm doing is none of your business. I paid my way. I'm only cutting a hole under my seat." What the man will not accept, what you and I cannot forget, is that all of us are in the same boat.
>
> —Elie Wiesel, winner of the
> Nobel Peace Prize in 1986

SUMMARY

The four basic determinants of health are: hereditary (biological) factors, medical care, lifestyle, and environment. Examples of biologically inherited diseases are hemophilia and juvenile diabetes. Medical care now includes advanced technologies such as electrocardiographs, CAT scans, kidney dialysis, artificial organs, and many others.

Among lifestyle contributors to disease are inadequate rest and sleep; smoking; heavy drinking; high-fat, high-sugar, high-salt, low-fiber diet; sedentariness; and stress. Conversely, sound nutrition, regular exercise, adequate rest and sleep contribute to a healthy life.

The causative agents of disease can be classified as biological, chemical, and physical agents. These enter the body via the skin, reproductive organs, respiratory tract, and digestive tract. Thus, diseases can be spread by air, water, food, insects and other animals, and fomites. Environmental measures concentrate on controlling these factors while they are still in the environment and before they enter the human body. Leading environmental practices that promote health include water quality management, sanitary waste disposal, rodent and insect control, milk sanitation, air and water pollution control, and others.

KEY TERMS

Aerobic, p. 15

Anaerobic, p. 15

Causative agents, p. 18

Environmental health practice, p. 14

Epidermis, p. 23

Facultative, p. 15

Hypertonic, p. 17

Hypotonic, p. 16

Immunity, p. 20

Isotonic, p. 16

Mesophilic, p. 16

Microbes, p. 16

Phagocytosis, p. 21

Plasmolysis, p. 17

Plasmoptysis, p. 17

Psychrophilic, p. 16

Resistance to disease, p. 13

Thermophilic, p. 16

REFERENCES

Earth Journal. 1993. Buzzworm Books, Boulder, CO.

Floyd, P. A., S. E. Mimms, and C. Yelding-Howard. 1995. *Personal Health: A Multicultural Approach.* Morton Publishing, Englewood, CO.

Morgan, M. T. May/June 1975. "Environmental Health Practice and Medicine." *Journal of Environmental Health.* Vol. 37, No. 6.

————. 1988. "The Role of Environmental Health in the Health Care System." Proceedings, Inaugural World Congress of Environmental Health, Sydney, Australia.

Ng, Lorenz, and D. L. Davis. 1981. *Strategies for Public Health: Promoting Health and Preventing Disease.* Van Nostrand Reinhold, New York.

Prescott, P. M., J. P. Harvey, and D. A. Klein. 1996. *Microbiology.* Wm. C. Brown. Dubuque, IA.

3

CHRONIC AND COMMUNICABLE DISEASES

OBJECTIVES

- Discuss and give examples of chronic diseases.
- Define communicable diseases and explain their significance.
- Discuss disease transmission.
- Explain how communicable disease is transmitted by intestinal discharges.
- Explain how diseases are spread by nose and throat discharges.
- Define zoonoses and explain them.
- Discuss the diseases spread by vectors.

Until about 1950, infectious diseases—typhoid fever, cholera, the dysenteries, bubonic plague, the typhus fevers, and tuberculosis—were major killers in the United States and throughout the world. As a result of advances in public health, environmental health, and medicine in developed countries, these diseases have come under control. Yesterday's success, however, often brings tomorrow's challenge. As we enjoy a longer life span—a mark of progress—we also face another group of basic health problems, the chronic degenerative diseases.

CHRONIC DISEASES

Chronic diseases are those that linger. They are degenerative because they cause progressive destruc-

tion of human tissue. Whereas many of the **communicable** diseases have a sudden onset, chronic diseases usually have a poorly defined beginning. Many times their causes are unclear, and often they develop over a long time. Usually they reduce the body's function for a long time and their treatment is costly because those afflicted require long-term care.

COMMUNICABLE DISEASES

Throughout history communicable diseases have caused much suffering and millions of deaths. They still comprise the leading causes of death in most underdeveloped countries of the world. Communicable diseases are those that are contagious. An individual

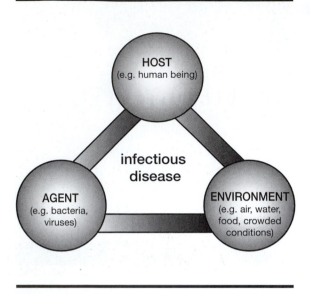

HOST
(e.g. human being)

infectious disease

AGENT
(e.g. bacteria, viruses)

ENVIRONMENT
(e.g. air, water, food, crowded conditions)

FIGURE 3.1 Conditions for communicable diseases.

■ **TABLE 3.1** ■

COMPARISON OF CHRONIC AND COMMUNICABLE DISEASES

	Chronic Diseases	Communicable Diseases
Causes	Often lifestyle- or environmentally related	Exposure to a biological agent
Timeline	Slow, insidious onset; long-lasting	Usually acute; sudden onset
Outcome	Often no recovery, gradual deterioration or degeneration	Relatively rapid recovery in most cases

with cancer is not a threat to others because the population will not catch the causative agent of cancer directly from the afflicted individual. Cancer is not communicable. In contrast, an individual with a communicable disease can transmit the causative agent to the surrounding population via the respiratory tract. The cold virus, for example, exits the body of one individual and another can contract it. The disease is communicable. We can avoid the transmission of many communicable diseases by understanding their modes of transmission and by controlling the causative agents in the environment before they reach humans. Figure 3.1 illustrates the conditions necessary for infectious or communicable diseases.

· · · · · · · · · · · · · · ·

COMPARING CHRONIC AND COMMUNICABLE DISEASE

Chronic and infectious diseases may be differentiated along at least three dimensions. One consists of their causes. Although some causes can be shared—for instance, genetic, nutritional, economic, and social factors—they more often are different. The onset of infectious diseases requires exposure to a biological agent such as a virus. In

contrast, the major causes of chronic diseases are related to lifestyle. These factors include exercise level, nutritional intake, and use of tobacco and alcohol. In recent years we have learned that the environment, particularly the occupational environment, plays a major role in the initiation and aggravation of certain chronic diseases.

A second dimension is the timeline associated with chronic and infectious diseases. Infectious diseases usually are **acute**. They have sudden onset and last for a relatively brief time. Chronic diseases, on the other hand, often have a slow and insidious onset and last for a long time. Sometimes the person never recovers.

A third dimension consists of the outcomes associated with chronic and infectious diseases. Given proper treatment, most persons with infectious diseases recover within a relatively brief time. In contrast, people with chronic diseases usually remain ill for a long time—often the remainder of their lives. Because getting people to change their lifestyles is difficult, chronic diseases associated with lifestyle are more difficult to control than communicable diseases, for which the person may be administered medication to control the causative agent. Table 3.1 gives a comparison of chronic and communicable diseases.

Health professionals, particularly health educators, strive to motivate people to alter their lifestyles so as to enhance their health. They stress the benefits of walking, running, biking, hiking, stress control, stopping smoking, and reducing alcohol consumption.

Industries follow guidelines of the Environmental Protection Agency (EPA) to prevent air and water pollution.

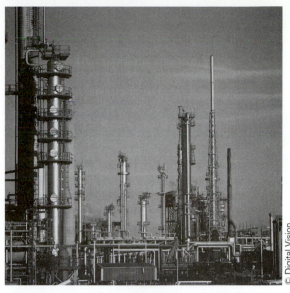

Industries follow guidelines of the Environmental Protection Agency (EPA) to prevent air and water pollution.

ENVIRONMENTAL INFLUENCES

The chronic diseases for which the causative agent is environmentally induced by outdoor pollution or in the occupational setting, along with the "lifestyles diseases," are a particular challenge in the United States and other developed nations today. In 1964 the World Health Organization first stated that, on the basis of the available evidence, 60% to 80% of all cancer was caused, at least in part, by natural and man-made carcinogens in the environment (Higginson and Muire, 1976). More recent research has supported the accuracy of that conclusion.

Most experts agree that human health and longevity are determined to a great extent by the "health" of the environment in which we live. Russell Train, former administrator of the Environmental Protection Agency, commented:

> Today we are plagued with chronic diseases that an increasing number of health experts believe are largely caused by environmental factors—where we work or live, our habits, diets, or lifestyles. The more sophisticated and sensitive our monitoring devices become, the more data we accumulate on health effects of pollutants and other agents in the environment, the worse things look. The battle against disease must increasingly be fought, not simply in the hospitals and doctors offices, but in our streets, homes, and work places; in our air and water; in our food and products; and in our habits and lifestyles. Such a shift in emphasis will require a searching re-examination, and radical revision of popular understanding of, and public approach to, health care and disease. If environmental disease is becoming "the disease of the century," as it appears to be, then environmental protection must become the most important ingredient in our national health programs. (Willgoose, 1979, p. 1)

Individuals do not have as much control over environmental influences on health as they do on lifestyle. Instead, environmental control is the responsibility of everyone, but environmental agencies such as the Environmental Protection Agency (EPA) and state health and environmental departments. The chapters in this book address environmental management as it relates to the prevention and control of infectious diseases as well as the chronic and degenerative diseases.

Throughout history, communicable diseases have been feared as much as anything including war. They have killed more people than any other cause of death. Now they reappear as a great cause of fear. Anthrax, as used by terrorists, has killed several people. Plague, cholera, yellow fever, typhus fever, smallpox, and others are possible biological agents of war.

METHODS OF DISEASE TRANSMISSION

Let's look at some methods of spreading diseases, the foremost of which are via air, water, food, **fomites**, animals, and insects (see Chapter 8). We have been taught to cover our mouth whenever we cough, to reduce the transmission of disease (such as the common cold) through the air. Nature provides its own defense against airborne diseases. Ultraviolet radiation from sunlight physically destroys some causative agents. Lack of humidity reduces the amount of moisture required for some organisms to reproduce.

Humans always have deposited many of their waste products in surface water as a means of sweeping the waste "out of sight and out of mind." Over time the concentration of wastes has increased and overloaded the ability of many water bodies to cleanse themselves, and **epidemics** of cholera, typhoid, and others have been the result. Today, virtually all surface water supplies used for human consumption require some form of treatment for removing disease-causing agents prior to consumption.

Some foods provide excellent growth media for biological causative agents. Salmonellosis is a good example. By controlling the factors required for growth, one can limit food's ability to transmit food-borne diseases. Food also can transport chemical and physical agents such as arsenic and radioactive materials.

Fomites are any inanimate objects that provide a "resting place" for causative agents of disease. We often observe people with a pencil or ink pen in the mouth. Transferring such objects between people can transmit infectious agents of disease like tuberculosis. Common examples of fomites are money, paper, countertops, and doorknobs, among any number of others.

Animals also can transmit disease to humans. The rabies virus and the bacillus of bovine tuberculosis are examples. A few of the many other diseases transmitted by animals are tularemia, brucellosis, anthrax, and psittacosis.

Because these organisms spread in the variety of ways listed above, they are difficult to control. In some cases the same agent may be spread in a combination of ways. For example, cholera can be spread via water, food, flies, or feces. Thus, environmental control has to be a multiple-defense control effort—covering the spectrum of water, food, air, insects, personal hygiene, and sewage disposal. In the remainder of the chapter we will group com-

municable diseases by causative agent, mode of transmission, how they affect the body, **incubation period**, and desired environment (chain of infection), with emphasis on methods of control.

· · · · · · · · · · · · · · · ·

COMMUNICABLE DISEASES TRANSMITTED BY INTESTINAL DISCHARGES

Some diseases spread by the intestinal discharge of humans are typhoid, paratyphoid, cholera, dysentery (amoebic), polio, bacillary dysentery (Shigellosis), and infectious hepatitis, campylobacteriosis, and Giardiasis.

Typhoid Fever

Causative agent: *Salmonella typhi* (about 106 types)

Methods of spreading:

- direct and indirect contact with patient or **carrier**
- contaminated water or food
- raw fruit and vegetables
  milk and milk products
- shellfish (especially oysters)
- other foods and liquids contaminated by carriers of the diseases
- under certain conditions, flies and other vectors

Effects on the body: Systemic bacterial infection characterized by insidious onset of fever, headache, malaise, anorexia, enlarged spleen, rose spots on the trunk, nonproductive cough, constipation, involvement of lymph system.

Incubation period: 1 to 3 weeks (2 weeks average).

Chain of infection: Susceptible animal → causative agent → water, food, flies, roaches.

Control measures:

- sanitary disposal of human excrement
- control of flies

- pasteurization of milk
- chlorination of water supplies
- shellfish sanitation
- education of public concerning personal cleanliness
- prevention of overcrowded living conditions
- proper handling of food, water, and human waste

Paratyphoid Fever

Causative agent: *Salmonella paratyphi*, *S. Schottmuelleri*, *S. hinschfeldi*

Methods of spreading: Same as typhoid.

Effects on the body: Bacterial enteric infection, abrupt onset of fever, malaise, headache, enlarged spleen, rose spots on trunk, diarrhea, involvement of lymphoid tissue.

Incubation period: 1 to 10 days for gastroenteritis; 1 to 3 weeks for enteric fever.

Chain of infection: Susceptible animal → causative agent → water, food, fomites, flies, roaches.

Control measures: Same as for typhoid.

Cholera

Causative agent: *Vibrio cholera*, including El Tor strain

Methods of spreading:

- ingestion of fecal-contaminated water
- sometimes food contaminated by carriers
- direct contact
- contaminated soiled hands and utensils
- flies
- raw uncooked seafood from polluted water

Effects on the body: Sudden onset, profuse watery stools, occasional vomiting, rapid dehydration, acidosis, circulatory collapse.

Incubation period: Few hours to 5 days (usually 2 to 3 days).

Chain of infection: Susceptible animal → causative agent → water, food, flies, roaches.

Control measures: Same as for typhoid.

Shigellosis (Bacillary dysentery)

Causative agent: Genus *Shigella* (27 types), a rod-shaped organism

Methods of spreading:
- direct contact, fecal-oral transmission
- indirect by objects soiled by feces
- consumption of contaminated foods, water, milk
- flies

Effects on the body: Diarrhea, fever, nausea, vomiting, cramps, tenesmus, convulsions (in children); stools may contain blood, mucus, pus.

Incubation period: 1 to 7 days (usually 1 to 3 days).

Chain of infection: Susceptible animal → causative agent → humans → water or flies, roaches.

Control measures:

- sanitary disposal of human feces
- public health education
- protection of water and food supplies and shellfish
- surveillance of food
- control of flies and roaches

Amoebic Dysentery

Causative agent: *Entamoeba histolytic* (protozoan)

Methods of spreading:

- direct contact with water
- mouth-to-mouth transfer of feces
- contaminated vegetables (especially raw vegetables)
- flies
- contaminated hands of food handlers

Effects on the body: Acute fever, chills, bloody or mucoid diarrhea, mild abdominal discomfort, diarrhea containing blood or mucus.

Incubation period: Varies, few days to several months or years (usually 2 to 4 weeks).

Chain of infection: Susceptible animal → causative agent → water, food, flies, roaches.

Control measures:

- sanitary disposal of human feces
- protection of public water supplies
- public health education
- personal hygiene
- fly and roach control
- food quality management

Poliomyelitis (polio)

Causative agent: Polio viruses Types 1, 2, and 3 (Type 1 is most common)

Methods of spreading:

- direct contact through association with infected persons
- sometimes milk
- water suspected at times
- fecal-oral route (major route of transmission)
- nasal discharges

Effects on the body: Fever, malaise, headache, nausea, vomiting, excruciating muscle pain and spasms, stiffness of neck and back with or without flaccid paralysis (hallmark of the disease).

Incubation period: 7 to 14 days (range of 3 to 35 days).

Chain of infection: Susceptible animal → causative agent → humans → water or food.

Control measures:

- active immunization (successful in U.S.)
- health education
- prevention of crowded conditions
- isolation in some cases

Infectious Hepatitis

Causative agent: Hepatitis A virus (a filtering agent has not been demonstrated)

Methods of spreading:

- intimate person-to-person contact by fecal or oral route with respiratory spread possible
- blood transfusions
- contaminated syringes
- contaminated water, milk, or food (including oysters and clams)

Effects on the body: Fever, malaise, anorexia, nausea, abdominal discomfort followed in a few days by jaundice.

Incubation period: 15 to 20 days, depending on dose (average 8 to 21 days).

Chain of infection: Susceptible animal → causative agent → humans, food, water, fomites.

Control measures:

- health education
- management of water and food (especially shellfish)
- monitoring of blood and blood products
- proper disposal of syringes
- sanitary disposal of feces, urine, blood
- hand washing to minimize fecal-oral transmission

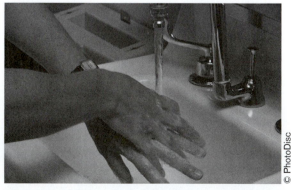

© PhotoDisc

Washing the hands is one of the most effective means of preventing infectious diseases.

Campylobacteriosis

Causative agent: *Campylobacter jejuni, Campylobacter fetus, Campylobacter coli* (rarely), *C. cinaedi, C. fennelliae*

Methods of spreading:

- found in human excreta and reservoirs
- found in cattle and poultry; puppies, kittens, other pets; swine, sheep, rodents, and birds
- transmitted by ingesting organisms in food, unpasteurized milk, and water
- contact with infected pets, wild animals, infected infants; infected children may transmit to puppies and kittens, which then may expose other children

Effects on the body: Acute bacterial disease of variable severity characterized by diarrhea, abdominal pain, malaise, fever, nausea, and vomiting; illness may be prolonged in adults; relapses may occur. Many infections are asymptomatic.

Incubation period: Usually 3 to 5 days (range of 1 to 10 days possible).

Occurrence: These organisms cause diarrheal illnesses in all parts of the world of all age groups (5% to 14% of diarrhea worldwide). In developed countries, children and young adults have the highest incidence of illness; in developing countries, illness is confined largely to children under age 2. Common sources of outbreak include chicken, unpasteurized milk, and unchlorinated water. Most cases occur in temperate areas in warmer months. This is an important cause of travelers' diarrhea.

Control measures:

- thoroughly cooking all foodstuffs derived from animal sources, especially poultry
- pasteurizing milk, chlorinating all water supplies
- recognizing, preventing, controlling campylobacter infections in domestic animals, pets (i.e., separate puppies, kittens with diarrhea)
- washing hands after contact with animals

- minimizing contact with poultry and their feces; washing hands as needed when this cannot be avoided
- avoiding mass feeding and poor sanitation

Giardiasis

Causative agent: *Giardia lamblia* (*G. intestinalis*), a flagellate protozoan

Methods of spreading: Human excreta, duodenal fluid, and small-intestine mucosa; hand-to-mouth transfer of cysts from feces of infected individual (especially in day-care centers, institutions, and the like); also occurs by ingesting fecally contaminated water. Contaminated food is less often implicated. Humans are the most common reservoirs, with beaver and other wild and domesticated animals implicated.

Effects on the body: May include **chronic** diarrhea, nausea, abdominal cramps, vomiting, weight loss, and fatigue lasting from a few days to several weeks; more often asymptomatic. Infection usually occurs in the upper small intestine. In severe cases duodenal and jejunal mucosal cells may be damaged.

Incubation period: 5 to 25 days or longer (average 7 to 10 days).

Occurrence: Worldwide, with children affected more frequently than adults; more prevalent in areas of poor sanitation, and where children are not toilet-trained (e.g., day-care centers). U.S. outbreaks (water-borne) occur mostly in mountain communities where streams or rivers are sources of drinking water without a water filtration system. It is also prevalent in certain temperate and tropical countries and often is associated with tour groups infected after drinking inadequately treated water.

Control measures:

- education of families, personnel, and inmates of institutions, especially day-care personnel, personal hygiene
- filtration of public water supplies that may be contaminated with human or animal feces (routine chlorination of water will not kill the giardia cysts, especially if the water is cold)

- protection of public water supplies from human and animal fecal contamination
- sanitary disposal of feces
- boiling of emergency water supplies

Ebola-Marburg Viral Diseases

Causative agent: Virons 80 nm in diameter and up to 970 nm in length. Ebola strains from Africa have been associated with human disease.

Method of spreading: Person-to-person transmission occurs by direct contact with infected blood, secretions, organs, or semen. Not thought to be airborne.

Effects on the body: Usually sudden onset of fever, malaise, headache followed by vomiting, diarrhea, and maculopapular rash. Also hepatic damage and renal failure often occur with a high fatality rate.

Incubation period: 3 to 9 days with Marburg and 2 to 21 days in Ebola virus disease.

Chain of infection: person to person

Control measures:

- education of the public
- avoid contact with secretions of infected people
- avoid sexual intercourse for 3 months or until semen is free of virus
- avoid vomit and feces of infected people

DISEASES SPREAD BY NOSE AND THROAT DISCHARGES

Tuberculosis

Causative agent: *Mycobacterium tuberculosis hominis* (human); *Mycobacterium bovis* (cattle)

Methods of spreading:

- exposure to bacilli in airborne droplet—sputum of infected persons
- indirect contact through contaminated articles or dust
- nasal secretions of infected cow
- consumption of unpasteurized milk from infected cow

Effects on the body: Primary infection usually goes unnoticed clinically, lesions commonly become inactive, leaving no residual changes except pulmonary or tracheobronchial lymph node calcification. Tuberculin sensitivity appears within a few weeks.

Incubation period: From infection to demonstrable primary lesion, about 4 to 12 weeks; to progressive pulmonary or extrapulmonary tuberculosis may be years.

Chain of infection: Susceptible person → causative agent → humans or cattle.

Control measures:

- improvement of poor social conditions that increase the risk of infection, such as overcrowding
- education of the public in mode of spread and method of control
- availability of medical, laboratory, and X-ray facilities for examinations of patients, contacts, and suspects; early treatment of cases
- pasteurization of milk
- TB control in cattle

Diphtheria

Causative agent: *Corynebacterium diphtheriae*

Methods of spreading:

- contact with a patient or carrier; or, rarely, with articles soiled with lesion discharges of infected persons
- raw milk (occasionally)

Occurrence: Diphtheria does not occur much any more in the United States because of DPT immunization given to children. (In the past, diphtheria killed many.)

Effects on the body: Acute infectious disease of tonsils, pharynx, larynx, nose, and, occasionally other mucous membranes or skin; sore throat; enlarged cervical lymph nodes.

Incubation period: Usually 2 to 5 days.

Chain of infection: Susceptible person → causative agent → humans → food.

Control measures:

- active immunization with diphtheria toxoid on a population basis, including an adequate program to maintain immunity
- immunization of adults subject to unusual risk, such as physicians, teachers, nurses, and other hospital personnel
- educational measures to inform the public, and particularly the parents of young children, of the hazards of diphtheria and the necessity and advantages of active immunization
- milk sanitation

Measles

Causative agent: Measles virus.

Methods of spreading: By droplet spread or direct contact with nasal or throat secretions or urine of infected persons by children who are not immunized.

Effects on the body: Fever, conjunctivitis, coryza bronchitis, Koplik spots on the buccal mucosa, dusky red blotchy rash appearing on the third to seventh day. A high percentage of children with the disease suffer brain damage.

Incubation period: About 10 days (varying from 8 to 13 days) after exposure to onset of fever; about 14 days until rash appears; uncommonly longer or shorter.

Chain of infection: Susceptible person → causative agent → humans.

Control measures:

- vaccination
- isolation
- education

Scarlet Fever

Causative agent: *Streptococcus pyogenes*

Methods of spreading:

- direct or intimate contact with patient or carrier

- indirect contact with patient or through transfer by objects or hands

Effects on the body: Fever, sore throat, tonsillitis, pharyngitis, leucocytosis. Can cause a heart murmur if the infection becomes systemic.

Incubation period: 1 to 3 days.

Chain of infection: Susceptible person → causative agent → humans → fomites → food or milk.

Control measures:

- lab tests for recognition of group A hemolytic streptococci
- education of the public in modes of transmission
- boiling or pasteurization of milk likely to be contaminated
- disinfection of soiled handkerchiefs, bed clothing

Whooping Cough

Causative agent: *Bondetella pertussis*

Methods of spreading: Primarily by direct contact with discharges from respiratory mucous membranes of infected persons, airborne by droplets, and indirect contact. (Whooping cough once was prevalent, but incidences have dropped since introduction of DPT vaccine.)

Effects on the body: Irritating cough, sore throat.

Incubation period: Commonly 7 days; almost always uniformly within 10 days.

Chain of infection: Susceptible person → causative agent → humans → air or fomites.

Control measures:

- active immunization with vaccine
- education of the public, particularly parents of children and infants
- control of fomites and indoor air

Smallpox

Smallpox was a worldwide problem until the 1960s. It is one of the first diseases eradicated using medical and public health technology.

Pneumonia

Causative agent: *Diplococcus pneumoniae*

Methods of spreading: Droplet; by direct oral contact; or indirectly, through articles freshly soiled with respiratory discharges. It is a major problem in hospitals and nursing homes, where it kills older persons.

Effects on the body: Chills, fever, pain in chest; cough productive of "rusty" sputum.

Incubation period: Believed to be 1 to 3 days.

Chain of infection: Susceptible person → causative agent → humans → air or fomites.

Control measures:

- avoidance of crowding in living quarters whenever practical, particularly in institutions, barracks, and on ships
- control of patient's respiratory discharges
- good personal and institutional hygiene

Influenza

Causative agents: Viruses

Methods of spreading: Direct contact, through droplet infection; also spread by nose and throat discharges and doorknobs infected people have touched.

Effects on the body: Fever, chills, headache, myalgia, prostration.

Incubation period: 24 to 72 hours.

Chain of infection: Susceptible person → causative agent → humans → air → fomites.

Control measures:

- active immunization when vaccine is potent
- avoidance of discharges from infected persons
- good personal and institutional hygiene

- education of the public in basic personal hygiene
- disinfection of eating and drinking utensils

Common Cold

Causative agent: A variety of viruses

Methods of spreading:

- by direct oral contact or by droplet
- indirectly by articles freshly soiled by discharges from nose and mouth

Effects on the body: Lacrimation (secrete tears), irritated nasopharynx, chilliness, malaise, fever.

Incubation period: 12 to 72 hours.

Chain of infection: Susceptible person → causative agent → humans → air or fomites.

Control measures:

- good personal health and hygiene
- disinfection of eating and drinking utensils and articles soiled by secretions and excretions of patients
- avoidance of articles and areas where infections are or have been

. . . .

DISEASES OF ANIMALS TRANSMITTABLE TO HUMANS (ZOONOSES)

Rabies

Causative agent: Lyssavirus type I (a neurotropic virus of family *rhabdoviridae*)

Methods of spreading:

- bite of rabid animal; rarely, by saliva of rabid animals entering a scratch or other fresh break in skin
- airborne transmission from bats to humans (possible in caves where bats are roosting)

Effects on the body: Onset with a sense of apprehension, headache, fever, malaise, and indefinite sensory changes. Disease progresses to paresis or paralysis, with muscle spasms or deglution (thickening of saliva cavity, choking) on attempt to swallow. Delirium and convulsions follow. Death is from respiratory paralysis. Rabies is almost invariably fatal by acute encephalitis.

Incubation period: Usually 4 to 6 weeks; occasionally shorter or longer, depending upon the extent and site of laceration or wound and other factors.

Chain of infection: Susceptible agent → causative agent → bite of dog or other rabid animal.

Control measures:

- specific prevention by vaccination. Protection depends upon how quickly vaccination is started after injury. Vaccine is usually given for 14 consecutive days. Vaccination often is supplemented by passive immune serum.
- prevention measures include the following:
  a. If the animal is apprehended, confined, and observed for 10 days, vaccination is started in affected person at the first physical sign or laboratory evidence of rabies in the observed animal.
  b. If the animal is not apprehended and rabies is known to be present in the area, vaccination in the affected person is started immediately.
  c. In severe bites, particularly in the region of head, face, and neck, with any likelihood that the animal is rabid, a dose of hyperimmune serum is given immediately, followed promptly by a full course of vaccine.
  d. Rabies vaccine is not given unless the skin is broken, as it may cause postvaccinal encephalitis.
- prompt cleansing of wounds caused by bite or scratch of rabid or suspected rabid animal with soap or detergent solution. Hyperimmune serum may be infiltrated beneath the bite wound.
- education of people regarding pet vaccinations, seeking immediate medical attention for any bites, confinement and observation of animals that have inflicted bites, reporting incidents promptly

- observation of dogs or other animals known to have bitten a person and knowing signs of rabies (change in behavior, with excitability and paralysis, followed by death)
- laboratory examination of brain from iced intact heads of animals dying of suspected rabies to search for Negri bodies, demonstration of which confirms rabies
- immediate destruction or detention of unvaccinated dogs or cats bitten by animals known to be rabid
- registration/licensing/vaccination of dogs and cats; destruction of stray animals

Brucellosis (Undulant fever)

Causative agent: *Brucella melitensis*; *Brucella abortus*; *Brucella suis*

Methods of spreading: Contact with infected animals' tissues and secretions; by ingestion of milk and dairy products from infected animals.

Effects on the body:

- may have acute or insidious onset; continued, intermittent, or irregular fever of variable duration; headache, weakness, profuse sweating, chills or chilliness, generalized aching
- disease may last several days, months, occasionally even years; recovery is usual, with a fatality rate of 2% or less of all cases

Incubation period: Highly variable; usually 5 to 21 days, occasionally several months.

Chain of infection: Susceptible agent → causative agent → fluid or tissue of diseased animal.

Control measures:

- education of farmers and workers in slaughterhouses, packing plants, and butcher shops about the nature of the disease and the dangers in handling carcasses and products of infected animals
- search for infection among animals by agglutination reaction and elimination of infected animals by segregation and slaughter
- calf immunization in enzootic areas

- pasteurization of milk and dairy products from cows, sheep, and goats; boiling of milk when pasteurization is impossible or unavailable

Bovine Tuberculosis

Causative agent: *Mycobacterium tuberculosis*

Methods of spreading: Ingestion of unpasteurized milk or dairy products from tuberculous cows, by airborne infection in barns, and from handling contaminated animal products.

Effects on the body: Fatigue, fever, weight loss; infection may spread to any part of the body through lymph and bloodstream and then cause manifestations in the specific locality.

Incubation period: Variable, from a few weeks to even years.

Chain of infection: Susceptible agent → causative agent → fluids and/or tissue of diseased animal.

Control measures:
- health education of the public regarding the importance of pasteurized milk
- BCG vaccination of uninfected persons
- elimination of tuberculosis among dairy cattle by tuberculin testing and slaughter of diseased animals
- pasteurization of milk and milk products

Q-fever

Causative agent: *Rickettsia burnetti* (*Coxiella burnetti*)

Methods of spreading: Commonly by airborne dissemination of rickettsiae in or near contaminated premises, in establishments processing infected animals or their by-products, and at necropsy (post mortem examination); also, raw milk from cows or direct contact with infected animals or other contaminated materials.

Effects on the body: Sudden onset of chilly sensation, headache, weakness, malaise, severe sweats; also, in most cases, pneumonitis with mild cough, scanty expectoration, chest pain, minimal physical findings and little or no upper respiratory involvement.

Incubation period: 2 to 3 weeks.

Chain of infection: Susceptible agent → causative agent → tissue fluid or hair of diseased animal or ticks.

Control measures:
- immunization of laboratory workers and others in exposing occupations
- pasteurization of milk from cows, goats, sheep, to inactivate rickettsiae
- public health education on sources of infection and the importance of pasteurizing milk
- control of infection in animals by vaccination and by regulating movement of infected livestock

Anthrax

Causative agent: *Brucella anthracis* (a spore-forming organism)

Methods of spreading:
- infection of skin by contact with contaminated hair, wool hides, and manufactured products such as shaving brushes, or by direct contact with infected tissues
- inhalation anthrax (below) from aspiration of spores
- gastrointestinal anthrax (below) from ingestion of contaminated undercooked meat

Effects on the body:
- Skin anthrax: An initial papule or vesicle at the site of inoculation develops into a depressed black eschar (spot), often followed by hard, edematous (watery) swelling of deeper and adjacent tissues. Pain is unusual. Untreated infections may spread to regional lymph nodes and bloodstream, with overwhelming septicaemia (blood poisoning) and death.
- Inhalation anthrax: Initial symptoms are mild and nonspecific upper respiratory infections.

Acute symptoms of respiratory distress, fever, and shock follow in 3 to 5 days, with death 7 to 25 hours thereafter. The fatality rate is very high.

Incubation period: Within 7 days, usually less than 4 days.

Chain of infection: Susceptible animal → causative agent → contact with tissue, wool, hair, etc., of diseased animal.

Control measures:

- immunization by cell-free vaccine, especially of veterinarians and persons handling potentially contaminated industrial raw materials
- for employees handling potentially contaminated articles, education in personal cleanliness, modes of transmission, and care of skin abrasions
- dust control and proper ventilation in hazardous industries; continuous medical supervision of employees, and prompt medical care of all suspicious skin lesions; adequate facilities for washing after work
- thorough washing, disinfection, or sterilization when possible, of hair, wool, or hides, and bone meal or other feed of animal origin, prior to processing
- ban on selling hides of animals infected with anthrax and carcasses used as food supplement
- postmortem examinations of animals dying of suspected anthrax
- noncontamination of soil or environment with blood and infected tissues
- incineration of carcasses or burial deeply with quicklime, preferably at the site of death
- prompt isolation and treatment of animals suspected of anthrax
- annual vaccination of animals when indicated

Leptospirosis (Weiel's disease, hemorrhagic jaundice)

Causative agent: More than 80 serotypes of leptospira

Methods of spreading:

- contact with water contaminated with urine of infected animals, as in swimming or accidental or occupational immersions
- direct contact with infected animals (infection presumably results from penetration of abraded skin or mucous membrane, or possibly through ingestion)

Effects on the body: Acute fever, headache, chills, severe malaise, vomiting, muscular aches, meningeal irritations, conjunctivitis; infrequently, jaundice, renal insufficiency, hemolytic anemia, hemorrhage in skin and mucous membrane. Clinical illness lasts 1 to 3 weeks; fatality is low.

Incubation period: 4 to 19 days.

Chain of infection: Susceptible animal → causative agent → animal urine.

Control measures:

- protection of workers in hazardous occupations with boots and gloves
- education of the public on mode of transmission and the need to avoid swimming or wading in potentially contaminated waters
- rodent control in rural and recreational human habitations
- segregation of domestic animals and prevention of contamination of living and working areas of people by urine of infected animals
- same as Campylobacteriosis and Giardiasis—see earlier listings

Salmonellosis

Causative agents: *Salmonella typhimurium, S. heidelberg, S. newport, S. oranienburg, S. infantis, S. enteritidis, S. derby*

Methods of spreading: Foods including meat pies, poultry products, raw sausages, lightly cooked foods containing egg or egg products, unpasteurized milk or dairy products, foods contaminated with rodent feces or by an infected food handler, or even through utensils, working surfaces, or tables used previously for contaminated foods such as egg products.

Effects on the body: Sudden onset of abdominal pain, diarrhea, and vomiting; fever nearly always. Deaths are uncommon, though anorexia and bowel looseness may continue for several days.

Incubation period: 6 to 48 hours; usually 12 to 24 hours.

Chain of infection: Susceptible person → causative agent → animals, eggs, meat, etc.

Control measures:

- thorough cooking of all foodstuffs derived from animal sources
- prevention of recontamination within kitchen after cooking turkey and other poultry
- not eating raw eggs
- refrigeration of prepared food before use
- education of food handlers and cooks in the necessity of protecting prepared food against rodent and insect contamination, in refrigeration of foods, and in hand washing before and after food preparation
- control of salmonella infection among domestic animals

Hantaviral Diseases

Causative agent: Hantaviruses

Methods of spreading: Aerosol transmission from rodent excreta presumed. Virus is present in urine, feces, and saliva with the highest concentration in the lungs.

Effects on the body: Abrupt onset of fever, lower back pain, varying degrees of hemorrhagic manifestations, and renal involvement. Severe illness with high fever, headache, malaise, and anorexia.

Incubation period: As short as a few days, or as long as two months, but usually 2 to 9 weeks.

Chain of infection: Rodent to humans.

Control measures: As described in Chapter 8, Rodent Control.

ARTHROPOD-BORNE DISEASES

Typhus Fever (epidemic typhus, louse-borne typhus)

Causative agent: *Rickettsia prowazeki*

Methods of spreading: Body louse *Pediculus humanus* is infected by feeding on the blood of a patient with acute typhus fever. Infected lice excrete rickettsia in their feces and usually defecate at the time of feeding. Humans are infected by rubbing feces or crushed lice into the bite or into superficial abrasions. Inhaling infective louse feces as dust may account for some infection.

Effects on the body: Variable onset; often sudden and marked by headache, chills, prostration, fever, general pains. A macular (spot) eruption appears on the fifth to sixth day, initially on the upper trunk.

Incubation period: 1 to 2 weeks; commonly 12 days.

Chain of infection: Susceptible person → causative agent → body louse → poor hygiene.

Control measures:

- at appropriate intervals, application of an effective residual insecticide powder to clothes and persons living under conditions favoring lice
- improved living conditions with provisions for bathing and washing clothes.

Murine Typhus Fever (endemic typhus fever, flea-borne typhus)

Causative agent: *Rickettsia typhi* (*Rickettsia mooseri*)

Methods of spreading: Infective rat fleas (usually *Xenophylla cheopsis*) defecate rickettsia while sucking blood, contaminating the bite site and other fresh skin wounds.

Effects on the body: Similar to louse-borne typhus, but milder.

Incubation period: Usually 10 to 12 days (varies from 6 to 21 days).

Chain of infection: Susceptible person → causative agent → fleas.

Control measures:

- preventing contact with infected mites by personal prophylaxis against the mite vector, by impregnating clothes and blankets with miticidal chemicals (benzyl benzoate) and applying mite repellents
- spraying with lindane or malathion.

....

MOSQUITOES

Yellow Fever Mosquito (*Aedes aegypti*)

Diseases spread by: Urban yellow fever, dengue fever, encephalitis, filariasis, dog heartworm.

Biological characteristics: The life cycle of all mosquitoes has four stages: egg, pupa, larva, and adult, with the first three stages occurring in water. Semidomesticated, mosquitoes can breed in artificial containers in and around human habitations. Eggs are laid singly on the side of containers at or above the waterline and are able to withstand drying for several months. When containers are filled with water again, they hatch quickly. If temperatures are high, hatching can take place in 2 or 3 days. Under favorable conditions the larvae can complete development in 6 to 10 days. The pupal period lasts about 2 days. The entire life cycle can be completed in 10 days, or it may vary as long as 3 weeks or more.

Identification: Small dark species with lyre-shaped, silver-white lines on the thorax and white bands on the torsal segments.

Desired environment: Prefers warm temperatures; susceptible to cold and usually does not survive the winter in northern U.S. Found in artificial containers in and around human habitations, such as: flower vases, tin cans, jars, discarded automobile tires, unused privies, cisterns, rain barrels, sagging roof gutters, and tree holes. *Aedes aegypti* prefers to live near human habitats.

Control measures: Keeping the habitat clean and free of objects that serve as breeding places for the mosquito (artificial containers such as cans, bottles, birdbaths, stopped-up gutters, old tires, automobiles, catch basins, watering containers, old appliances) to prevent mosquitoes from having a place to lay their eggs.

Malaria Mosquito
(*Anopheles quadrimaculatus*)

Diseases spread by: Malaria; have been found infected with encephalitis viruses and may have a role in the transmission of filariasis as well. This species was the most important vector of malaria in the United States.

Biological characteristics: The eggs of anophelines are always laid singly on the water surface and are supported by lateral floats. The female lays her eggs in batches of 100 or more. The eggs hatch in 2 to 6 days; the larval stages last 6 to 7 days to several weeks, depending on the species and environmental conditions, especially the water temperature. Most *anopheles* need a blood meal before they can produce fertile eggs. They usually winter as hibernating, fertilized females. A single female may deposit more than 3,000 eggs in as many as 12 batches. Hibernating females may survive 4 to 5 months.

Identification: Fairly large, dark brown with four dark spots near center of each wing. Palpi and tarsi are entirely dark.

Desired environment: Breeds chiefly in permanent freshwater pools, ponds and swamps that contain aquatic vegetation or floating debris. It is most abundant in shallow waters. This species shows a preference for clear, quiet waters neutral to alkaline. Common habitats are lime-sink ponds, burrow pits, sloughs, bayous, sluggish streams, shallow margins, and backwater areas of reservoirs and lakes. Production is greatest in waters with aquatic vegetation or flotage of twigs, bark, and leaves. The most favorable temperature for development is between 85° and 90°F. An improperly constructed farm pond could be the desired environment for *Anopheles quadrimaculatus*.

Control measures: Altering the favorable environment described and creating an unfavorable environment for breeding: filling potholes, depressions, swamps, and marshes with soil or other media; deepening trenches to remove standing water; placing tile under the ground for drainage; fluctuating the water level of farm ponds, reservoirs, and other water impoundments (used to control mosquitoes in TVA lakes).

Northern House Mosquito (*Culex pipiens pipiens*) and Southern House Mosquito (*Culex pipiens quinquefasciatus*)

Diseases spread by: St. Louis encephalitis, filariasis.

Biological characteristics: These species lay eggs in clusters of 50 to 400. These clusters, known as egg rafts, float on the water surface. In warm weather the eggs hatch within a day or two. Eight to 10 days are required to complete the larval and pupal stages. These mosquitoes can survive and produce fertile eggs without a blood meal. They are active only at night.

Identification: Brown mosquitoes of medium size with cross bands of white scales on the abdominal segments but without other prominent markings.

Desired environment: Develop prolifically in rain barrels, tires, tanks, tin cans, and practically all types of artificial containers; also live in storm-sewer catch basins, poorly drained street gutters, polluted ground pools, and cesspools. Heavy production is found in water with high organic content. Faster development occurs in warm environment.

Control measures: Same as those listed for *Aedes*.

· · · · · · · · · · · · · · ·

TICKS

American Dog Tick (*Dermacentor variabilis*) and Wood Tick (*Dermacentor andersoni*)

Diseases spread by: Rocky Mountain spotted fever (tick-borne typhus), tularemia, Colorado tick fever, possibly Q-fever, anaplasmosis, tick paralysis.

Biological characteristics: The life history has four stages: egg, six-legged larva, eight-legged nymph, adult. "Hard" ticks usually mate while they are on the host animal. The female drops to the ground and, after a brief pre-oviposition period (usually 3 to 10 days), begins to deposit eggs on or near the earth. The female feeds once and lays one large batch of eggs, sometimes numbering in the thousands. The eggs hatch in 2 weeks to several months depending on temperature, humidity, and other environmental factors. The larvae, or "seed ticks," possess only six legs and are not distinguishable as to sex. Their chance of attaching to a host is precarious, sometimes making prolonged fasts obligatory. After a blood meal, the engorged larvae usually drop to the soil and molt to the eight-legged nymph stage. This stage also requires a critical waiting period for a suitable host. After engorgement, the nymph drops from the host, molts, and becomes an adult. Although the life cycle of some species of hard ticks is completed in less than 1 year, it may require 2 years or longer.

Both male and female hard ticks are blood suckers, and both require several days feeding before copulation. After the male hard tick becomes engorged, he usually copulates with one or more females and then dies. Following copulation, the female tick drops to the ground. The eggs require several days to develop. She then begins oviposition. After a few more days, the female hard tick also dies.

Identification: Dorsal shield; tapered anteriorly.

Desired environment: Climatic factors, particularly temperature, are important. The several tick species are extremely variable in their ability to withstand temperature extremes, some surviving frigid winters as hibernating adults, nymphs, or larvae, and others surviving high temperatures and arid conditions. In most species the higher temperatures of spring and summer accelerate tick development and activity.

Control measures (for humans):

- buttoned clothing, trouser legs tucked into socks, shirttail tucked into trousers
- no sitting on ground or logs in brushy areas

- clearing or burning brush along paths and keeping weeds and grass cut in recreation areas
- in residential areas, closely cut lawns and well-kept yards
- tick repellents to the skin impractical but the military treats clothing with repellents

Control measures (for animals):

- dusting the animal
- using flea and tick collars (may be ineffective on large dogs)
- Ronnel, an organic phosphorus insecticide (in pill form), prescribed by veterinarian
- insecticides (dust or spray) in vegetated areas
- removing the hosts (dogs can be put outside)
- for cattle tick infestation, rotation of pastures

Deer tick (*Borrelia burgdorferi*)

Disease spread by: Lyme disease.

Method of spreading: Bite from tick belonging to genus *Ixodes*: *Ixodes dammini* or *Ixodes ricinus*.

Effects on the body: Lyme disease; clinical manifestations vary, mimicking several disorders, but affecting primarily the skin, nervous system, heart, and joints. The disease typically occurs in three stages. A patient can have one or all of the stages, and the infection may not become symptomatic until Stage 2 or 3.

- Stage 1: The first stage is characterized by localized erythema chronicum migrans, a rapidly expanding skin lesion, usually occurring in a circular radiating pattern. This lesion occurs in 60% to 80% of the patients and may be accompanied by flulike symptoms and/or regional lympadenopathy. Secondary lesions may develop within several days of the initial lesion, but they are smaller, less radiating, and are not indurated or in the area of the tick bite. Other clinical manifestations at this stage can be conjunctivitis (eye infection), hives, and a malar (spot) rash.
- Stage 2: The second stage consists of disseminated infections including neurologic and/or cardiac abnormalities. The most common neurological problem is Bell's palsy, which can be unilateral or bilateral and sometimes occurs in conjunction with radiculopathic syndrome, a condition of the small nerves caused by the disease. Aseptic meningitis often occurs without fever and may begin as recurring headaches, stiff neck, photophobia, nausea, and vomiting. Various encephalitic symptoms may include lethargy, fatigue, poor memory, dementia, personality changes, and psychoses with auditory hallucination. Less commonly reported are neurologic syndromes including pseudotumor cerebri and chorea—jerky movement.

  Carditis, which occurs in 4% to 10% of Lyme disease cases, manifests with varying degrees of atrioventricular block. This transient myocarditis usually occurs 3 to 6 weeks after the initial illness and generally resolves completely with antibiotic therapy. Complete heart block rarely persists more than a week, and the long-term prognosis is excellent. In more severe cases, hospitalization with continuous monitoring and temporary cardiac pacing may be required, as death is a possibility. Lyme carditis usually affects otherwise healthy young men. Prompt recognition and treatment is crucial to avoid unnecessary, permanent pacemaker implantation or death.

- Stage 3: This stage is rheumatologic, lasting months rather than weeks. Symptoms may arise within weeks of the secondary stage or within a gap of several years. Symptoms begin as migratory musculoskeletal discomforts that involve the joints, bursae, and tendons. The knee, the most commonly affected joint, usually is more swollen than painful. In severe cases, chronic Lyme disease may lead to erosion of cartilage and bone, and rarely to permanent joint disability.

  Congenital infection through transplacental transmission of *B. burgdorferi* can cause adverse fetal outcomes, but this is not usually the case.

Incubation period: Anywhere from 3 to 30 days from the time of the bite, in some cases may be much longer.

Chain of infection: Susceptible animal → causative agent → *Ixodes* tick.

Control measures (for humans):

- buttoned clothing, trouser legs tucked into socks, shirttail tucked into trousers

- no sitting on ground or logs in brushy areas

- clearing or burning brush along paths and keeping weeds and grass cut in recreation areas

- in residential areas, closely cut lawns and well-kept yards

- tick repellents to the skin impractical but the military treats clothing with repellents

Control measures (for animals):

- dusting the animal

- using flea and tick collars (may be ineffective on large dogs)

- Ronnel, an organic phosphorus insecticide (in pill form), prescribed by veterinarian

- insecticides (dust or spray) in vegetated areas

- removing the hosts (dogs can be put outside)

- for cattle tick infestation, rotation of pastures

Treatment: Causative agent is susceptible to several antibiotics including penicillin, tetracycline, ampicillin, ceftriaxone, and imipenem. Erythromycin is effective against the spirochete in vitro but not as effective in vivo. Amoxicillin is the drug of choice for children. No appropriate treatment for pregnant women has been developed. In the past, high doses of penicillin have been introduced intravenously. Corticosteroids, which were used to treat the disease before antibiotics came into use, have been used with success in treating carditis in patients not responding to antibiotic therapy. Prophylactic antibiotic therapy remains unresolved, and no vaccine is yet available.

············
MITES

Scabies or Itch Mite (*Sarcoptes scabiei*)

Diseases spread by: *Sarcoptes scabiei* causes scabies. Other mites spread sheep scab, Texas itch of cattle, mange in dogs and horses, scrub typhus (not found in U.S.), rickettsial pox, encephalitis virus, dermatitis; infestation of the lungs, intestines, urinary passages.

Biological characteristics: Mites lay eggs that hatch into larvae that pass through two or more nymphal stages to finally become adults. Larvae have two pairs of legs, and the nymphal stages have four pairs. The females burrow beneath the outer layer of skin and lay their eggs in the sinuous tunnels that they excavate. The eggs hatch into larvae. Some believe that males have only one nymphal stage and complete their life cycle in 9 to 11 days, and that the females have two nymphal stages and take 14 to 17 days—perhaps longer in cold weather—to complete their life cycle. The adults live about a month.

Identification: No well-defined segmentation of the body. Females average 0.2 to 0.4 mm in length, and males are somewhat smaller. Oval sac-like body; body surface is finely wrinkled; long body hairs.

Desired environment: Most commonly in tiny papules, particularly in the webbing between fingers, and folds of the skin at wrist.

Control measures:

- trapping or poisoning rodents to eliminate the source of the blood meal essential for nourishment and reproduction of mites

- starving out rodents by storing garbage and food in rat-proof containers, rooms, buildings

- keeping rodents out of buildings

- removing vegetation near houses; pruning shrubs so they are at least one yard from buildings

- chigger (mite) control depends on modifying the environment to permit sunlight and air to circulate freely, drying out its usual damp habitat

- sulfur has been used for years as a chigger (mite) repellent

FLIES

House Fly (Musca *domestica*)

Diseases spread by: Bacillary dysentery, infantile diarrhea, typhoid fever, paratyphoid fever, cholera, amoebic dysentery, giardiasis and pinworm, roundworm and tapeworm infections.

Biological characteristics: The developmental stages of the house fly are: the egg, larva, pupa, and adult. This cycle requires 8 to 20 days under average conditions. The female begins laying eggs within 4 to 20 days after emergence as an adult. The small, white oval eggs are about 1 mm long and are deposited in batches in of 75 to 150. The average female lays five or six batches her lifetime. Eggs usually are placed in cracks and crevices in the breeding material, away from direct light. Hatching occurs in 12 to 24 hours during the summer months. The larval stage lasts from 4 to 7 days in warm weather. When ready to pupate, the larva contracts until the skin forms a case about 6 mm in length. The pupal stage ordinarily lasts 4 or 5 days. When the pupal period is complete, the fly breaks open the end of the puparium and works its way out. The wings unfold and the body expands, dries, and hardens. This requires about 1 hour under summer conditions. Adulthood is reached in about 15 hours. Mating then may take place. Two or more generations per month may be produced during warm weather.

Identification: Small species, 6 mm to 9 mm long with dull thorax and abdomen. The thorax has four longitudinal dark stripes, sides of the abdomen usually are pale basally, and the fourth wing vein is angled sharply, ending before the wingtip. The arista of the antenna has many fine hairs like a feather.

Desired environment:

- almost any type of warm, moist organic material, such as animal manure and garbage. Flies are inactive at temperatures below 45°F and are killed by temperatures slightly below 32°F.
- flight begins when air temperature is about 53°F and complete activity occurs at 70°F.

Maximum activity is reached at 90°F, with a rapid decline at higher temperatures until 112°F, which produces paralysis and death. Flies are phototropic.

Control measures:

- sanitary refuse storage and regular collection
- control of feces of warm-blooded animals
- elimination of open dumps and littering
- sanitary landfill (refuse is compacted and covered with dirt daily)
- garbage grinders and compactors
- incinerators
- proper sewage and industrial waste disposal
- elimination of any organic material accumulation that remains moist long enough to produce flies
- elimination of weeds
- screening, electrocution (very expensive)
- release of sterile flies
- chemical methods (such as larviciding, fly baits, space sprays, fly cords and resin strips, residual sprays, fly repellents, fly attractants)

Black Horse Fly (*Tabanus atratus*)

Diseases spread by: Several diseases of humans and animals caused by viruses (equine infectious anemia, vesicular stomatitis, hog cholera, and California encephalitis), bacteria (anthrax and tularemia), rickettsia-like organisms (Q-fever and anaplasmosis), trypanosomas (surra), and filarial worms (loiasis and elaephorosis). Black horse fly is a major pest of cattle and horses.

Biological characteristics: Many species deposit their eggs on vegetation near water, and their larvae develop in damp soil or water. Biting flies may take 2 to 3 years for development. Horse flies are vicious biters, inflicting wounds that can itch for days. Only the females suck blood; the males feed on plant nectar.

Identification: Large fly; five posterior cells on the wing and three-segmented antenna.

Desired environment: Moist soil in the shade of trees under dry or sparse grass, where standing water seldom or never occurs. Some larvae develop in dry pasture land.

Control measures: Difficult, though repellents are somewhat effective.

Stable Fly (*Stomoxys calcitrans*)

Diseases spread by: Probably a vector of surra (a disease of horses and mules) and infectious anemia (a viral disease of horses). Stable fly larvae have been reported as causing myiasis in humans and domestic animals. Because of its blood-sucking habits, it is suspected of transmitting a number of diseases.

Biological characteristics: Stable flies do not breed in human excrement and usually are not attracted to feces or garbage. Therefore, they are less likely to pick up germs of diarrhea and other intestinal diseases. Larval development takes 8 to 30 days or more, depending on temperature.

Identification: 5 mm to 6 mm long, dull thorax with four dark longitudinal stripes and a pale spot behind the head, dull-colored abdomen with dark spots. Both male and female are vicious biters. Distinguished from all other common domestic flies by its piercing proboscis that protrudes bayonet-like in front of the head.

Desired environment: For laying eggs—plant waste more so than manure, and in old straw stacks, piles of fermenting weeds, grass, peanut hay, or stable manure well mixed with straw or hay.

Control measures:
- careful disposal of plant waste
- control of piles of fermenting weeds, peanut hay waste
- control area where manure is mixed with straw
- good environmental sanitation

Black Fly (*Simulium venustum*)

Diseases spread by: Tularemia in North America, human onchocerciasis in Africa and Central America, and bovine onchocerciasis in Europe and Australia. Some black fly species transmit deadly protozoa to ducks and turkeys.

Biological characteristics: Both sexes suck nectar from flowers, and most females suck blood. The eggs are laid in or near flowing water, and the larvae and pupae are found attached to submerged rocks, sticks, and vegetation. The adult emerges from the pupa in a submerged cocoon and floats to the surface of the water in a bubble of air. Many species mate soon after emergence. Black fly bites are painless at first but later become swollen, hard, and painful, and sometimes infected from scratching. They swarm around exposed parts of the body, particularly the head, and get into the nose, eyes, ears, and mouth. Heavy attacks may be fatal to humans, cattle, horses, and poultry, possibly from toxemia, anaphylactic shock, or suffocation brought about by inhalation of large numbers of swarming insects.

Identification: 2 mm to 5 mm long, stout-bodied with short antennae, wings with well-developed anterior veins, and a "humped" thorax, bestowing the common name "buffalo gnats."

Desired environment: Flowing water with rock and vegetation to which they may attach eggs, larvae.

Control measures:
- creation of unfavorable environment
- application of insecticides into breeding area
- encouragement of natural predators, such as the rainbow eating crabs

Deer Fly (*Chrysops discalis*)

Diseases spread by: In the United States tularemia, known locally as deer fly fever; particularly in the southern United States, mechanical carriers of anthrax bacteria from domestic animals to humans.

Identification: Average 6 mm to 12 mm long, spotted wings, two spurs on hind tibiae. Similar to horse fly characteristics.

Desired environment: Moist soil in the shade of trees under dry to sparse grass where standing water seldom or never occurs. Some larvae develop in dry pasture land.

Control measures: Difficult, though repellents are somewhat effective.

. . . .

LICE

Body Louse ("cooties")
(*Pediculus humanus humanus*)

Diseases spread by: Louse-borne typhus, trench fever, relapsing fever, pediculosis.

Biological characteristics: Life cycle has three stages: eggs, nymphs, adults. Eggs are yellowish and about 0.8 mm long by 0.3 mm wide. The egg (called a "nit") is cemented to fibers of underclothing. The eggs are incubated by heat from the body and hatch in about a week. Hatching of eggs is greatly reduced or completely prevented by exposure to temperatures above 100° F or lower than 75° F. Thus, the body louse is controlled readily when the same articles or apparel are worn intermittently. If clothing were stored for a month, even without treatment, all eggs would hatch or die, and any young that hatch would die. After emerging from the egg, the louse nymph molts three times before becoming a sexually mature adult. The nymphal stages require 8 to 9 days for lice re-maining in contact with the human body but may require 2 to 4 weeks when the clothing is removed at night. The total life cycle of body lice may be completed in about 18 days. The adult body louse differs little from the nymph except in size and sexual maturity. The male is smaller than the female. Mating occurs frequently and at any time in the adult's life, from the first 10 hours until senescence. Eggs are laid 24 to 48 hours later, depending upon temperature conditions. Body lice may deposit 9 to 10 eggs each day and a total of 270 to 300 eggs in a lifetime. See Figure 3.2.

Body lice can move fairly rapidly and will pass from host to host, or from one host to bedding, by simple contact.

Identification: 2 mm to 4 mm long; elongated abdomen, without hairy lateral processes; legs are three pair approximately equal; grayish-white in color; legs have hook-like claw for grasping. (Body louse rests on clothing except when feeding.)

Desired environment: Inner surface of the clothing, next to the skin—their blood meal. Hatching of eggs is greatly reduced or prevented by exposure to temperatures above 100° F and below 75° F. These lice depend upon human blood for sustenance. It is difficult to find human lice away from humans.

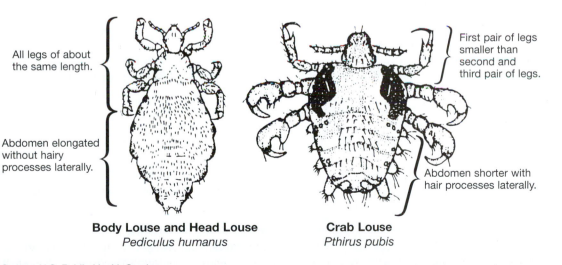

All legs of about the same length.

Abdomen elongated without hairy processes laterally.

First pair of legs smaller than second and third pair of legs.

Abdomen shorter with hair processes laterally.

Body Louse and Head Louse
Pediculus humanus

Crab Louse
Pthirus pubis

Source: U.S. Public Health Service

FIGURE 3.2 Lice commonly found on humans.

Control measures:

- examination of clothing along seams and folds
- ordinary laundering with hot water
- dry cleaning to destroy lice on wool garments
- treated shampoos and lotions
- insecticide powders for dusting
- bathing with emulsifiable concentrates (requires a physician's prescription)

Head Lice (*Pediculus humanus capitis*)

Diseases spread by: Pediculosis.

Biological characteristics: Metamorphosis same as body lice. Head lice live on head and neck region. Eggs are cemented to hairs of the scalp, where they incubate. Head lice are less prolific than body lice, depositing about four eggs per day, for a total of about 88 in a lifetime.

Identification: 1 mm to 2 mm; elongated abdomen without hairy lateral processes; three pairs of legs and approximately equal; grayish-white with dark margins (see Figure 3.2).

Desired environment: Most prevalent on back of neck and behind ears; head and neck region. Preferred temperatures same as body. Most abundant in children.

Control measures:

- very close haircut
- shampoo with emulsions
- not sharing personal belongings such as brushes or combs
- dusting of applications with DDT where permitted, or 1% lindane (kwell)
- preschool examination of children

Crab Lice (*Pthirus pubis*)

Diseases spread by: Pediculosis.

Biological characteristics: Life cycle is similar to that of head and body lice; eggs are glued to hairs. It is not known definitely how many eggs are laid in nature, but one female confined under a stocking laid 26 eggs, averaging three per day.

There are three nymphal stages. In a few specimens that have been studied, it took 13 to 17 days for them to become adults. Adult life apparently lasts less than a month. Legs are adapted for grasping large hairs, and adult prefers widely spaced hairs. These insects survive only a short time away from hosts because they are blood-sucking lice.

Identification: Small, 0.8 mm to 1.2 mm, grayish-white with short abdomen bearing hairy lateral tufts and large second and third pairs of legs (Figure 3.2).

Desired environment: Most commonly on hair in pubic and anal areas. May be found on hairy areas of chest and armpits. Infestations of eyebrows and eyelashes have been reported frequently. Crab lice are spread chiefly by sexual contact but may be acquired by other means such as infested toilet seats and beds, and by close personal contact.

Control measures:

- shaving or cutting infested hair to remove adults, immature stages, and eggs glued to hairs
- dusting with 1% lindane or malathion
- ophthalmic ointment for eyelashes and brows
- sanitization of restrooms, beds, self

·············

ROACHES

American Cockroach (sometimes called "water bug") (*Periplaneta americana*)

Diseases spread by: Organisms causing enteric diseases (diarrhea, dysentery, typhoid fever, food poisoning, cholera). American cockroaches may carry many strains of salmonella and staphylococcus bacteria that can cause food poisoning. They often visit sewers, garbage cans, then people's food.

Biological characteristics: The life cycle has three stages: egg, nymph, adult. The eggs are deposited in an egg capsule shaped like a clam shell. Tiny wingless nymphs emerge. Growth occurs during a succession of molts in which the body covering and some interior body linings are cast away. New characters, such as wing buds and eventually wings, appear after these molts. Males mature more rapidly than females and have fewer molts during their development. Average about a year developing from egg to adult. Females lay 14 to 16 eggs per case.

Identification: Largest species, 35 mm to 40 mm in length, reddish or dark brown with variable amount of yellowish color on pronotum.

Desired environment: Almost worldwide in distribution, preferring a warm, humid environment, as in sewers, boiler rooms, basements, kitchens, and cracks of homes. Also found in tree hollows, wood piles, and accumulations of trash. Has an appetite for beer and sweets but will eat starch and glue, damaging books and pictures.

Control measures:

- basic sanitation (deprives them of food, water, harborage)
- proper refuse storage (trash bags) and litter control (clean up litter)
- proper food storage
- insecticides

German Cockroach (*Blattella germanica*) (most common pest in homes and restaurants)

Diseases spread by: Organisms causing enteric diseases (diarrhea, dysentery, typhoid fever, food poisoning, cholera). They often visit sewers, garbage cans, then people's food.

Biological characteristics: Life cycle has three stages: egg, nymph, adult. Develops from egg to adult in 2 to 3 months. Female differs from females of most other species by carrying the egg case (ootheca) protruding from the abdomen until shortly before the young emerge. The young may emerge from the egg case even before the female drops it. The adults can fly but rarely do. Females lay 37 to 44 eggs per case.

Identification: Small, 10 mm to 15 mm long, grayish color with two blackish bars on pronotum covering the head.

Desired environment: Most abundant in kitchen and pantry; also bathroom and sometimes throughout buildings.

Control measures: Same as American cockroach.

SUMMARY

In recent years, people in developed countries enjoy health as a result of the ability to control communicable diseases that are still the major problem in many developing countries. However, we face a new group of diseases—chronic diseases. To a certain extent they are a result of one's lifestyle and environmental influences.

Communicable diseases are divided into four groups based on how they are spread. The four groups are as follows: (1) communicable diseases transmitted by intestinal discharges; (2) diseases spread by nose and throat discharges; (3) diseases of animals transmittable to humans (zoonoses); and (4) arthropod-borne diseases.

West Nile Fever As this book goes to press, West Nile Fever is becoming a problem in the United States. The disease is caused by a virus and spread by mosquitos. The control of West Nile Fever is like that for yellow fever and malaria. The West Nile virus is discussed further on p. 145.

KEY TERMS

Acute, p. 28	Epidemics, p. 30
Carrier, p. 30	Fomites, p. 29
Chronic, p. 33	Incubation period, p. 30
Communicable, p. 27	Zoonoses, p. 36
Endemic, p. 40	

REFERENCES

Altman, Lawrence K. 1996, April 2. "Mad Cow Epidemic Puts Spotlight on Puzzling Human Brain Disease (research into the causes of Creutzfeldt-Jakob disease) (Medical Science Pages)." *New York Times.* v. 145 p. B8 (N) p. C3 (L) col 4.

Barbour, Alan G. 1989, April 1. "The Diagnosis of Lyme Disease: Rewards and Perils." *Annals of Internal Medicine.* v. 110 n. 7. pp. 501–502.

Benenson, Abram. 2000. *Control of Communicable Diseases in Man.* 17th ed. American Public Health Association, Washington, DC.

———. 1989, Jan. "The Continuing Saga of Lyme Disease." *American Journal of Public Health.* v. 79 n. l. pp. 9–10.

"Changes in National Notifiable Diseases Data Presentation." 1996, Jan 19. *Morbidity and Mortality Weekly Report.* v. 45 n. 2. p. 41.

"Diagnosis of Lyme Disease." 1989, July 22. *Lancet.* v. 2 n. 8656 pp. 198–199.

Falco, Richard C., and Darland Fish. 1989, Jan. "Potential for Exposure to Tick Bites in Recreational Parks in a Lyme Disease Endemic Area." *American Journal of Public Health.* v. 79 n. l. pp. 12–14.

Finkel, Michael F. 1988, Jan. "Lyme Disease and Its Neurologic Complications*." Archives of Neurology.* v. 45 n. l. pp. 99–104.

Garrett, Laurie. 1996, Jan–Feb. "The Return of Infectious Disease." *Foreign Affairs.* v. 74 n. l. p. 66 (14).

Lederberg, Joshua. "Infection Emergent." 1996, Jan 17. *Journal of the American Medical Association.* v. 275 n. 3. pp. 243.

McAlister, Hugh F., et al. 1989, March 1. "Lyme Carditis: An Important Cause of Reversible Heart Block." *Annals of Internal Medicine.* v. 110 n. 5. pp. 339–345.

Morse, Stephen S. 1995, Oct. "Controlling Infectious Diseases." *Technology Review.* v. 98 n. 7. p. 54.

"National Surveillance for Infectious Diseases, 1995." 1995, Oct 6. *Morbidity and Mortality Weekly Report.* v. 44 n. 39. pp. 737.

Patlak, Margie. 1996, April. "Book Reopened on Infectious Diseases." *FDA Consumer.* v. 30 n. 3. p. 19.

Prescott, P. M., J. P. Harvey, and D. A. Klein. 1996. *Microbiology.* Wm. C. Brown, Dubuque, IA.

"Rising Toll from Infectious Diseases." 1996, April. *American Journal.* v. 96 n. 4. p. 11.

Seachrist, Lisa. 1996, Jan 20. "Infections Make Deadly Comeback." *Science News.* v. 149 n. 3. p. 38.

Steere, Allan C. 1989, Aug. 31. "Lyme Disease." *New England Journal of Medicine.* v. 321 n. 9. pp. 586–596.

Winker, Margaret A., and Annette Flanagin. 1996, Jan 17. "Infectious Diseases: A Global Approach to a Global Problem." *Journal of the American Medical Association.* v. 275 n. 3. p. 245.

WATER SUPPLIES

David McSwane, H.S.D.

Indiana University

OBJECTIVES

- Explain the hydrologic cycle.
- Identify the various types of wells.
- Discuss water quality.
- Explain water distribution.
- Discuss community and noncommunity supplies.
- Explain the basic water treatment processes for surface water and groundwater.

Water may well be the most valuable natural resource on our planet. There could be no life on earth without water. Water makes up two-thirds of our bodies, and humans can live only a few days without it. Civilizations have always located their communities close to water sources. Nearly 71% of the earth's surface is covered with water. Yet less than 1% of this water is fresh surface water and groundwater that is available for human use. Figure 4.1 shows the earth's distribution of water.

The water we consume can transport microorganisms that cause a variety of diseases including cryptosporidiosis (from which approximately 400,000 people in Milwaukee, Wisconsin, became ill in 1993), shigellosis, cholera, amebic dysentery, Hepatitis A, acute gastrointestinal illness, and many others. Table 4.1 gives a synopsis of reported cases of water-borne disease in the United States over nearly three decades.

In addition, many harmful chemicals—arsenic, pesticides, fertilizers, lead from pipes—are dissolved in and conveyed to humans by water. Physical agents such as the radionuclides Iodine-131, Phosphorus-32, and Strontium-90 may concentrate in surface waters after nuclear weapons testing. Radioactivity also is found naturally in some waters.

Data from the Centers for Disease Control and Prevention (CDC) show that water-borne disease outbreaks reported in community water systems between 1974 and 1996 were caused by bacterial pathogens (12%), parasites (33%), viruses (5%), chemical contaminants (18%), and unknown

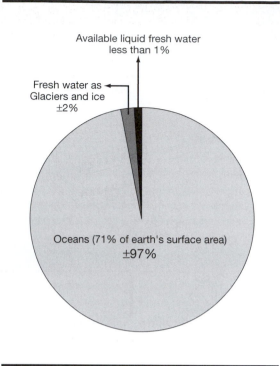

Available liquid fresh water
less than 1%

Fresh water as
Glaciers and ice
±2%

Oceans (71% of earth's surface area)
±97%

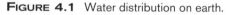

FIGURE 4.1 Water distribution on earth.

sources (31%). The number of reported outbreaks in the United States has declined over the past 25 years. Nevertheless, some of the more recent outbreaks have been very serious, causing many people to become ill or even die as in Milwaukee in 1993.

The availability of water can have a great impact on an area's economy and health. The presence of an abundant water supply can increase property values and provide incentives for agricultural, industrial, and overall community growth. **Potable** (water that has good taste, odor, and microbiological quality and is suitable to drink) water helps prevent economic hardship resulting from water-related illnesses affecting individual and community health. The critical importance of a potable drinking water supply cannot be overemphasized.

CRYPTOSPORIDIUM CAUSES MASSIVE WATER-BORNE DISEASE OUTBREAK IN MILWAUKEE, WISCONSIN

Cryptosporidium came to national attention in the spring of 1993 when 400,000 people became ill and over 50 people died in Milwaukee, Wisconsin, due to contaminated drinking water. Cryptosporidium is a single-celled protozoan that lives in the intestines of warm-blooded animals and humans. The organism is excreted in the feces of an infected person or animal.

Cryptosporidiosis is the disease caused by the Cryptosporidium parasite. This disease in humans is characterized by nausea, diarrhea, abdominal pain, low-grade fever, and weight loss. In a healthy adult the symptoms usually last for only 10 to 14 days. The disease will usually run its course in about two weeks. However, for individuals who have suppressed immune systems due to AIDS, cancer treatment, or organ transplant the disease can be life-threatening.

The Cryptosporidium parasite was traced to a water filtration plant that served a portion of the people of Milwaukee with drinking water. An investigation found there was a strong likelihood the organism passed through the filtration process and entered the water supply distribution system. The parasite is resistant to the chlorine used in water purification.

The actual source of the organism is believed to be animal operations located along the tributaries of the Milwaukee River. Rain and the spring thaw probably washed the parasite in manure from farm pastures and barns into the tributaries. The Milwaukee River drains directly into Lake Michigan, just north of where the intake for the city's water treatment plant is located.

Cryptosporidium is resistant to the chlorine used in water purification. The only protection from the parasite is proper filtration. Cities that draw drinking water from rivers or lakes—such as Milwaukee—are required to chemically treat their water but not to filter it.

The 800,000 people who used Milwaukee's municipal water supply were urged to boil the water they used for drinking and cooking or buy bottled water for several days until the problem could be corrected. If they did not, there was a high risk of getting sick.

SUMMARY OF REPORTED CASES OF WATER-BORNE DISEASE IN THE UNITED STATES, 1970–1996

Disease	1970–1979	1980–1989	1990–1996
U.S. Resident Population (in thousands)	2,121,804	2,374,749	2,814,219
Acute Gastrointestinal Illness			14,546
Amebiasis	30,586	48,282	
Cholera	18	71	11
Cryptosporidium			406,882
Giardiasis			1,967
*Hepatitis	421,787	258,112	158
Leptospirosis	716	656	Nonreportable disease
Shigellosis	180,859	207,801	566
Typhoid Fever	4,493	4,476	625

*Reported cases include both infectious and serum hepatitis in one combined figure.

Source: U.S. Environmental Protection Agency, Office of Water

· · · · · · · · · · · · · ·

THE HYDROLOGIC CYCLE

The amount of available water is finite. There is essentially the same amount of water today as there was at the time our planet was formed. The water may be altered in form and distribution, but the quantity always stays the same. Just think—the last water you consumed was as old as the earth!

Water is recycling continuously through what is called the hydrologic cycle (Figure 4.2). Atmospheric moisture—rain, snow, sleet, and the like—contains water that has been drawn from the earth by evaporation. Water evaporates from oceans, streams, ponds, soil, moisture on leaves, transpiration of plants, and precipitation falling to earth. This is a natural process. As the sun draws the moisture into the atmosphere, any existing pollutants are left behind.

Many students have done a simple experiment in science class in which salt is placed into a dish of water. The water is heated and evaporates. The salt remains behind in the dish. A similar process occurs in nature on a much larger scale. This natural cleansing of water allows atmospheric moisture to be water in its purest, most natural state. The atmospheric moisture then condenses and falls back to the earth as some form of precipitation.

As the precipitation falls toward earth, the water's naturally pure quality is influenced by the atmosphere through which it passes. Air pollutants, such as carbon dioxide and the oxides of nitrogen and sulfur from transportation and industrial processes, change the qualities of falling water. Acid rain is one direct result.

Once the precipitation reaches the earth, several situations may occur. Some water may land in an existing reservoir; some will run over the surface of the ground toward lakes, streams, rivers, and oceans; and some water may be absorbed into the soil. In short, when water hits the ground, it will become either surface water or groundwater. The ground surface, topography, soil type, and the like influence whether it will become surface water or groundwater.

Surface water picks up the characteristics of the surface over which it passes. If water flows across a parking lot, gasoline, oil, and other contaminants may be carried by or dissolved into the water. Water may pick up fertilizers, road salts, radioactivity from fallout, and biological contamination from farms, as well as countless other biological, physical, and chemical pollutants.

The same principle holds true for **groundwater**. As the water enters the ground, it picks up the characteristics of the formation through which it

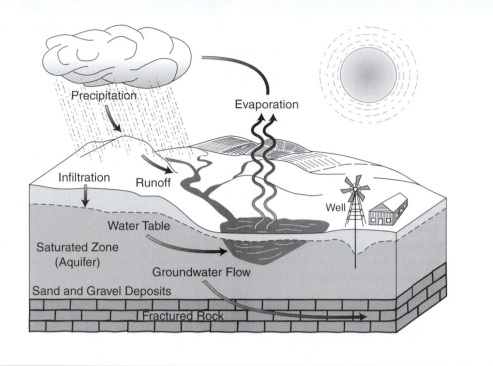

FIGURE 4.2 The hydrologic cycle.

passes. Water may pick up disease-causing agents from subsurface sewage systems, and many minerals from the soil dissolve in the water. As the water moves through the ground, the soil often filters out biological contaminants. The soil type and geological structures can have a great effect on the extent of biological filtration. For example, water moving slowly through a fine, sandy, clay soil will be filtered much better than water moving through a fractured rock formation. Water can move for miles through cracks in a limestone formation with very little filtration. For this reason, stabilization ponds are not permitted in limestone areas.

Usually, the deeper an underground water source is located, the better is the biological quality, because of filtration. On the other hand, theoretically, the deeper the water source is located, the poorer the chemical quality. Generally, deep water has been in the ground for a longer time, allowing prolonged contact with the underground strata. The increased contact time may cause additional minerals to dissolve

into the water, changing the chemical quality. Examples are calcium and magnesium compounds, which dissolve in groundwater and cause hardness.

Once above ground, spring water may flow directly to lakes, rivers, or oceans, or may evaporate directly. Then the hydrologic cycle starts all over again.

. . . .

SURFACE WATER SUPPLIES

Water supplies come either from the surface or below the ground. If a water supply comes to the surface naturally, it constitutes a surface water supply. Examples of surface water supplies are cisterns, ponds, lakes, and rivers. Large rivers are important sources of water for public water supplies. Although water from some lakes and rivers is clean, surface water must frequently be treated to remove sediment and disease-causing organisms before it will be safe to drink.

A **cistern** is a tank for storing rainwater from a catchment area, such as the ground's surface or a

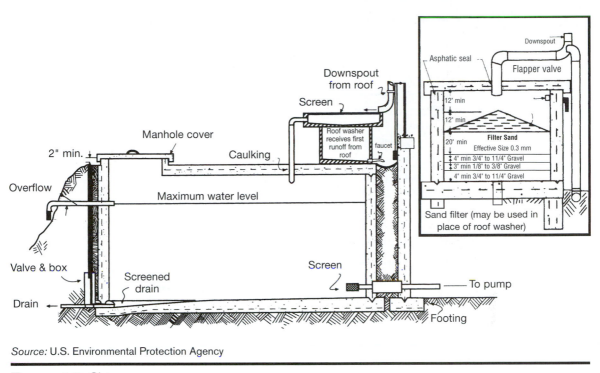

Downspout from roof

Screen

Manhole cover

2" min.

Caulking

Overflow

Maximum water level

Valve & box

Screened drain

Drain

Screen

To pump

Footing

Roof washer receives first runoff from roof

faucet

Downspout

Asphatic seal

Flapper valve

12" min

12" min

20" min

Filter Sand
Effective Size 0.3 mm

4" min 3/4" to 1 1/4" Gravel
3" min 1/8" to 3/8" Gravel
4" min 3/4" to 1 1/4" Gravel

Sand filter (may be used in place of roof washer)

Source: U.S. Environmental Protection Agency

FIGURE 4.3 Cistern.

rooftop, or for storing water that has been hauled in from some outside source. Although cisterns are rarely used in the United States, they still find application in developing countries where more advanced water treatment systems are not available. The cistern as a water source is limited greatly by the amount of rainfall an area receives. The catchment area and the size of the storage tank for a cistern should be large enough to hold enough water to meet the needs of users during the driest periods of the year.

The biggest factor affecting the quality of the water collected in a cistern is the type of material used on the roofs, and the condition of the gutter system. The roof and gutter system should be constructed of weather-resistant materials such as galvanized steel, aluminum, or plastic. Debris from trees and brush should not be allowed to collect on the roof and accumulate in the gutter system.

Imagine the amount of pollutants on a rooftop in an area where no rain has fallen for an extended time. Raindrops flowing across such a surface introduce

bird droppings, decaying leaves, soot, and many other contaminants into the water. Thus, the first flow of water off a roof's surface should be prevented from entering the cistern. This can be accomplished by using a flow diversion valve at the downspout of the gutter prior to the cistern entrance. Once the rooftop has been adequately rinsed, the operator will divert the water toward the cistern (see Figure 4.3).

The influent is filtered to remove any suspended particles prior to entering the cistern. The cistern should be constructed solidly to prevent entrance of any surface water that has not been filtered. A screened drain and manhole allow draining, entering, and cleaning of the cistern. The manhole should extend beyond the surface of the ground and be covered with a shoebox-type lid or another type of lid to prevent surface water from entering. Because water does not run upward, the shoebox lid prevents surface water from entering.

A **spring** appears where the natural flow of groundwater rises to the surface. The two types of

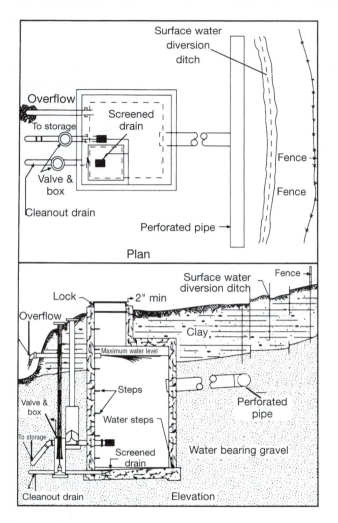

Source: U.S. Environmental Protection Agency

FIGURE 4.4 Spring protection.

springs are gravity and artesian. When a spring is chosen for a water supply, it is necessary to determine that the water quality is acceptable, the quantity of water available is adequate to meet the needs of the water system, and the spring is protected from contamination. Before a spring is used as a drinking water source, it is necessary to:

1. Note whether the spring has a relatively constant flow throughout the year. The spring should provide enough water to supply needs even during the driest time of the year. The flow rate should not be affected by slight precipitation.

2. Observe the effluent from the spring after rainfalls and note whether the water supply is more turbid or "muddy" at that time.

A substantial variation in the rate of flow coupled with increasing turbidity could indicate surface water or shallow groundwater intrusion. Springs often are located in low areas and get contaminated from pollution sources at higher elevations. For instance, a spring located directly down slope from a farmyard, septic tank system, or parking lot, or one that becomes muddy or has increased flow after a rain, is not a desirable water source.

If the spring has an adequate flow rate to meet consumption needs and is not affected greatly by precipitation, it may be used as a water source. The overall objective is to collect the water flowing from the water table and at the same time prevent any surface water intrusion. This is achieved by various construction techniques (Figure 4.4). Special care must be taken to prevent contamination of the spring during construction of the improvements necessary to supply the source of water.

Like a cistern, a spring storage tank should have some means of access for cleaning. A manhole extended above the surface of the ground with a shoebox lid is suitable.

· · · · · · · · · · · · · · ·

GROUNDWATER SUPPLIES

Many areas of the world do not have access to adequate springs, cannot rely on precipitation to fill a cistern, or do not have available surface water. If surface water is not readily available, we may dig or drill into the earth in an attempt to locate undergroundwater-bearing formations. Shallow holes will produce water in some places, while in others it may be necessary to drill hundreds of feet through earth and rock to reach a suitable supply of groundwater.

Although groundwater can be found in most areas, the quantity of water may not be enough to meet all water supply needs. While the amount of water available at some locations can supply individual home wells, it may not be enough to serve the needs of a public water system that serves a large number of customers.

A portion of the water that falls on the earth as rain or snow seeps into the soil and flows downward by gravity until it contacts a layer of rock or other impervious material. It then moves in a general downhill direction, taking the path of least re-

sistance. The layer of soil, sand, gravel, and rock through which the water moves is called an **aquifer**. An aquifer can be thought of as a layer of saturated soil or rock. The level of the water surface in the aquifer is called the **water table**. The movement of water through an aquifer is generally quite slow. Water may travel 20 feet or more a day in coarse sand. In fine sandstone it may move only a few feet in a year.

Wells are used to get groundwater to a distribution system that delivers it to the point of use. A major concern in the design of a well is preventing contaminants from entering the aquifer. Before constructing a well, the builders must conduct a survey of the proposed construction area to determine the presence of any pollution sources. In particular, these include feedlots, underground on-site sewage disposal systems, deep well injection facilities for hazardous wastes, underground storage tanks, and sewage stabilization ponds. Also, they are on the alert for any chemical contamination of the soil, which may result from application of insecticides, spraying of herbicides near overhead power lines, leaks in underground storage tanks, and others. Future uses of the area should also be considered to assure the well is placed in a location that will protect it from various sources of contamination.

Health departments and environmental agencies impose minimum separation distances between drinking water wells and pollution sources. For instance, at a private residence, the well and on-site sewage disposal system must be at least 50 and preferably 100 feet apart. For public water systems, the well must be at least 100 feet from sewers and other sources of contamination. A well should not be located in a flood plain or areas that receive large amounts of surface water runoff. Flooding is a natural source of contaminants in the water supply source. Surface runoff, which is a major contributor to flooding, will transport sediment, oil, pesticides, fertilizers, and other contaminants that might be found in the watershed. Surface waters should flow away from, rather than toward, a well.

The four major types of wells are dug, bored, driven, and drilled. The type of well to be constructed is often dependent upon the geological formations in an area.

Dug Wells

In many cases groundwater collects over the surface of the bedrock or some other dense formation, which creates a water source over the top of the rock. If this condition exists and enough water is available, the site may be appropriate for a dug well (see Figure 4.5). A **dug well** is constructed by dig-ging straight down into the earth until reaching water. The depth of a dug well can be limited by the depth of dense bedrock. With conventional tools it is difficult for workers to dig manually into the bedrock. The walls of dug wells are lined with rock, brick, wood, or concrete to prevent them from caving in and to prevent the entry of surface water. Dug wells are usually shallow, and because of the

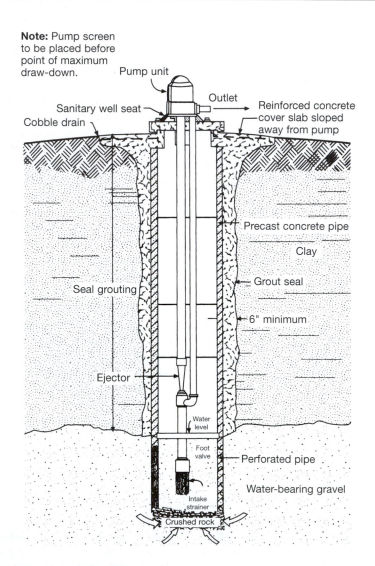

Source: U.S. Environmental Protection Agency

FIGURE 4.5 Dug well with two-pipe jet pump installation.

type of construction, may be subject to surface contamination.

Bored Wells

A **bored well** is constructed where the earth is soft and the aquifer is less than 40 or so feet deep. A bored well is similar to a dug well. The main difference between a dug well and a bored well lies in the methodology used to reach the water. Whereas a dug well is constructed by hand, a mechanical device such as a power-operated auger is used to dig a bored well. The hole is then lined with brick, concrete, plastic, or another suitable material. A bored well has the same limitations as a dug well in that its depth usually is no deeper than the underlying consolidated bedrock or impervious strata. Like a dug well, the water collected from a bored well has moved down from the surface and has ponded on some confining layers. The depth of the well has to be adequate to allow for soil filtration of any microorganisms that may have collected in the air or on the surface. Bored wells may also be subjected to reduced flow rates from the water table in times of drought, because of their dependency on precipitation for recharge.

Driven Wells

To dig a **driven well**, a pipe-end is fitted with a sharp point and a screen. The point is then driven into the ground until locating water. The pipe remains in place to carry water. Driven wells are limited to areas where soil particles are large, such as sands, sandy loams, and dense layers where rock and compacted soils do not exist.

Driven wells are often found in coastal regions where there are shallow water tables. Operators drive the pipe into the ground manually or with a machine. The pipe driven into the ground has a diameter too small to allow a submersible pump to be lowered to the water table. For that reason, operators place a pump at the top of the well that cannot draw water from more than approximately 25 feet (7.6 m) of pipe, thus limiting the depth of the well. The shallow depth of the driven well, along with its location in sandy soils, may make its water undesirable for human consumption.

Drilled Wells

Drilled wells (Figure 4.6) are used where a larger diameter pipe is needed, where hard ground and rock may be encountered, or where the well must be deep. Operators construct drilled wells to hundreds of feet in depth by mechanically drilling through rock and compacted areas. The drilling bit is forced through the earth and rock by being repeatedly lifted and dropped on the end of a cable or by being rotated on the end of a shaft. Drilled wells are most commonly installed for public water systems because it is necessary to tap deeper aquifers to assure an adequate quantity of water and to obtain the highest quality water. Drilled wells are commonly constructed with a large diameter to facilitate the installation of large capacity pumps. The water collected from a deep-drilled well is often less subject to reduced flows in times of drought and is not as vulnerable to contamination.

Several different types of pumps are available for lifting water out of wells. The selection of the method and equipment is primarily dictated by the water depth and the quantity of water to be pumped.

Suction pumps work on the principle of creating a vacuum and allowing atmospheric pressure to push the water up to the pump level. This type of pump can only be used with relatively shallow wells.

Ejector pumps are operated by a centrifugal pump at the ground surface that forces water at high pressure down a drop pipe into the well. At a point below the water level, the water is directed through a venturi tube and into a riser pipe back to the surface. The jet action of the venturi carries additional water with it to the surface. A portion of the water is drawn off for use, and the remainder is pumped back down the drop pipe.

Turbine well pumps have a vertical shaft motor located at the ground surface and a long drive shaft extending down the well to operate the pump suspended below the water level. The pump unit must be relatively small in diameter in order to fit down the well casing. Turbine pumps are widely used by public water systems because they are available in a wide variety of capacities and can be designed to produce almost any desired water pressure (Figure 4.5).

Submersible pumps combine a turbine pump with a waterproof motor that can be dropped into a

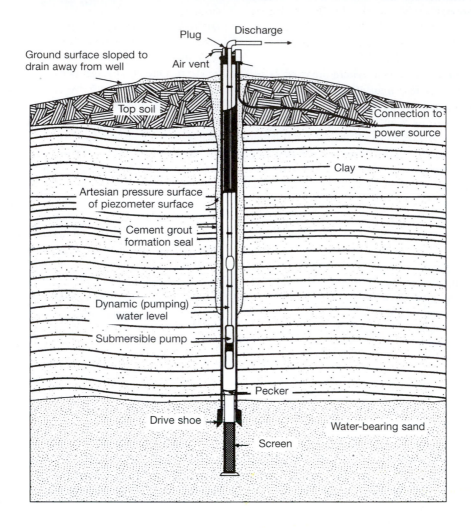

Plug

Discharge

Ground surface sloped to
drain away from well

Air vent

Top soil

Connection to
power source

Clay

Artesian pressure surface
of piezometer surface

Cement grout
formation seal

Dynamic (pumping)
water level

Submersible pump

Pecker

Drive shoe

Water-bearing sand

Screen

Source: U.S. Environmental Protection Agency

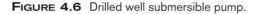

FIGURE 4.6 Drilled well submersible pump.

well as a single unit. Submersible pumps are made in sizes ranging from small pumps used for private home wells to very large units that pump hundreds of gallons per minute for public water systems (Figure 4.6).

Protecting the Water Supply

One feature all wells have in common is that a hole is constructed from the earth's surface down to the aquifer. Without some means of protection, surface water could flow across the top of the ground, picking up contaminants, and flow directly into the well.

A well is started by making a hole in the ground down to a water-bearing aquifer. The hole is supported by a solid, watertight pipe (casing) installed to just below the water table. The casing should extend high enough above the ground to prevent intrusion from floodwater. Screen material is installed below the casing to allow water into the casing while keeping sand and silt out. The screen should be constructed of corrosion-resistant material that is strong and allows the free flow of water.

The space between the hole and the casing is filled with grout or bentonite clay to prevent surface water and undesirable groundwater from getting into the well and contaminating the aquifer.

The well also needs to be sealed at the surface to prevent contamination from entering the well. This seal is usually a concrete pad poured around the casing and sloping away from the well. A cap, whether it is a shoebox lid or a sanitary seal, must be placed over the top of the casing to prevent any surface water from entering. This lid for a dug well should have some overhang beyond the outside of the casing to allow precipitation and contaminants to drop on the exterior rather than the interior of the casing. Figure 4.5 shows an example of casing, grout, and protective lid.

The sanitary seal for a drilled well should have a vent to permit air to enter the well shaft; the well pump creates a negative pressure, allowing atmospheric pressure to push the water out of the well. This vent should be screened to prevent the entrance of insects as shown in Figure 4.6.

Well drillers can "build out" surface pollution by using the proper casing, grout, and well cap. After completing the well's construction, a water sample is collected to determine the quality of water in the well. In most cases a bacteriological analysis should be done using the coliform group as an indicator. The **coliform group** consists of two different gram-negative bacillus species: *Escherichia coli* and *Aerobacter aerogenes*. *E. coli* is found widely in the intestinal tract of all warm-blooded animals. *A. aerogenes* is found widely in the soil, on our hands, and in the air. Presence of the coliform group indicates that fecal contamination is entering the water supply. The contamination or pollution may not be limited to just coliform organisms. Many types of pollutants including pathogens may be present. The coliform group merely indicates the presence of pollution.

After construction of a new well, collection of a positive (contaminated) coliform sample is almost inevitable. The mere handling of the well's piping and pump is enough to introduce pollutants into the water supply. The pipes also may have been stored in an area subject to surface contamination prior to installation. For this reason, the well should be disinfected prior to being put into service. Disinfection is typically achieved by placing a chlorine solution of at least 50 (and preferably 100) milligrams per liter (ppm) into the well to kill any organisms that may be present. After the disinfectant has been poured into the well, the plumbing faucets in the building served by the well should be opened to allow the water to flow until a faint odor of chlorine can be smelled at the faucet. The chlorine solution is then left in the well for at least a few hours and preferably overnight. The next day the plumbing faucets should be turned on allowing the water to flow. Let the water run until all odor of chlorine disappears. After disinfection, a water sample should be collected in a sterile bottle that contains sodium thiosulfate to chemically reduce any chlorine that may still be present.

The water sample that has been collected should be sent to a certified laboratory for bacteriological analysis. Lab technicians commonly use two techniques when conducting a coliform analysis: (a) the multiple-tube fermentation test, and (b) the membrane filtration technique, which is the usual choice today. If the results of either of these techniques are positive, the well must be disinfected a second time and another sample collected. If the results continue to be positive and a physical area where pollutants may be entering the well is not found, the water source may require more extensive treatment. A common procedure is to chlorinate the well continuously. Unlike the disinfection described previously, this chlorination is the continuous mechanical application of chlorine in proportion to flow for the purpose of killing any pathogens that may be present.

· · · · · · · · · · · · · · ·

WATER QUALITY

As discussed earlier, the ground's surface and the ground through which water flows can influence its quality. The characteristics of water easily can be changed biologically, physically, or chemically. Biological quality is altered any time living organisms enter the water. Some organisms are pathogenic and cause illnesses in humans. Removing all disease-causing organisms in water enhances its quality and reduces the chance of illness.

Water has many physical parameters. One of these is **pH**. When the pH of water becomes too alkaline (far above neutral pH 7), many dissolved materials settle out of the water. These materials can clog pipes and affect the taste of the water.

Water with very low pH, on the other hand, can leach metals from pumps, piping, and fixtures. Water that is too acidic (below pH 7) has the capability of "eating away" plumbing systems. Metals that can be leached include copper, lead, cadmium, and zinc.

Another physical parameter is the *color of water*. Imagine drawing a glass of water from a faucet and having it appear the color of tea. The water may be safe to drink (although this is unlikely), but the color makes it unappealing. In laundering, water color also can stain clothing. The color of water is altered by the natural breakdown of organics within it. These organics (such as tannin) produce a yellowish-brown color if untreated. Iron in water causes a reddish color, and manganese a black color. Copper produces green stains. Other materials may affect a water's color as well.

Turbidity is another physical parameter. Whereas water color often results from substances dissolved into the water, turbidity is a result of particles suspended in the water. Waters that have high turbidity may also stain clothes. If allowed to stand in a sink or tub, the particles suspended in turbid water will settle to the bottom and form sediments. Much turbidity, however, comes from a colloid, which will not settle easily.

Taste and *odor* also can affect a water's physical quality. Water that has a foul taste and/or odor may be safe to drink. However, consumers will likely find the water offensive and avoid drinking it. Some common contributors to foul taste and odor problems in water are tannic acid produced from decaying vegetation, dissolved gases such as hydrogen sulfide, and salts that can produce objectionable taste if present in high concentrations.

Many *chemicals* have the capability to alter water quality greatly. For example, nitrites and nitrates can cause methemoglobinemia, commonly known as "blue baby syndrome." The list of chemicals detrimental to human health is long. Only a chemical laboratory can detect their presence in most cases.

Water hardness is a common problem in many areas. The cause of hard water is dissolved minerals. These minerals are usually calcium and magnesium that dissolve in rainwater as it passes through soil and rock formations. Other minerals, such as iron, may contribute to hardness of water, but in natural water they are generally present in small amounts. Hard water interferes with almost every cleaning task from laundering and dishwashing to bathing and personal grooming. Clothes laundered in hard water may look dingy and feel scratchy. Dishes and glasses may be spotted when dry. Hair washed in hard water may look dull and feel sticky. Hard water may cause a film on glass shower doors, shower walls, and bathtubs. Cooking with hard water can also be difficult. Hard water can produce scale on pots and affect the performance of household appliances. When hard water is heated, a hard scale is formed that can plug pipes and coat heating elements. This reduces the efficiency of the heating unit and may cause the appliance to overheat.

················

WATER DISTRIBUTION

The water distribution system is the collection of pipes, valves, storage tanks, and other devices that carry water from the water source and deliver it to consumers (Figure 4.7). In private water systems, the pipes in the distribution system must be large enough to meet the maximum need of the family. In public water systems the distribution system must be large enough to meet the needs of residential, commercial, and industrial customers.

The amount of water needed to fight fires always creates the largest demand. Therefore, it usually determines the pipe sizes required in the system. Occasionally, fire flow capacity can not be provided for economic reasons. This exists in rural areas where homes are far apart and can only be served by small-diameter pipes that furnish only domestic needs. In these situations, fire departments will have to bring water with them when fighting fires.

Small-diameter pipes are used to carry water to sinks, toilets, and other plumbing fixtures throughout a building. These pipes are generally made of

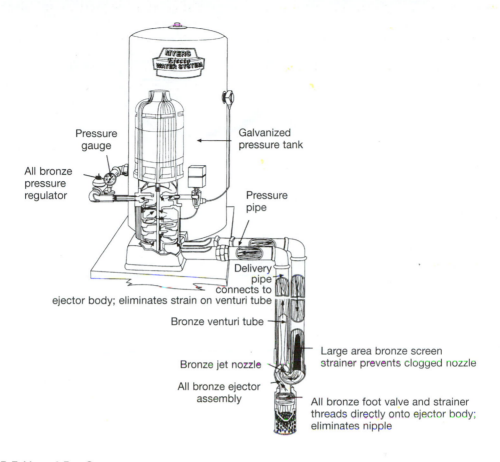

Pressure
gauge

Galvanized
pressure tank

All bronze
pressure
regulator

Pressure
pipe

Delivery
pipe
connects to
ejector body; eliminates strain on venturi tube

Bronze venturi tube

Large area bronze screen
strainer prevents clogged nozzle

Bronze jet nozzle

All bronze ejector
assembly

All bronze foot valve and strainer
threads directly onto ejector body;
eliminates nipple

Source: F. E. Myers & Bro. Company

FIGURE 4.7 Deep well jet pump system.

copper or plastic. Copper pipe came into use in the early 1900s and gradually became the preferred material in many areas of the country. Copper is flexible, rather easy to install, resistant to corrosion, and highly durable under most water and soil conditions. The major disadvantage of copper pipe is cost.

Plastic pipe has been used in many buildings since the late 1940s. Plastic is lightweight and easy to install. It is moderately priced and resistant to corrosion. In some areas, plastic pipe has been used almost exclusively for years. There are many types of plastic, but only certain types and grades are approved for potable water use. Plastic pipe must be

tested for durability and freedom from constituents that cause taste, odor, or release toxic chemicals. Only pipe that has the seal of an accredited testing agency printed on the exterior should be used for potable water purposes.

In distribution systems, it is necessary to prevent cross-connections and backflow. A cross-connection is a physical connection between a potable water line and a line that contains a source of contamination such as sewers and drains. Backflow is the backward flow of contaminated water into a potable water supply. Two examples of backflow are a garden hose attached to a mop sink, with the open end of the hose submerged in the sink below

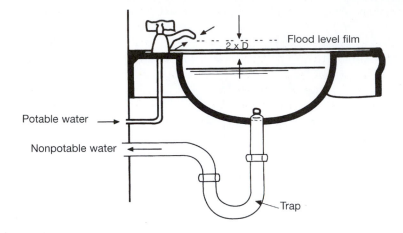

Source: Basic Housing Inspection, a U.S. Public Health Service training manual

FIGURE 4.8 Details of an air gap at a wash basin.

Housing

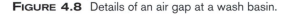

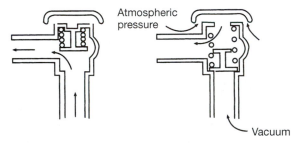

Normal Flow   **Vacuum Condition**

Source: Water Supply and Plumbing Cross Connections, U.S. Public Health Service

FIGURE 4.9 Operational details of a pressure-type vacuum breaker.

contaminated water; and a wash basin with the hot and cold water lines below the flood-level rim.

The wash basin cross-connections can be corrected, as shown in Figure 4.8 by providing an air gap between the faucet and the flood rim of the sink. An air gap is a physical separation of the potable and nonpotable system by a vertical air space. The vertical distance between the supply pipe and the flood rim of the sink must be at least two times the diameter of the supply pipe, but never less than one inch. Cross-connections can also be prevented by providing a vacuum breaker as shown in Figure 4.9. Other methods of preventing backflow are check valves and reduced pressure backflow preventers.

· · · · · · · · · · · · · · ·

MUNICIPAL WATER DISTRIBUTION

Thus far we have concentrated on individual water supplies obtained from wells, springs, and cisterns. Now we will discuss **public water systems** serving at least 25 people or 15 service connections for at least 60 days per year. There are two main types of public water systems. **Community water systems** provide drinking water to the same people all year long. According to the Environmental Protection Agency (EPA) there are approximately 54,000 community water systems that serve more than 250 million residences in the United States. All federal drinking water regulations apply to these systems.

Noncommunity water systems serve customers less than 12 months per year. The EPA has created two categories of noncommunity water systems. One category serves 25 or more people for more than six months each year but not the entire year. Schools and factories that have their own water source are examples of facilities that fall within this category. Most drinking water regulations apply to this category. The second category of noncommunity water system provides water to campgrounds, roadside rest stops, and other facilities where people stay only short periods of time. Only regulations of contaminants posing immediate health risks apply to the systems in this category.

We will focus on community water systems and the water treatment techniques they use to remove contaminants from drinking water. According to the EPA's Office of Water, 80% of the nation's community water systems used groundwater and 20% used surface water as their water source in 1998.

The specific treatment processes and facilities at a water treatment plant depend on the quality of the source water and the regulatory requirements that must be met. Some common steps in a water treatment process for surface water sources are:

- Presedimentation
- Rapid mix
- Coagulation/Flocculation
- Sedimentation/Clarification
- Filtration
- Disinfection

Presedimentation basins are typically used at treatment plants with raw water sources that are highly turbid. In such cases, the presedimentation process allows the removal of larger suspended matter (i.e., silt and clay) and provides a more uniform quality of raw water. The presedimentation process is sometimes supplemented with aeration equipment that injects air into the water to help control taste and odor problems.

After leaving the presedimentation basin, water enters the rapid-mix basin. At this point in the treatment process, primary coagulants such as aluminum sulfate (alum) or ferric sulfate are added to the water. The coagulant helps draw the suspended solids together, allowing them to settle out of the water. The purpose of the rapid-mix unit is to provide a thorough and complete mixing of the raw water and coagulant chemicals. Mixing can be achieved by the use of mechanical mixers, diffusers, or baffles in the basin(s).

After leaving the rapid-mix basin, the water flows into flocculation basins. These basins gently stir the water, allowing the alum or other coagulant to mix thoroughly with the suspended solids. These solids, which cause turbidity, clump together with the aid of the alum, forming large particles that are heavy enough to settle out from the water.

Once the particles of small solids have combined and formed larger particles, or **floc**, the water flows into a settling basin. The water flows very slowly through the settling basins, allowing the floc to settle from the water. The coagulation/flocculation process is essential to properly condition raw water for effective particle removal through sedimentation and filtration.

Most of the removable turbidity should be settled from the water before it reaches the next treatment step—filtration. The filtration process is the final barrier for physical removal of particles at the treatment plant. Without it, the suspended particles that remain in the water following the sedimentation/clarification process would be delivered to customers. Activated carbon often is added to the water after sedimentation and prior to filtration. The activated carbon absorbs color and some radioactivity and removes taste and odor. The water then passes through filters that remove most of the remaining suspended solids and the added activated carbon. The filters are important in that they filter out bacteria and turbidity as the water passes through.

After flowing through the filters, the water enters a clear well where approximately 1 milligram per liter (ppm) of chlorine is introduced to kill pathogens that may not be physically removed during sedimentation and filtration. Disinfection has proven to be one of the most important advances in reducing the incidence of water-borne disease. Chlorine is the most widely used disinfectant for drinking water. The two major advantages of chlorine are its effectiveness and low cost. Free chlorine provides a high level of disinfection at the treatment plant and a measurable residual in the distribution system. Unfortunately free chlorine also combines with natural organic materials that may be present in the source water to form **disinfection by-products (DBPs)** called **trihalomethanes (THMs)**. Two examples of THMs are chloroform and bromoform. THMs can cause cancer and other chronic health effects. Many treatment plants use chlorine in combination with ammonia to establish a chloramine residual and minimize THM formation. Some water treatment plants have chosen to use chlorine dioxide, ozone, or ultraviolet (UV) light as alternatives to chlorine for disinfection purposes.

As a final step, approximately 1 milligram per liter (ppm) of fluoride is added in water supplies that are fluoridated, and pH adjustments will take place if necessary. The water is now potable, palatable, and ready for distribution to the consumer. Pumps take the water from the plant into large, elevated tanks that store it and provide gravity flow pressure. From these tanks the water simply flows downhill through the distribution system and to homes, businesses, and industries that are served by the system.

Water treatment plants have a quality control laboratory in which technicians perform bacteriological, physical, and chemical tests on the raw and finished water to see if the water meets standards. In the lab, a pH meter determines the pH, a colorimeter determines the color, a turbidimeter determines the amount of turbidity, and so on. The tests done on the finished product are critical to the public health.

Before 1974 the United States had no enforceable national standard for drinking water. The **Safe Drinking Water Act (SDWA)** required the EPA to regulate contaminants that present health risks and are known, or are likely, to occur in public drinking water supplies. For each contaminant requiring federal regulation, EPA sets a nonenforceable health goal, or **maximum contaminant level goal (MCLG)**. This is the level of a contaminant in drinking water below which there is no known or expected risk to health. EPA is then required to establish an enforceable limit, or **maximum contaminant level (MCL)**, which is as close to the MCLG as is technologically feasible, taking cost into con-

sideration. Where analytical methods are not sufficiently developed to measure the concentrations of certain contaminants in drinking water, EPA specifies a treatment technique, instead of an MCL, to protect against these contaminants. All federal drinking water regulations apply to community water systems and most drinking water regulations apply to noncommunity water systems that serve at least 25 of the same people for more than six months per year. Each state sets its own standards that cannot be less stringent than the levels prescribed in the Safe Drinking Water Act. Generally, these standards are not enforced for private wells because of the cost of water quality determination. Table 4.2 presents a summary of the national primary drinking water regulations that are imposed to protect public health.

In 1979, the EPA added nonenforceable guidelines called national secondary drinking water regulations to the Safe Drinking Water Act. These voluntary standards were created to control contaminants that affect the taste, color, odor, or appearance of drinking water. A list of the contaminants for which secondary drinking water standards were created is provided in Table 4.3.

The Safe Drinking Water Act has been amended several times since 1974. Significant changes to the law occurred when the SDWA was reauthorized in 1986. The 1986 amendments required EPA to set MCLGs and MCLs for 83 named contaminants and to regulate 25 additional contaminants every three years beginning in 1991. The 1986 amendments also required EPA to set policies that required disinfection of all public water supplies, specific filtration requirements for nearly all water systems that use surface water sources, programs to protect groundwater supplies (Wellhead Protection and Sole Source Aquifer programs), and a ban on lead-based solder, pipe, and flux materials in distribution systems. The EPA used the Total Coliform Rule, Surface Water Treatment Rule, Lead and Copper Rule, and others to bring drinking water systems into compliance with the 1986 amendments of the Safe Drinking Water Act.

The Safe Drinking Water Act was also amended in 1996. These amendments emphasized the importance of protecting public health through risk-based standard setting, increased funding, reliance on best

NATIONAL PRIMARY DRINKING WATER REGULATIONS

Contaminants	MCLG[1] (mg/L)*	MCL[2] (mg/L)*	Health Effects	Sources
Microorganisms				
Cryptosporidium	zero (as of 01/01/02)	TT[3] (as of 01/01/02)	Gastrointestinal illness (e.g., diarrhea, vomiting, cramps)	Human and animal fecal waste
Giardia lamblia	zero	TT[3]	Gastrointestinal illness (e.g., diarrhea, vomiting, cramps)	Human and animal fecal waste
Heterotrophic plate count	n/a	TT[3]	Used as an indicator of how effective treatment is at controlling microorganisms	Bacteria that are naturally present in the environment
Legionella	zero	TT[3]	Legionnaire's Disease	Found naturally in water
Total Coliforms (including fecal coliform and *E. coli*)	zero	5.0%[4]	Used as an indicator that other potentially harmful bacteria may be present	Coliforms are naturally present in the environment; fecal coliforms and *E. coli* come from human and animal fecal waste
Turbidity	n/a	TT[3]	Used to indicate water quality and filtration effectiveness	Soil runoff
Viruses (enteric)	zero	TT[3]	Gastrointestinal illness	Human and animal fecal waste
Disinfectants & Disinfection By-Products				
Bromate	zero	0.010	Cancer	By-product of drinking water disinfection
Chloramines (as Cl_2)	MRDLG=4[4]	MRDL=4.0[5]	Eye/nose irritation; stomach discomfort, anemia	Water additive used to control microbes
Chlorine (as Cl_2)	MRDLG=4	MRDL=4.0	Eye/nose irritation; stomach discomfort	Water additive used to control microbes
Chlorine dioxide (as ClO_2)	MRDLG=0.8	MRDL=0.8	Anemia; nervous system effects	Water additives used to control microbes
Chlorite	0.8	1.0	Anemia; nervous system effects	By-product of drinking water disinfection
Haloacetic acids (HAA5)	n/a	0.060	Cancer	By-product of drinking water disinfection
Total Trihalomethanes (TTHMs)	n/a	0.080	Liver, kidney, central nervous system problems; cancer	By-product of drinking water disinfection
Inorganic Chemicals				
Antimony	0.006	0.006	Increased blood cholesterol; decreased blood glucose	Petroleum refineries; fire retardants; ceramics; electronics; solder
Arsenic	none	0.05	Skin damage; circulatory system problems; cancer	Natural deposits; glass & electronic production wastes

(continued)

NATIONAL PRIMARY DRINKING WATER REGULATIONS

Contaminants	MCLG[1] (mg/L)*	MCL[2] (mg/L)*	Health Effects	Sources
Asbestos (fiber >10 micrometers)	7 million fibers per liter	7 million fibers per liter	Benign intestinal polyps	Asbestos cement in water mains; natural deposits
Barium	2	2	Increased blood pressure	Drilling wastes; metal refineries; natural deposits
Beryllium	0.004	0.004	Intestinal lesions	Metal refineries, coal-burning factories; electrical aerospace, and defense industries
Cadmium	0.005	0.005	Kidney damage	Galvanized pipes; natural deposits; metal refineries; waste batteries and paints
Chromium (total)	0.1	0.1	Allergic dermatitis	Steel and pulp mills; natural deposits
Copper	1.3	Action Level=1.3	Gastrointestinal distress. liver or kidney damage.	Household plumbing systems; natural deposits
Cyanide (as free cyanide)	0.2	0.2	Nerve damage or thyroid problems	Discharge from steel/metal factories; discharge from plastic and fertilizer factories
Fluoride	4.0	4.0	Bone disease (pain and tenderness of the bones); children may get mottled teeth.	Water additive that promotes strong teeth; erosion of natural deposits; discharge from fertilizer and aluminum factories
Lead	zero	Action Level=0.015	Delays in physical or mental development of children. Kidney problems; high blood pressure	Household plumbing systems; natural deposits
Mercury (inorganic)	0.002	0.002	Kidney damage	Natural deposits; refineries and factories; runoff landfills and cropland
Nitrate (measured as Nitrogen)	10	10	"Blue baby syndrome" in infants under six months	Fertilizer use; leaching from septic tanks, sewage; natural deposits
Nitrite (measured as Nitrogen)	1	1	"Blue baby syndrome" in infants under six months	Fertilizer uses; leaching from septic tanks, sewage; natural deposits
Selenium	0.05	0.05	Hair or fingernail loss; numbness in fingers or toes; circulatory problems	Petroleum refineries; natural deposits; mines
Thallium	0.0005	0.002	Hair loss; changes in blood; kidney, intestine, or liver problems	Ore-processing sites; electronics, glass, and pharmaceutical companies

(continued)

NATIONAL PRIMARY DRINKING WATER REGULATIONS

Contaminants	MCLG[1] (mg/L)*	MCL[2] (mg/L)*	Potential Health Effects from Ingestion of Water	Sources of Contaminant in Drinking Water
Organic Chemicals				
Acrylamide	zero	TT[6]	Nervous system or blood problems; cancer	Added to water during sewage/wastewater treatment
Alachlor	zero	0.002	Eye, liver, kidney or spleen problems; anemia; cancer	Herbicide
Atrazine	0.003	0.003	Cardiovascular system problems; reproductive difficulties	Herbicide
Benzene	zero	0.005	Anemia; decrease in blood platelets; cancer	Factories; gas storge tanks, and landfills
Benzo(a)pyrene (PAHs)	zero	0.0002	Reproductive difficulties; cancer	Linings of water storage tanks and distribution lines
Carbofuran	0.04	0.04	Problems with blood or nervous system; reproductive difficulties	Soil fumigant
Carbon tetrachloride	zero	0.005	Liver problems; cancer	Chemical plants, industrial activities
Chlordane	zero	0.002	Liver or nervous system problems; cancer	Residue of banned termiiticide
Chlorobenzene	0.1	0.1	Liver or kidney problems	Chemical and agricultural chemical factories
2,4-D	0.07	0.07	Kidney, liver, or adrenal gland problems	Herbicide
Dalapon	0.2	0.2	Minor kidney changes	Herbicide
1,2-Dibromo-3-chloropropane (DBCP)	zero	0.0002	Reproductive difficulties; cancer	Soil fumigant
o-Dichlorobenzene	0.6	0.6	Liver, kidney, or circulatory system problems	Industrial chemical factories
p-Dichlorobenzene	0.075	0.075	Anemia; liver, kidney, or spleen damage; changes in blood	Industrial chemical factories
1,2-Dichloroethane	zero	0.005	Cancer	Industrial chemical factories
1,1-Dichlorethylene	0.007	0.007	Liver problems	Industrial chemical factories
cis-1,2-Dichloroethylene	0.07	0.07	Liver problems	Industrial chemical factories
trans-1,2-Dichloroethylene	0.1	0.1	Liver problems	Industrial chemical factories
Dichloromethane	zero	0.005	Liver problems; cancer	Pharmaceutical and chemical factories
1,2-Dichloropropane	zero	0.005	Cancer	Industrial chemical factories
Di(2-ethylhexyl) adipate	0.4	0.4	General toxic effects or reproductive difficulties	PVC plumbing systems; chemical factories
Di(2-ethylhexyl) phthalate	zero	0.006	Reproductive difficulties; liver problems; cancer	Rubber and chemical factories

(continued)

NATIONAL PRIMARY DRINKING WATER REGULATIONS

Contaminants	MCLG[1] (mg/L)*	MCL[2] (mg/L)*	Potential Health Effects from Ingestion of Water	Sources of Contaminant in Drinking Water
Dinoseb	0.007	0.007	Reproductive difficulties	Herbicide use
Dioxin (2,3,7,8-TCDD)	zero	0.00000003	Reproductive difficulties; cancer	Waste incineration and other combustion; chemical factories
Diquat	0.02	0.02	Cataracts	Herbicide use
Endothall	0.1	0.1	Stomach and intestinal problems	Herbicide use
Endrin	0.002	0.002	Nervous system effects	Banned insecticide
Epichlorohydrin	zero	TT	Stomach problems; reproductive difficulties; cancer	Industrial chemical factories; added to water during treatment process
Ethylbenzene	0.7	0.7	Liver or kidney problems	Petroleum refineries
Ethelyne dibromide	zero	0.00005	Stomach problems; reproductive difficulties; cancer	Petroleum refineries
Glyphosate	0.7	0.7	Kidney problems; reproductive difficulties	Herbicide use
Heptachlor	zero	0.0004	Liver damage; cancer	Banned termiticide
Heptachlor epoxide	zero	0.0002	Liver damage; cancer	Breakdown of heptachlor
Hexachlorobenzene	zero	0.001	Liver or kidney problems; reproductive difficulties; cancer	Metal refineries and agricultural chemical factories
Hexachlorocyclopentadiene	0.05	0.05	Kidney or stomach problems	Chemical factories
Lindane	0.0002	0.0002	Liver or kidney problems	Insecticide used
Methoxychlor	0.04	0.04	Reproductive difficulties	Insecticide used
Oxamyl (Vydate)	0.2	0.2	Slight nervous system effects	Insecticide used
Polychlorinated biphenyls (PCBs)	zero	0.0005	Skin changes; thymus gland problems; immune deficiencies; reproductive or nervous system difficulties; cancer	Landfills; waste chemicals
Pentachlorophenol	zero	0.001	Liver or kidney problems; cancer	Wood preserving factories
Picloram	0.5	0.5	Liver problems	Herbicide runoff
Simazine	0.004	0.004	Problems with blood	Herbicide runoff
Styrene	0.1	0.1	Liver, kidney, and circulatory problems	Rubber and plastic factories; landfills
Tetrachloroethylene	zero	0.005	Liver problems; cancer	Factories and dry cleaners
Toluene	1	1	Nervous system, kidney, or liver problems	Petroleum factories

(continued)

NATIONAL PRIMARY DRINKING WATER REGULATIONS

Contaminants	MCLG[1] (mg/L)*	MCL[2] (mg/L)*	Potential Health Effects from Ingestion of Water	Sources of Contaminant in Drinking Water
Toxaphene	zero	0.003	Kidney, liver, or thyroid problems; cancer	Insecticide used
2,4,5-TP (Silvex)	0.05	0.05	Liver problems	Banned herbicide
1,2,4-Trichlorobenzene	0.07	0.07	Changes in adrenal glands	Textile finishing factories
1,1,1-Trichlorethane	0.20	0.2	Liver, nervous system, or circulatory problems	Metal degreasing sites and other factories
1,1,2-Trichloroethane	0.003	0.005	Liver, kidney, or immune system problems	Industrial chemical factories
Trichlorethylene	zero	0.005	Liver problems; cancer	Petroleum refineries
Vinyl chloride	zero	0.002	Cancer	PVC pipes; plastic factories
Xylenes (total)	10	10	Nervous system damage	Petroleum factories; chemical factories

Radionuclides

Contaminants	MCLG[1] (mg/L)*	MCL[2] (mg/L)*	Potential Health Effects from Ingestion of Water	Sources of Contaminant in Drinking Water
Alpha particles	zero (as of 12/08/03)	15 picocuries per Liter (pCi/L)	Cancer	Natural deposits
Beta particles and photon emitters	zero (as of (12/08/03)	4 millirems per year	Cancer	Natural and man-made deposits
Radium 226 and Radium 228 (combined)	zero (as of 12/08/03)	5pCi/L	Cancer	Natural deposits
Uranium	zero (as of 12/08/03)	30ug/L (as of 12/08/03)	Cancer, kidney toxicity	Natural deposits

*Units are in milligrams per liter (mg/L) unless otherwise noted.

[1] Maximum Contaminant Level Goal—The level of a contaminant in drinking water below which there is no known or expected health risk.

[2] Maximum Contaminant Level—The highest level of a contaminant that is allowed in drinking water.

[3] Drinking water systems using surface water or groundwater under the direct influence of surface water must disinfect their water and filter their water or meet prescribed microbial limits to avoid filtration.

[4] Maximum Residual Disinfectant Level Goal—The level of a drinking water disinfectant below which there is no known or expected risk to health.

[5] Maximum Residual Disinfectant Level—The highest level of a disinfectant allowed in drinking water.

[6] Treatment Technique—A required process intended to reduce the level of a contaminant in drinking water.

Source: U.S. Environmental Protection Agency, Office of Water

NATIONAL SECONDARY DRINKING WATER REGULATIONS

Contaminant	Secondary Standard
Aluminum	0.05 to 0.2 mg/L
Chloride	250 mg/L
Color	15 (color units)
Copper	1.0 mg/L
Corrosivity	noncorrosive
Fluoride	2.0 mg/L
Foaming Agents	0.5 mg/L
Iron	0.3 mg/L
Manganese	0.05 mg/L
Odor	3 threshold odor number
pH	6.5–8.5
Silver	0.10 mg/L
Sulfate	250 mg/L
Total Dissolved Solids	500 mg/L
Zinc	5 mg/L

Source: U.S. Environmental Protection Agency, Office of Water

available science, prevention tools and programs, strengthened enforcement authority of EPA, and public participation in drinking water issues. The 1996 amendments improved the existing regulatory framework for drinking water safety in two important ways. First, they emphasized setting contaminant regulation priorities based on data about the adverse health effects of the contaminant, the occurrence of the contaminant in public water systems, and the estimated reduction in health risk that would result from regulation. Second, states were given greater flexibility when implementing the SWDA to meet their specific needs while arriving at the same level of public health protection.

"Right-to-know" provisions were also included in the 1996 amendments. These requirements assured that consumers were given the information they needed to make informed health decisions. These provisions also provided for increased participation in drinking water decision making and promoted accountability by drinking water systems and the state and federal agencies that regulate them.

MUNICIPAL GROUNDWATER SUPPLIES

Approximately 80% of the community water systems in America use wells to get their water from groundwater sources. For example, Memphis, Tennessee, though located on the Mississippi River, obtains most of its water from wells of varying depths. The quality of its groundwater depends upon many factors, such as depth of the well, existing geological formations, distance from sources of pollution, and demand for groundwater in the vicinity.

The extent of treatment required by community water systems using groundwater varies greatly depending upon the quality of the source water. In some areas, the source water needs only to be disinfected before use. In other areas, where water is of poor chemical, physical, and biological quality, the water must be treated using processes like those described for surface water supplies. For example, hard water may have to be softened, iron and manganese may have to be removed, fluoride may have to be added, or aeration may have to be used to remove hydrogen sulfide (H_2S). In all cases, public water supplies must disinfect their water to destroy pathogens that may be present in the groundwater.

When a public water supply uses wells, the wells must be designed, constructed, and located to protect them from sources of contamination. In addition, groundwater must meet the same drinking water standards that surface water supplies must meet.

CONSUMPTION AND CONSERVATION

Americans drink more than 1 billion glasses of tap water per day. On average, 50% to 70% of residential water is used outdoors for watering lawns and gardens. The American Water Works Association estimates that indoor water use in the typical single family home with no water-conserving fixtures is nearly 73 gallons per day. A breakdown of residential usage is presented in Table 4.4.

**DAILY PER CAPITA WATER USE
IN SINGLE FAMILY HOMES WITHOUT
WATER-CONSERVING FIXTURES**

Type of Use	Gallons per Capita	Percentage of Total Daily Use
Showers	12.6	17.3%
Clothes Washers	15.1	20.9%
Toilets	20.1	27.7%
Dishwashers	1.0	1.3%
Baths	1.2	2.1%
Leaks	10.0	13.8%
Faucets	11.1	15.3%
Other Domestic Uses	1.5	2.1%
TOTAL	72.6	100%

Source: 1999 Residential Water Use Summary, American Water Works Association

■ TABLE 4.5 ■

**DAILY PER CAPITA WATER USE
IN SINGLE FAMILY HOMES WITH
WATER-CONSERVING FIXTURES**

Type of Use	Gallons per Capita	Percentage of Total Daily Use
Showers	10.0	20.2%
Clothes Washers	10.6	21.5%
Toilets	9.3	18.9%
Dishwashers	1.0	2.0%
Baths	1.2	2.4%
Leaks	5.0	10.1%
Faucets	10.8	21.9%
Other Domestic Uses	1.5	3.0%
TOTAL	49.4	100%

Source: 1999 Residential Water Use Summary, American Water Works Association

The American Water Works Association estimates that the average household in the United States could decrease its water use by approximately 30% by installing water-saving devices and checking for leaks. This would save more than 5.4 billion gallons per day and produce a cost savings of more than $4 billion per year. A summary of water use for households using conservation measures is presented in Table 4.5.

WATER AND THE WORLD POPULATION

Water shortages and contaminated drinking water supplies pose serious problems for people in developing countries. Water is essential to sustain life. Yet, people in many countries do not have an adequate supply of water for drinking, bathing, cooking, and other purposes. To alleviate water shortages it will be necessary to manage water resources carefully to ensure proper use of available supplies and to avoid conflicts over access to fresh water.

The World Health Organization estimates that 1.1 billion persons (one-sixth of the global population) do not have access to safe drinking water. Lack of improved domestic water supply leads to disease through two principal transmission routes:

- Water-borne diseases that are transmitted by drinking contaminated water
- Diseases that are spread when there are insufficient quantities of water for washing and good personal hygiene

Water-borne disease outbreaks pose a serious health threat because a high proportion of a community can be infected at one time. The water-borne diseases of international significance include diarrhea, typhoid, hepatitis A, cholera, and dysentery. According to the World Health Organization there are approximately 4 billion cases of diarrhea each year that cause 2.2 million deaths. Most of these deaths involve children under the age of five.

When there is not enough water, people cannot keep their hands, bodies, and domestic environments clean and hygienic. Without an adequate supply of potable water, fecal-oral diseases are easily spread as are skin and eye infections including trachoma.

Lack of access to basic water and sanitation is often associated with poverty and the poor often pay more for small quantities of water of doubtful quality. Serious illness can be caused by drinking water that is contaminated with human and animal wastes. These wastes frequently contain bacteria, viruses, and parasites that can cause illness. Failure to provide adequate protection and effective treatment of water sources will expose the community to the risk of outbreaks of intestinal and other infectious diseases. Those at greatest risk of water-borne disease are infants and young children, the elderly, people who are ill, and those who are debilitated or living under unsanitary conditions. For these people, infective doses are significantly lower than for the general adult population. The potential consequences of drinking contaminated water are so significant for these individuals that control of these hazards is of paramount public health importance and must never be compromised.

SUMMARY

In the hydrologic cycle, water evaporates from surface water into the atmosphere, where it falls to the earth again in some form of precipitation. Some impurities enter the water while it is in the atmosphere—called air pollution—and others contaminate the surface water or groundwater after it reaches the earth.

Surface water supplies are obtained from cisterns, ponds, lakes, and rivers. Groundwater is obtained from aquifers located below the surface of the earth.

The quality of water is considered in two ways: the presence of contaminants that might cause illness and the presence of contaminants that affect the aesthetic properties of water such as color, taste, and odor. The Safe Drinking Water Act contains primary drinking water standards that community water supplies must comply with to protect public health.

The United States has one of the safest drinking water supplies in the world, and the quality of our drinking water has improved over the last 25 years. Nevertheless, the future will be full of challenges for water industry professionals. Given the national increase in population, urbanization, and development, it will be necessary for all communities to participate in water conservation measures and source water protection activities to lessen the negative impacts that these trends can have on the availability and quality of drinking water.

As a global society, we have learned a great deal about drinking water quality. However, there is still much to learn about the health effects of drinking water contaminants, the treatment technologies required to remove contaminants, and ways to protect our water resources. This will require a commitment by our society to invest in the research, technology, and protection programs needed to achieve the highest quality drinking water possible.

KEY TERMS

Aquifer, p. 57

Bored well, p. 59

Cistern, p. 54

Coliform group, p. 61

Community water system, p. 64

Disinfection by-products, p. 66

Drilled well, p. 59

Driven well, p. 59

Dug well, p. 58

Floc, p. 65

Groundwater, p. 53

Maximum contaminant level (MCL), p. 66

Maximum contaminant level goal (MCLG), p. 66

Noncommunity water system, p. 65

pH, p. 62

Potable, p. 52

Public water system, p. 64

Safe Drinking Water Act, p. 66

Spring, p. 55

Surface water, p. 53

Trihalomethanes (THMs), p. 66

Turbidity, p. 62

Water table, p. 57

REFERENCES

Barzilay, Joshua I. M.D., Winkler G. Weinberg, M.D. and J. William Eley, M.D. 1999. *The Water We Drink: Water Quality and Its Effects on Health*. Rutgers University Press, New Brunswick, NJ.

Craun, Gunther F. 1999. "Water-borne Outbreaks in Community Water Systems, 1971–1996." *Journal of Environmental Health*. July–August 2002. pp. 16–25.

Droste, R. L. 1996. *Theory and Practice of Water and Wastewater Treatment*. John Wiley & Sons, New York.

Environmental Protection Agency. 1999. *25 Years of the Safe Drinking Water Act: History and Trends*. EPA

Office of Groundwater and Drinking Water. EPA 816-R-99–007. Washington, DC.

Environmental Protection Agency. 1982. *Manual of Individual Water Supply Systems*. U. S. Government Printing Office, Washington, DC.

Friedman, Mel. 1996, March. "Troubled Waters." *Parents Magazine*. v. 71 n. 3. p. 50.

Frost, Floyd J., Rebba L. Calderon, and Gunther F. Craun. 1995, Dec. "Waterborne Disease Surveillance." *Journal of Environmental Health*. v. 58 n. 5. p. 6.

Grimes, Deanna E. 1991. *Infectious Diseases*. Mosby-Year Book, St. Louis.

Hammer, Mark. 1988. "Water and Wastewater." *Environmental Engineering*. Butterworth Publishers, Stoneham, MA.

Isaac-Renton, Judith. 1996, Jan. "Longitudinal Studies of Giardia Contamination in Two Community Drinking Water Supplies: Cyst Levels, Parasite Viability, and Health Impact." *Applied and Environmental Microbiology*. v. 62 n. l. p. 47.

Jones, Keith. 1994, July 9. "Water-borne Diseases." *New Scientist*. v. 143 n. 1933. p. A1.

Letterman, Raymond D. (ed.). 1999. *Water Quality and Treatment*. 5th ed. McGraw-Hill Inc., New York.

New York State Dept. of Health. *Manual of Instruction for Water Treatment Plant Operators*. n.d., n.p.

Pickford, John. 1987. *Developing World Water*. Grosvenor Press International, Hong Kong.

Rhyner, Charles R., Leander J. Schwartz, Robert B. Wenger, and Mary Kohrell. 1995. *Waste Management and Resource Recovery*. CRC, Boca Raton, FL.

Sawyer, Clair N., and Perry L. McCarty. 1994. *Chemistry for Environmental Engineering*. 4th ed. McGraw-Hill Book Company, New York.

Silverstein, Kenneth. 1994, March. "Everything in the Kitchen Sink (nonpoint pollution threatens city water supplies)." *American City & County*. v. 109 n. 3. p. 26.

Smith, Richard A. 1994, Jan. "Water Quality and Health: A Global Perspective." *Geotimes*. v. 39 n. l. p. 19.

Roizman, Bernard. 1995. *Infectious Diseases in an Age of Change: The Impact of Human Ecology and Behavior on Disease Transmission*. National Academy Press, Washington, DC.

Vesiland, Aarne. 1997. *Environmental Engineering*. PWS Publishing Company, Boston.

5

ENVIRONMENTAL HEALTH IN RECREATIONAL AREAS

Franklin B. Carver, Ph.D.

North Carolina Central University

OBJECTIVES

- Identify health and safety risks common to most types of recreational areas.
- Identify the major environmental concerns that should be addressed in the planning, development, operation, and maintenance of recreational areas.
- Identify the environmental health concerns that must be addressed in planning and conducting a mass gathering.
- Identify and discuss the safety issues and precautions specific to snowmobiling and snowskiing.
- Discuss physical and biological safety in water-oriented recreational areas.
- Understand the basics of swimming-pool construction, maintenance, and water quality.
- Discuss the operation, maintenance, and safety of two specific types of special pools.
- Discuss the most common playground equipment-related dangers.

In the 1990s, there was a growing trend toward the development and enjoyment of lifetime recreational activities. These leisure pursuits in the year 2000 and beyond are now being geared toward the individual; that is, to be active and enjoy recreational activities without depending on others. Individuals no longer have to compete against someone else. They are participating in recreational activities that can be as demanding as the person chooses.

This new millennium recreational trend that seems to be evolving has some disturbing implications: enjoying recreational activities at the expense of taking maximum risks. A phrase that describes this approach to recreation is "taking it to the limit."

In a society that continues to offer the workers more comfort, fewer challenges, and more leisure time, most people find it necessary to fulfill themselves in other ways. A person whose job is to input data into a computer 8 hours a day, 5 days a week, 50 weeks a year can get rather bored. There is no challenge. Therefore, on Saturdays and Sundays, driving a snowmobile becomes the challenge. But it's not just driving the snowmobile; instead, the person "takes it to the max" by driving faster and in locations beyond where the manufacturer recommends.

This chapter provides a broad overview of a number of recreational activities that are both challenging and enjoyable. Major aspects that should be considered when planning, developing, operating, and maintaining selected recreational environments will be addressed. Emphasis will be placed on how to receive the maximum challenge and enjoyment with a minimum of risk. As you cover each of these recreational activities, keep in mind the four factors that one must consider in attaining a safe level of performance: (1) knowledge and understanding of the risks involved, (2) skill development, (3) the state of the performer, and especially (4) the condition of the environment. The recreational environments covered in this chapter were chosen because of their continually expanding and innovative use by the public, coupled with increased public health and safety concerns. They are: mass gatherings, winter recreation, water-oriented recreation, and playgrounds.

. . . .

PROBLEMS ASSOCIATED WITH ALL RECREATIONAL AREAS

Recreational areas and activities have many problems in common. These problems often are related directly to the public's increased use and misuse of recreational areas. Therefore, public behavior in recreational settings is a growing concern. Problems caused by public behavior are attributed mainly to irresponsibility and a carefree attitude by consumers of all age groups. Lack of respect for rules and regulations in recreational areas has become all too common. Complaints about vandalism and other lawless acts against people, property, and the environment continue to show significant increases. Alcohol use and illegal drug use in recreational areas have been identified as major factors contributing to irrational public behavior. Most recreational areas have banned the use of alcohol and increased protection against illegal drugs.

Another growing concern for recreational areas is site selection. Sites selected for recreational areas should be well drained, gently sloping, free from topographical, biological, chemical, and physical hazards. Marshes, swamps, and water containing domestic, industrial, or agricultural waste should not be near recreational areas. Swamps and marshes breed mosquitoes that spread diseases and annoy people with their bites. Agricultural waste (cattle urine and feces) in water can spread disease in addition to being unacceptable aesthetically.

Traffic and noise are additional considerations when selecting sites. Recreational facilities should be far enough away from main thoroughfares to minimize accidents. A facility's access road design should exclude sharp curves and other potential traffic hazards. The site should be away from railroads, airports, truck routes, factories, and other sources of noise and accidents. In addition, recreational sites should be as far removed as possible from sources of pollution such as manufacturing plants, refineries, oil and coal burning power plants, and industrial establishments that produce noise pollution plus smoke, fumes, dust, objectionable odors, and other forms of air pollution.

It stands to reason that a recreational site should not be located near a nuclear power plant, farmyard, swamp, wastewater treatment plant, or bombing range. With such extensive site selection criteria and the immense development of industrial and residential areas over the past decade, new recreational sites are difficult to locate. This has brought about intense scrutiny of environmental impact studies, including the preservation of **wetlands**, during the site selection process. Risk assessments commonly are done to determine the suitability of proposed sites.

Because of the seasonal nature of certain activities, various problems arise in relation to purchasing expensive equipment for use during short periods of time, hiring and maintaining trained personnel, and conducting inspection and enforcement procedures over a 3- to 4-month period. Managers of recreational areas have tried to compensate for seasonal economic losses by turning ski resorts into year-round vacation sites or extending prime months for skiing by using more sophisticated snow-making equipment. Others have opted to develop multi-use facilities that will accommodate indoor or outdoor recreational activities.

MASS GATHERINGS

Mass gatherings for recreational purposes are defined differently by individual states. Some states define a mass gathering as an assembly of 1,000 or more people. Other states consider it an assembly of 5,000 or more people, with or without overnight accommodations. Some states also define a **mass gathering** by the number of hours an activity will continue and whether it is sponsored by the government or any of its agencies, along with the proposed site of the activity. Regardless of the definition, when large numbers of people come together and interact closely, the likelihood for transmitting diseases increases.

Specific types of mass gatherings that require various permits from local and state enforcement and planning agencies, including health departments, are rock concerts, fairs, carnivals, jamborees, auctions, and many other similar-type festive occasions. The planning stages for events such as these are important and should include all significant parties involved, especially promoters and local government officials, state and local police, public health officials, fire, transportation, and emergency medical personnel. All planning activities should be coordinated by one individual with distinct preparation for activities that are to occur before, during, and after the event. Some of the major environmental health concerns that have caused significant public health problems at mass gatherings in the past are the lack of:

- potable water from approved sources
- adequate sewage disposal systems
- proper solid waste collection, storage, and disposal
- noise levels in excess of 70 dBA* at perimeter of site
- proper food sanitation practices

---

*dBA = decibels in A scale.

WINTER RECREATION

Winter recreational activities have extended outdoor recreation into a year-round industry and are growing faster than any other recreational activities. This activity has brought about major environmental health and safety concerns. Some of the most common and current winter recreational environmental health and safety concerns are discussed next.

Ice Safety

With every winter season come stories of accidents and deaths resulting from falls through breaking ice. These incidents could be prevented by taking a few basic precautions including supervising children, avoiding certain locations of icy areas, and knowing how to react in case of an ice emergency.

During the winter months when temperatures are near freezing, children never should be allowed to play outside without supervision if the area has bodies of water, no matter how large or small. The water body does not have to be a pond or lake for an accident to occur. A drainage ditch or even standing water in a field can be the site of a catastrophe.

A major principle of ice safety is respect for the ice. When ice is safe depends on the activity. The same ice could be safe for a person on skis but unsafe for someone on foot. Generally, a 2-inch depth of ice is considered safe for someone on foot, and 4 inches to 6 inches will support groups of people or vehicles. Ice 8 inches thick is considered safe for loads up to 1,000 pounds per square foot.

Basic to all ice and water safety is the ability to swim. Beyond this, the two key rules are:

1. If something happens, do not panic. This alone has saved many lives.

2. If you feel you are breaking through an icy surface, throw yourself forward and out flat. If you fall through the ice and have your arms outstretched on the ice, use your feet as a propeller and edge yourself up onto the ice.

If an accident happens to a companion, a rope is the best means of rescue. If a rope is not available, a long branch or a pole can be used. Without these, and if several people are on hand, a "human chain" can be used for an effective rescue. To do this, individuals lie face down on the ice with another person holding their ankles and slowly propel across the ice to the victim.

Once rescued, frostbite precautions must be taken, along with seeking shelter and warmth immediately because the victim's clothes will quickly freeze.

Generally, activities on ice are relatively safe. One 25-year study found that **recreation** on ice is 20 times safer than other recreational sports on water and 50 times safer than highway travel. With the proper knowledge and precautions, ice can be a safe and enjoyable source of winter recreation.

Frostbite

David L. Bever's 1996 book, *Recreational Safety*, defines **frostbite** as "a localized cold weather injury characterized by freezing with ice crystal formation." Frostbitten tissues typically are pale, firm or hard, and often lose sensation. Freezing of the body's fluids and soft tissue of the skin is a result of reduced blood flow. The two most common sites of frostbite are the toes and the fingers. The nose and ears also can be damaged. Hypothermia (see below) and restrictive clothing can invite frostbite. Either may restrict blood flow, leading to frostbite.

Frostbite can be prevented by wearing protective clothing to keep the skin warm and by not wearing restrictive clothing. Also, people should be aware that smoking restricts blood flow and that alcohol dulls the nervous system, providing a false sense of warmth and security.

Hypothermia

Hypothermia occurs mostly when the body is exposed to outside temperatures between 30°F and 50°F. and the internal body temperature is reduced to 95°F or lower. The four major ways of reducing the body temperature are convection, conduction, evaporation, and radiation.

Convective and conductive loss of body heat both occur when air, water, or other elements around the body are cooler than the body and, by absorbing heat from the body, decrease the body's temperature. **Convection** can be defined as the transfer of heat from one location to another via movement in any "fluid," be it liquid (e.g., water) or gas (e.g., air). When convection takes place, the air or water around the body gains heat via transfer from the body, then the warmed fluid (air or water) circulates away from the body, loses the heat gained from the body, and is replaced next to the body by unheated fluid, which begins the convective process all over again. Although convection occurs in both air and water, water removes heat from the human body more readily than does air.

Conduction is defined as the transfer of heat from the body through substances with which the body may have direct contact. Unlike convection, conduction can occur with any solid substance, as well as any fluid, and the human body can gain heat through conduction from a warmer substance—for example, from hot water while bathing, or from contact with a heating pad.

Evaporation occurs when water escapes from the skin during respiration. It is responsible for 20% to 30% of heat loss in temperate climates.

Radiation is the largest source of heat loss. The human body gives off heat that cooler objects absorb. The body, too, absorbs radiant heat from the sun and from fires.

The human body is affected greatly by heat loss. The body's first defense against cold is shivering, which generates heat. As the body continues to lose heat, hypothermia decreases the brain's need for oxygen. This leads the victim into a disoriented and confused state. The circulatory system slows down, reducing the flow of blood, causing heat to leave areas of the body, notably the fingers and toes.

Protection from hypothermia is the same as for frostbite: wearing proper protective clothing. The best fabric is wool because of its insulating properties. Wool also is known to continue insulating even when fully saturated. Mittens, headgear, and footgear are the most significant protective clothing items. Mittens are better than gloves because they provide better insulation. Headgear is necessary because heat loss from the head can be great. For footgear, leather is the best material to use.

Snowmobiling

One of the fastest-growing winter recreational activities is snowmobiling. The state of Ohio defines a **snowmobile** as a self-propelled vehicle steered by skis, runners, or caterpillar treads, and designed to be used principally on snow or ice. Most state laws require the registration of snowmobiles every 3 years, and the annual registration of dealers who sell or furnish these vehicles for hire. An accurate account of the number of snowmobiles in use cannot be determined because many states still do not require the registration of snowmobiles if used on private property. Snowmobilers must obey all operating regulations for motor vehicle traffic, with most state officials authorizing the use of snowmobiles for winter travel in the following situations: (a) to cross a highway other than a limited-access highway or freeway; and (b) on the berm or shoulder of any highway, other than a limited-access highway, or freeway when the terrain is such that the vehicle can be used safely.

When attempting to cross ice, the snowmobiler must be extra careful. It is best to stay off the ice unless local or state officials deem it safe. To support the weight of a driver as well as the snowmobile, the ice must be at least 4 to 6 inches thick. It also is necessary to watch out for areas between two or more big lakes or other bodies of water. This situation often indicates that fast-moving water is in the area, which can make the ice thinner in certain spots.

Most state officials enforce a law that allows the operation of snowmobiles only during specific hours of the day, usually between one-half hour before sunrise and one-half hour after sunset. Snowmobiles operating before sunrise and after sunset and during periods of poor visibility must be equipped with proper lighting. Officials also warn snowmobilers about operating their vehicles during **winter white-outs**, when an overcast sky or snow precludes shadows and thus causes the horizon to be indistinguishable from the terrain.

Over the last several years fatal and nonfatal injuries related to snowmobile use continue to increase. This, in part, reflects the rising popularity of individual sports along with winter recreational activities in general. Most snowmobile accidents have involved operators between 20 and 30 years of age, and alcohol and excessive speed have played predominant roles. More than half of all fatal accidents have been attributed to head injuries, and a significant number of other fatalities have occurred as a result of operating on frozen bodies of water or hypothermia and drowning as a result of falling through the ice.

Snowmobile injuries range from hand trauma from engine belts to head injuries and open fractures caused by colliding with stationary objects. Data on snowmobile injuries are statistically irrelevant in comparison to other motor vehicle injuries mainly because most snowmobile accidents are not reported. Based on the analysis of fatalities, however, the following regulations would improve snowmobile safety if uniformly implemented:

- Increased and more accurate accident reporting by medical personnel, snowmobile operators, and winter-resort property owners
- Registration of all snowmobiles for tags at the time of purchase
- Requirement of a course in safety for owners and all prospective drivers. The course should involve training in handling the snowmobile and familiarization with the safety hazards before operation.
- Required licensure for snowmobile operation, including mandatory successful completion of a safety course, for individuals 16 years of age and older, regardless of a valid automobile driver's license
- Application of the same alcohol-use penalties to snowmobile operators as are applied to drivers of automobiles who use alcohol
- Strict prohibition of individuals under 16 years of age from operating snowmobiles
- Requirement of safety-designed footwear for operation of snowmobiles

- Mandatory use of safety helmets for all drivers and passengers
- Yearly public awareness efforts, through the media, on safety requirements for the use of snowmobiles
- Enforceable speed limits according to various terrain and conditions

Skiing

Skiing has evolved through the years to become one of the favorite winter outdoor activities throughout the entire Northern Hemisphere. As a recreational sport, it can be enjoyed by most age groups and does not require special skills or elaborate training. Skiing, however, has earned the reputation of being a relatively dangerous activity.

For many years efforts have been made to improve ski safety by changes in boots, bindings, and skis, and in trail design, trail grooming, and crowd control. Many of the hazards of skiing never will be removed completely from the sport. To do so would be impossible and would take from skiing much of its aesthetic beauty as well as its appeal as a vigorous mountain or cross-country experience.

Some hazards at ski areas are operational necessities. For example, groups of trees strategically placed on specific trails can be hazardous, but these same trees provide necessary reference points to skiers when weather conditions cause poor visibility. Ski-lift towers are also essential, but when they stand alone in the middle of ski runs, they become serious hazards.

Many of the hazards once considered inherent in recreational skiing are no longer acceptable. As accidents and failures have pointed out flaws in systems, equipment, and machines, new technologies have been employed to remedy the problems. The result has been a steady improvement not only in equipment quality and performance but, more important, a reduction in the number and types of hazards and the resulting injuries they cause.

One of the most life-threatening natural environmental phenomena for skiers is a snow avalanche. No one can predict **avalanche** occurrence with certainty, and not even the experts fully understand their causation.

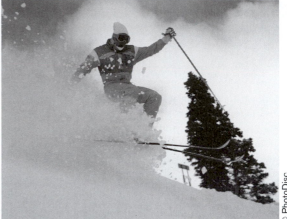

Though fun and popular, snow skiing has inherent risks.

© PhotoDisc

The two main types of snow avalanches are:

1. A **loose-snow avalanche**, which starts at the point or side of a slope when unattached snow crystals slide downward. It grows in size, and the quantity of snow increases as it descends. Loose snow moves as a formless mass with little internal cohesion.

2. **Slab avalanche**, which starts when a solid area of snow breaks away all at once. There is a well-defined fracture line where the moving snow breaks away from the stable snow. Slab avalanches are characterized by the tendency of snow crystals to stick together. The slide may contain angular blocks or chunks of snow. Slab avalanches often are triggered by the victims themselves. Their weight on the stressed snow slab is enough to break the often fragile bonds that hold it to the slope or to other snow layers. Loose-snow slides that trap victims usually are triggered naturally or by other members of the ski party.

Many other ski hazards are triggered by natural phenomena or environmental surroundings; however, most ski accidents and injuries have been directly correlated with the skier's behavior. Individual skiers have sole, personal, and final responsibility for knowing the range of their own abilities and skiing within the limits of those abilities. Each skier is responsible for judging whether he or she has the skills necessary to safely negotiate any slope or trail. Other responsibilities for which skiers are accountable, which commonly lead to accidents and injuries when disregarded are the following:

1. Each skier must maintain control of his or her speed and course at all times when skiing, and maintain a proper lookout so as to be able to avoid other skiers and objects.

2. The primary responsibility should be on the person skiing downhill to avoid colliding with any person or objects on the ski trail.

3. No skier should ski on any slope or trail that has been posted as "closed" or "off limits."

4. Skiers should stay clear of snow-grooming equipment, all vehicles, lift towers, signs, and any other equipment on the ski slopes and trails.

5. Skiers have the responsibility to heed all posted information and other warnings and to refrain from acting in a manner that may cause or contribute to the injury of the skier or others.

6. Skis used by downhill skiers while skiing should be equipped with a strap or other device capable of stopping the skis should they become detached from the skiers. (This requirement does not apply to cross-country skiers.)

7. Before beginning to ski from a stationary position, or before entering a ski slope or trail from the side, skiers are responsible for avoiding moving skiers already on the ski slope or trail.

8. Skiers should not move uphill on any passenger tramway or use any ski slope or trail while impaired by alcohol or by illicit drugs.

9. No skier should knowingly enter public or private lands from an adjoining ski area when the land has been posted as being closed by its owner or by the ski-area operator.

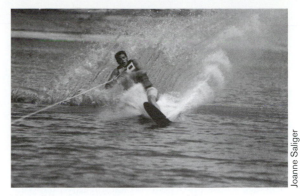

Joanne Saliger

Waterskiing is a very popular water activity.

WATER-ORIENTED RECREATION

More than half of all outdoor recreation is related to water. This form of recreation ranges from sheer aesthetic appreciation to the excitement of jet skiing and includes activities in the water and along the shore. Examples are boating (rowing, sailing, canoeing, kayaking, float trips, scenic river trips), water skiing, swimming, diving, snorkeling, surfing, scuba diving, fishing, hunting, studying and observing water birds and aquatic life, sunbathing, camping on the shore, and collecting shells, driftwood, and rocks. Theme parks featuring water-related activities such as water slides also have become extremely popular over the past few years.

Regardless of how water is used, the quality of the water historically has been the number-one concern in relation to recreational activities. Contamination from any substance that may pose a hazard to human health through ingestion, skin absorption, or entrance through body openings (such as the ear) is due cause for public health authorities to restrict a body of water to nonswimming recreation or, in severe cases, to prohibit the use of a body of water for recreation altogether.

Classification of Bathing Places and Water Quality

People swim in a variety of different settings. When swimming in any body of water, the person should be aware of the depth and quality of the water.

Every swimming area should be free of debris such as glass, cans, logs, and rocks. The swimmer must know what kind of bottom is present, as slope and footing are important in preventing unintentional injuries and fatalities. Each specific bathing place requires unique safety knowledge and practices.

NATURAL WATERS

One classification of bathing places consists of natural outdoor ponds, rivers, lakes, tidal waters, and beaches. These all depend on natural flow, temperature, and sunlight for sanitation, making this type of swimming area extremely difficult to manage from a public health standpoint. Usually there is a large volume of water per bather, which reduces the chances of water becoming contaminated. Nevertheless, one must be sure that no pollution from outside sources is present such as household waste piped to a stream, or a sewer outfall nearby, because of the possibility of contacting a pathogen. Natural bathing waters and their surroundings can be contaminated by waste from septic tanks, cesspools, privies, or sewage treatment plants entering the bathing water by any means. When polluted, the bathing area is condemned to protect the health of the people. This can be determined by a sanitary survey and coliform testing.

Studies have been made in an attempt to determine reasonable bacterial standards for this class of bathing place. Years ago, some states made extensive surveys of physical characteristics of saltwater beaches and correlated those with *E. coli* counts. Table 5.1 gives sample bacteriological standards. Beaches where the coliform organism density exceeded 1,000 per 100 ml were considered unsafe.

Results of sanitary surveys were correlated with the bacteriological findings. The final classification of the bathing place is not made upon the basis of the bacterial test alone, but also upon sanitary-survey finding.

Whenever one swims in a river or at the seashore, dangers can arise from the various currents and tides. The current of a flowing stream or river can catch swimmers by surprise and pull them under the water or dash them against rocks before they have time to react.

In an **undertow**, the wave breaks over the beach and then recedes toward the lake or ocean. If

■ TABLE 5.1 ■

AVERAGE COLIFORM INDEX

Class	Per 100 ml	Standard
A	0 to 50	Good
B	50 to 500	Fair
C	500 to 1,000	Doubtful
D	Over 1,000	Poor

the waves are large enough and the beach has a slope, the undertow has a force great enough to pull a person out into the water. A swimmer who is caught in such a current should not "fight" the water but, rather, be led by the current until reaching an object such as a tree limb that can be grasped or until the current recedes.

OUTDOOR POOLS

Another classification of bathing consists of outdoor pools that are partly artificial and partly natural. These are found in camps where a stream is utilized for a constant flow and change of water. The stream often is widened with masonry but seldom is chlorinated. These pools are difficult to control from a sanitary standpoint because turnover of water depends on the flow of the stream. If no disinfectant, such as chlorine, is used to kill pathogens, it would not take long to transmit a pathogen from person to person. Also, a sanitary survey and bacteriological test should be made on the contributing stream.

ARTIFICIALLY CONSTRUCTED POOLS

A third classification of a bathing place encompasses indoor and outdoor pools that are entirely of artificial construction. These are of three types.

1. *Fill and draw pools*, which depend on frequent emptying and refilling to maintain sanitary conditions. If the water is not changed frequently, these pools can be as unsanitary as a communal bathtub. This type is rarely used today.

2. *The flow-through pool*, which gets its water from natural sources such as streams. In areas where water is cheap, water from the municipal supply or a private well may flow

through the artificial pool; however, this latter type is rare, especially in arid regions.

3. *Recirculatory pools*, which are the most satisfactory from a public health standpoint. The water is recirculated through the filtering equipment by pumps, and chemicals are used to control the water quality. Disinfecting agents are added before the water reenters the pool. Some recirculating pools are filled only once a year, and the water is used, treated, filtered, and reused. The water should be recirculated at least every 8 hours, and preferably every 6 hours. If properly maintained, the recirculated water is relatively clear at all times to prevent accidents and to lower the amount of disinfectant needed. The water quality should be such that a 6-inch (15 cm) black disk painted on a white background is visible from the side of the pool at the deepest point.

pH

The pH of swimming-pool water is the single most important factor in maintaining pool water quality. Every other chemical balance in swimming pool water is affected by pH. Water with a low pH irritates the eyes, ears, and mucous membrane. Most state bathing codes require that pool water pH be maintained between 7.2 and 8.2, though the ideal range is between 7.4 and 7.6. If the pH is allowed to drop below 7.2, metal surfaces such as the filter tank, pipes, and heater coils can corrode. Skin irritation and excessive chlorine odor also may result.

High pH readings, above 7.6, also must be avoided. As readings approach 8.0, iron and calcium can form a precipitate (solid particles suspended in the water), causing turgidity or unclear water. In addition, scale can form on the filters and in the plumbing and heater. Precipitates also form from chemical conditions, such as hardness and alkalinity.

Another undesirable effect of high pH is that it reduces the efficiency of chlorine added to the water for disinfectant purposes. High pH impedes the formation of **hypochlorous acid**, the bactericide that is formed when chlorine is added to the water. At pH 7.2, approximately 60% of the chlorine dissolved in water will convert to hypochlorous acid. By comparison, at pH 8.5, the conversion is limited to approximately 10%. The remainder is converted to hypochlorite ion, a useless acid. If the pH exceeds the recommended maximum of 7.6, more chlorine will be required to maintain the desired level of disinfectant in the water, resulting in a higher operating cost.

Recirculating Pools

Maintaining desired water quality requires the proper use of circulating and filtering equipment. A recirculating swimming pool is similar to a water treatment plant. In a water treatment plant, "new" water is treated; in a swimming pool, the pool is filled in the spring and the water is used (swimming), contaminated, treated, reused, retreated, and so on, all year. The equipment and chemicals used in water treatment plants and swimming pools in most cases are the same—chlorine, alum, filters, pumps, and so on. In fact, swimming pools are small water treatment plants. Figure 5.1 illustrates the path pool water takes as it is treated.

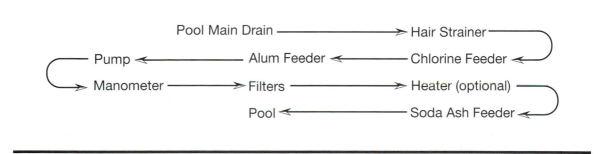

FIGURE 5.1 Path of swimming pool water.

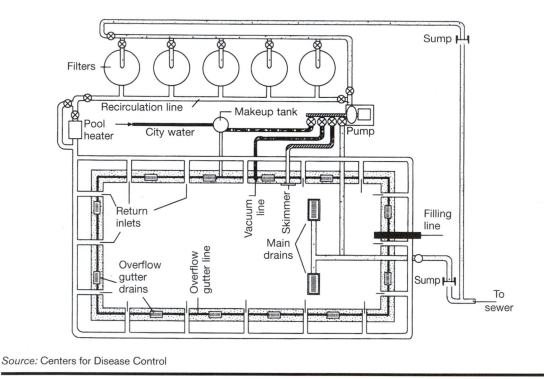

Figure labels within the diagram:

Filters

Sump

Recirculation line

Makeup tank

Pool heater

City water

Pump

Return inlets

Vacuum line

Skimmer

Filling line

Main drains

Overflow gutter drains

Overflow gutter line

Sump

To sewer

Source: Centers for Disease Control

FIGURE 5.2 Swimming pool piping system.

All pools should be equipped with either gutter drains, surface skimmers, or both (see Figure 5.2). The water pulled through these comes from the surface, where it is most contaminated because the material with specific gravity less than that of water will float. Therefore, this water is skimmed off the top to be filtered. The amount of water skimmed from the top can be controlled by opening or closing the valve to the surface skimmer; usually the gutter drains flow by gravity to the pump. Most of the water to be recirculated is pulled through the main drains. This is helpful in maintaining a chlorine residual throughout the pool. The water from the gutter drains through the make-up tank, which serves to replenish the water lost by splash, evaporation, and the like. There must be an air gap between the fresh water make-up line and the pool water to prevent **backsiphonage** (see Figure 5.3). Water from the make-up tank, surface skimmers,

line, and main drains goes through a hair strainer where lint, hair, and other extraneous materials are removed. At this point the water is still on the suction side of the recirculating pump.

Next, chlorine is added to the water as a disinfecting agent to kill pathogenic organisms. After chlorination, a filter aid (usually alum) is added to the water. Alum is a general term referring to aluminum compounds of sulfate or potassium, which aid in the flocculation (settling out) of small particles of impurities. The water now goes to the pump, which also serves as a rapid mixer. Once through the pump, the water passes by a manometer, used to measure the rate of flow to the filters.

Six filtration systems are commonly used in swimming pools. All six utilize some type of filter media (sand and gravel or diatomaceous earth). All are acceptable in their ability to remove dirt and impurities. The two basic filter types are classified

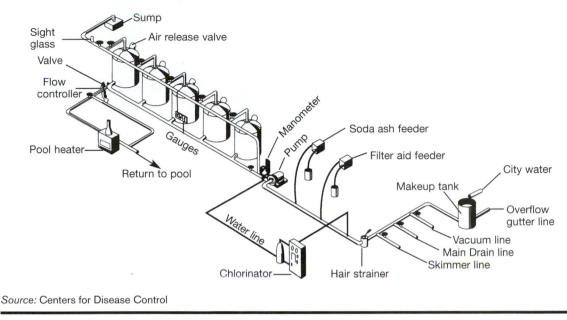

Source: Centers for Disease Control

FIGURE 5.3 Swimming pool filtration equipment.

as perpetual and temporary media. Filters in which the same media can be reused are of the perpetual media type and include the following:

- *Pressure sand*. Prior to 1950 this was the standard method of filtration. It employs one or more filter tanks filled with layers of sand and gravel. A motorized pump forces water down through the various layers of sand and gravel and back to the pool.

- *Vacuum sand (gravity sand)*. The oldest method of pool filtration, this was the most common until it was replaced by the pressure sand type. Once called the gravity sand method, it has undergone engineering changes and now is known as the vacuum sand method. The filter is a large, open bed consisting of several layers of gravel topped with sand. Water flows through the bed, with a combination of gravity and vacuum forces used to circulate it back into the pool.

- *High-flow sand*. In this more recent type of sand filtration (Figure 5.4), water is forced through sand that is kept in suspension by a rapid flow rate. The system requires half the filter surface area needed with the pressure sand method. Another advantage is that no coagulant (alum) is needed. Some question whether high-flow sand filters can deliver the same quality of water as the regular sand filters.

Filters that require new media after cleaning, the temporary media type, include the following:

- *Vacuum diatomaceous earth*. This method of filtration is also commonly referred to as the open pit or open tank method. Its filter medium consists of fossilized marine plants (diatoms) that form a 1/16 inch thick layer on the elements, which are visible in an open tank. The fossilized diatoms serve as a screen on the surface of filter elements and

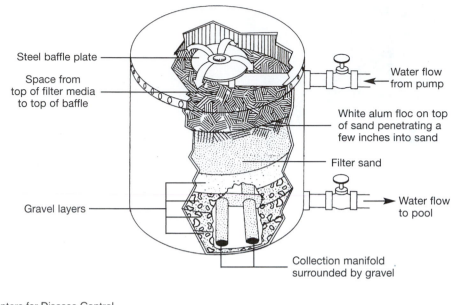

Steel baffle plate

Space from
top of filter media
to top of baffle

Gravel layers

Water flow
from pump

White alum floc on top
of sand penetrating a
few inches into sand

Filter sand

Water flow
to pool

Collection manifold
surrounded by gravel

Source: Centers for Disease Control

FIGURE 5.4 High-flow sand filter vessel.

strain dirt particles from the water. Water flows into the tank via gravity and is drawn through the elements and recirculated back to the pool. The advantage of this method is easier access for maintenance and cleaning.

- *Pressure diatomaceous earth.* D.E. pressure filtration was developed during World War II. The filter elements are housed in pressurized tanks, and water is pushed through the D.E.-coated elements and recirculated back to the pool (Figure 5.5).

- *Regenerative cycle diatomaceous earth.* Regenerative filters are a relatively recent adaptation of pressure D.E. filtration. The elements, several hundred per tank, are small tubes, usually made of spring stainless steel and covered with an acid- and base-resistant synthetic material. The main difference between the pressure and regenerative types is that the regenerative system automatically removes the previous D.E. coating and reapplies it to the elements, using the same filter

media several times a day. This system may require as few as eight 50-pound bags of D.E. per 12-month operating season.

Most of the filtering is done by gelatinous material, usually aluminum hydroxide, that forms on top of the filter media. From the bottom of the filters comes the filtered water that may or may not be heated as it reenters the pool. Soda ash then is added to raise the pH to the desired level. (Recent studies indicate it is best to introduce the soda ash after the filtration process.) Urine, body acids, alum, and gaseous chlorine have a tendency to lower the pH level.

Swimming Pool Construction and Maintenance

Pools obviously should be constructed of an impervious material. Concrete pools are common, and packaged steel panel units are available. The walls and bottom should be smooth and light-colored to facilitate cleaning. Water depth should vary from 3 feet (.9 m) to at least 6 feet (1.8 m) in every 15 feet (4.5 m) at the

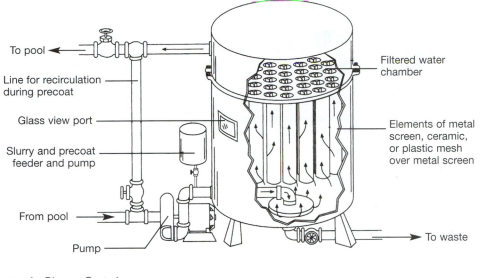

To pool

Line for recirculation
during precoat

Glass view port

Slurry and precoat
feeder and pump

From pool

Pump

Filtered water
chamber

Elements of metal
screen, ceramic,
or plastic mesh
over metal screen

To waste

Source: Centers for Disease Control

FIGURE 5.5 Pressure diatomaceous earth filter with cylindrical elements.

shallow end. The shallow area—that area less than 5 feet (1.5 m) deep—should comprise from 70% to 80% of the pool area. Areas less than 2 feet (.6 m) deep should be confined to wading pools. Surface area is based on approximately 2 square feet per person at maximum load on the assumption that one-third of the patrons will be outside the pool itself at any given time.

Pool shapes vary from square to bean-shaped and banjo-shaped. Rectangular-shaped pools in which the width is one-third the length probably are most common. Regardless of the shape of the pool, depth markers should be located around the periphery. These markers should be readily visible from the deck, and placed no more than 25 feet (7.5 m) apart, but preferably 10 feet (3.0 m) apart. Their purpose is to prevent nonswimmers from jumping into deep water and divers from diving into shallow water.

Pools should have a runway not less than 4 feet (1.2 m) wide, commencing with the edge of the pool. The deck or runway should slope away from the pool at about 1/4 inch per foot to prevent the water from draining back into the pool. A deck drain should be provided for approximately each 100 square feet of deck/runway surface. These drains may connect to a public sewer.

Where submersed lights are used, an electrical inspector should inspect them annually to assure that they are safe. This could prevent electrocution accidents.

The following are various parts of the pool, also shown in Figure 5.6, that must be understood for proper pool operation and maintenance.

Overflow gutter drains: drainage fittings used in the overflow gutter at the uppermost portion of the water.

Vacuum fitting: the place where a hose is connected to the suction piping to allow vacuuming of the pool. No other duty should be assigned to the pump when the pool is being vacuumed.

Return water inlets: located all around the pool and adjusted to control the amount of water entering the various areas of the pool.

Surface skimmer: a device that skims the water after storms, rain, etc. (less important in indoor

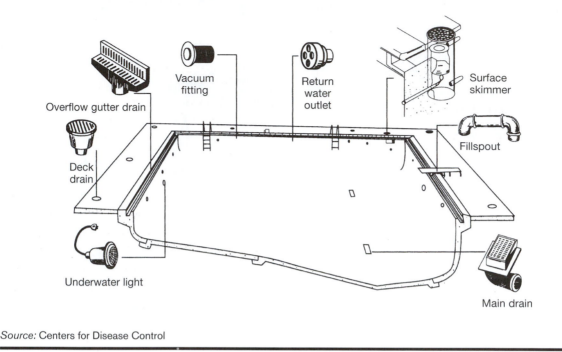

Overflow gutter drain

Vacuum fitting

Return water outlet

Surface skimmer

Deck drain

Fillspout

Underwater light

Main drain

Source: Centers for Disease Control

FIGURE 5.6 Longitudinal section through pool showing fittings.

pools). After each use the strainer basket in the skimmer is removed and cleaned.

Fillspout: located underneath the diving board for safety, its purpose is to fill the pool.

Main drain: outlet fittings at the bottom of a swimming pool through which water passes to the recirculating pump. During recirculation, three-fourths of the pool's total water volume leaves through the main drain and the other one-fourth leaves through overflow gutters or skimmers. The main drain opening should be protected and be at least four times the diameter of the pipe.

Other parts of a pool include:

Filter aid unit: in anthracite and sand filter systems, alum or another coagulant is added here.

Soda ash feeders: may be used to raise pH of pool water.

Pumps: serve three basic functions: to recirculate the pool water, to backwash the filters, and to agi-

tate alum so a large surface area is provided. Centrifugal pumps usually are used in swimming pools.

Manometer: a pressure device that measures volumetric flow to ensure that the desired turnover rate is being met. All pools must be recirculated three or four times daily or must be treated every 6 or 8 hours.

Make-up tank: contains fresh water to fill or refill the pool as a result of water loss. The water level here is the same as the pool's; therefore, it determines the water level in the pool. The make-up tank is connected to the city water supply. The disadvantage of this lies in provision of an air gap.

Gauges: two gauges that measure the pressure to ascertain when the filters should be backwashed. The difference in the pressure gauges indicates that the filters are dirty.

Sight glass: a device through which one can determine when the filter is clean by observing the water in the backwashing process as it passes through.

Special Pools

Many different types of pools currently are being manufactured. Most are confronted with the same maintenance and public health concerns, though. This discussion will be confined to two specific types, therapeutic and wading pools.

THERAPEUTIC POOLS

Therapeutic pools (public spas and hot tubs) are becoming almost as popular as swimming pools. They represent a relatively new development, and many of the new public pools are including a therapeutic pool as a separate system with its own circulating pump and filter. The turbulence and heated water in these pools have enhanced their "spa" effect. Because of the growing demand for therapeutic pools, the following requirements have become important:

- *Circulation.* The contents of a therapy pool should be recirculated quickly. The small volume of water in relation to the number of bathers necessitates rapid turnover to ensure water purity.
- *Surface skimmer and main drain.* Each therapeutic pool should have two main drains and at least one skimmer. The reason for this is to prevent suction and body entrapment accidents and to ensure rapid and complete water turnover.
- *Hydro-therapy system.* To achieve the "spa" or "jetting" effect, a properly sized pump and aid blower should be installed. The temperature of the water should not be higher than 104°F. The therapy pool always should have a thermometer so pool users can make an accurate check.
- *Chlorine/bromine feeding.* Because of the high water temperature in a therapy pool, chlorine/bromine dissipates rapidly. An automatic feeding device, properly sized to the therapy pool, must be installed and operated continuously.
- *Safety requirements.* Skid-proof decking and handrails for steps are necessary. In addition, all steps and seat edges should be delineated so that when the water is agitated, the edges are easily visible. The edges of steps and seats should be marked by installing a solid dark tile in a contrasting color.

WADING POOLS

Presenting the worst conditions of any swimming pool, shallow wading pools often are packed with small children who are most susceptible to waterborne diseases. The relative amounts of ammonia and organic nitrogens introduced into a wading pool (mainly by urine) are enormous. The chances of children being immune to diseases spread by pools are less than for older people, and the likelihood of their consuming pool water is greater. To keep a wading pool in good operating condition and as sanitary as possible, the following rules should be adhered to rigorously.

1. The circulation rate should be checked and maintained at the desired levels at least once an hour.
2. Chlorine and pH readings should be taken every hour and adjusted to maintain a minimum of 1.5 ppm of free chlorine and a pH of 7.2 to 7.6.
3. The pool should be vacuumed and skimmed as often as necessary and at least once a day.

A wading pool should not be made a part of another pool. It should be separated by a barrier and should have its own recirculating and chemical feeding systems.

Gas Chlorine Room

When chlorine gas is used as the means of disinfection, special precautions must be taken. There must be a separate room with an outside entrance for the chlorination equipment (see Figure 5.7). The room should have a door with louvers at the top instead of at the bottom, where they normally are located. The chlorine cylinders, both full and empty, must be fastened securely to prevent breaking. A self-contained breathing apparatus (SCBA) should be available in case of a chlorine gas leak. An exhaust fan, which switches on as the door to the chlorine room opens, should be installed and operative. This fan should be at floor level. If the chlorine room is below

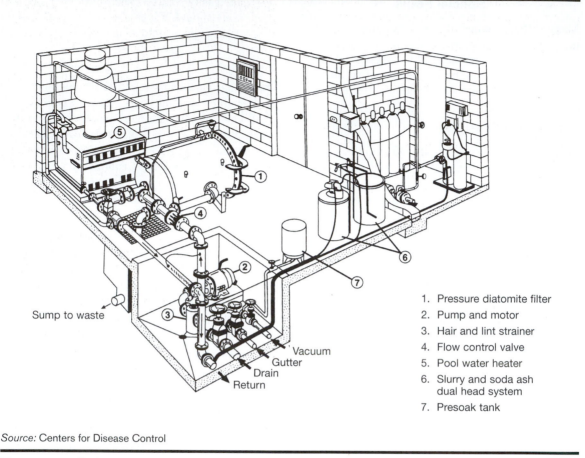

1. Pressure diatomite filter
2. Pump and motor
3. Hair and lint strainer
4. Flow control valve
5. Pool water heater
6. Slurry and soda ash dual head system
7. Presoak tank

Sump to waste

Vacuum
Gutter
Drain
Return

Source: Centers for Disease Control

FIGURE 5.7 Typical pressure diatomite filter system.

ground level, the fan duct should terminate above ground level. Chlorine gas is approximately two-and-one-half times as heavy as air and therefore will be near the floor. A stationary chlorine sniffer and alarm system are recommended. As a substitute, a can of ammonia should be kept in the chlorine room to check for chlorine leaks after cylinder changes and at other times when needed. Ammonia reacts with chlorine to form ammonium chloride, a white substance with a cloudlike appearance in air.

Chlorine is highly corrosive; therefore, either an inert metal tubing or rubber tubing must be used to transport the chlorine solution to the recirculating line. Another way of ascertaining a chlorine leak before entering the room is to have a glass panel in the door through which one can check pe-riodically to see if a highly polished brass object placed in the chlorine room shows corrosion. Chlorine is highly corrosive to brass, reacting with it in a few minutes.

Because chlorine is so corrosive and hazardous to people, the trend is away from chlorine gas and toward the use of calcium hypochlorite or some other disinfectant.

. . . .
PLAYGROUNDS

Playgrounds, whether in public locations—such as schools or parks—or in private backyards, are places that allow children to interact socially while they swing, slide, climb, or simply sit and talk.

These areas play a vital role in the development of children by providing challenges and testing their skills. The challenges presented should be stimulating and fun within a safe and healthful environment.

Design and Maintenance

When planning a new playground, it is important to consider hazards or obstacles to children traveling to and from the playground. A barrier around the playground site is recommended to prevent children from running into the street or roadway. Even when a barrier is present, however, children never should be left unattended or unsupervised. Playgrounds should be organized carefully into different areas to prevent possible injuries caused by conflicting games or activities, such as a playing field located too close to a swing set, in which a child runs in front of a swing in motion.

Active, physical activities always should be separated from more passive or quiet activities. Areas for play equipment, open playing fields, and sand boxes should be located in different sections of the playground. In addition, popular, heavy-use pieces of equipment or activities should be dispersed appropriately to avoid crowding in any area of the playground.

The layout of playground equipment and activities should provide for a clear line of sight to every area of the playground, enabling good supervision. All moving equipment on the playground, such as swings, teeter-totters and merry-go-rounds, should be located toward a corner or edge of the playground or play area. Slide exits always should be located in an uncongested area of the playground to prevent possible collisions between children.

Poor or inadequate maintenance of playground equipment can lead to severe injuries on the playground. Because the safety of playground equipment and its stability depend on good inspection and maintenance, the manufacturers' maintenance instructions and recommended inspection schedules should be strictly followed and enforced. A comprehensive maintenance program should be developed for each playground. All equipment should be inspected frequently for any potential hazards, for corrosion or deterioration from rot, insects, or weathering. The playground also should be checked frequently for broken

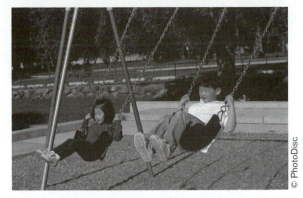

© PhotoDisc

Playground equipment should be inspected often for safety.

glass and other dangerous debris. Some manufacturers supply, with their maintenance instructions, a checklist for general or detailed inspections. These can be used to ensure that inspections are in compliance with the manufacturer's specifications.

Inspections alone do not constitute a comprehensive maintenance program. All hazards or defects identified during inspections should be repaired as quickly as possible using only replacement parts listed by or obtained from the manufacturer of the equipment. In addition to general maintenance inspections, more detailed inspections should be conducted on a regular basis depending upon the types and amount of equipment on the playground, level of use, local climate, and manufacturer's maintenance instructions.

Playground design and maintenance have been continuously improving, mainly because of the U.S. Consumer Product Safety Commission's (CPSC) publication of a *Handbook on Public Playground Safety*. Thanks to the CPSC guidelines, landscape architects and playground designers no longer are forced to rely solely on intuition and experience when trying to design and maintain a safe play environment. They also can follow specific guidelines for playground equipment established by the American Society of Testing Materials (ASTM) and be confident that new structures from top manufacturers will be unlikely to impale, entrap, cut, pinch, bruise, or otherwise cause serious injury to children. The discouraging side to playground safety is that not all playgrounds are inspected for safety, and few of the inspections that do occur are conducted by well-trained, certified environmental health and safety inspectors.

Equipment-Related Injuries

Approximately 170,000 children are injured on playgrounds throughout the United States each year. Most life-threatening injuries result from falls from equipment, impact with moving equipment, entanglement of clothing, and head entrapment. Many of these injuries can be prevented by the proper design and maintenance of playground facilities. The most common playground equipment-related dangers are as follows.

- *Pinch-crush parts.* Moving or sliding parts on equipment such as seesaws, gliders, and bending coiled springs can cause serious injury to extremities such as fingers and toes. When using these types of equipment, proper clothing (including shoes) should be worn at all times.

- *Rings.* When using this type of equipment, it must be the proper size. The ring should be bigger than 5 to 10 inches in diameter so a child cannot get his or her head entrapped within the ring. Any ring smaller than the specified minimum size should be discarded immediately.

- *Hooks.* This type of equipment is shaped like a large metal S. Hooks usually are used for attaching chains to swing sets. Large, open-ended S-hooks are the most dangerous, as they can easily grab clothing or contribute to pinching or cutting. With these hooks, the ends of the S always should be squeezed together tightly, which usually can be done with some type of pliers. If this is not possible, the local gym-set dealer should be consulted.

- *Hard, heavy swing seats.* This type of equipment can strike a hard blow to a child's head, inflicting trauma. Features to look for when choosing a swing seat include: light weight, sturdy, round edges, and a grip on the seat. If purchasing a seat made of aluminum or other metal, it should have rolled edges.

- *Inadequate spacing.* When installing a gym set, the set should be a minimum of 6 feet from fences, building walls, walkways, and other play areas such as sand boxes. This allows a safe margin. Adequate spacing of equipment from playground boundaries also is highly advisable for playgrounds near busy streets.

- *Exposed screws and bolts.* Two of the most common injuries to children in the playground are cuts and bruises. An uncapped or unprotected protruding screw is often the offender. Unprotected screws should be covered immediately, either with tape or some type of rubber cap.

- *Hard surfaces.* A gym set never should be installed over a hard surface such as concrete, blacktop, or cinders. Grass, rubber, wood chips, and sand are always better alternatives.

- *Sharp edges.* Some gym sets have sharp edges or points where the parts fit together. These areas should be taped over with heavy tape, and the taped areas inspected regularly for weather damage.

- *Improper anchoring.* Legs of equipment should be set in concrete for stability. All types of anchoring devices should be placed below ground level to avoid a tripping hazard.

- *Strangulation hazard with playground cargo nets.* The U.S. Consumer Product Safety Commission advises parents to check outdoor play equipment featuring cargo nets before allowing children to play on them. Nets having openings with a perimeter length (sum of the length of the four sides) of between 17 and 28 inches could allow head entrapment and possible strangulation. The CPSC cites incidents at fast-food restaurants playgrounds where a child's head was entrapped and an adult had to cut the net to release the child.

- *Strings and strangulation.* Clothing strings, loose clothing, and stringed items placed around the neck can catch on playground equipment and strangle children. When children are playing, they should not be wearing these.

- *Hot metal playground equipment.* A good rule of thumb is to always check for hot surfaces on metal playground equipment before allowing children to play on it. Solid steel decks, slides, and steps in direct sunlight may reach temperatures high enough to cause serious contact-burn injuries in a matter of seconds. Typically affected are the hands, legs, and buttocks.

Playground Surfacing

The CPSC has estimated that approximately 100,000 playground equipment-related injuries resulting from falls to the (ground) surface are treated annually in U.S. hospital emergency rooms. This represents about 60% of all playground equipment-related injuries. Injuries resulting from falls to the ground are potentially fatal, especially when the head is involved. According to the CPSC, about three-fourths of all fall-related deaths involve head injuries.

Until 1981, the preferred playground surfaces were concrete, asphalt, and grass. Schools liked asphalt because it was considered to be softer than concrete and was easily maintained. There was nothing to track into the school building (like sand), and it needed no raking or care. In public parks, grass and hard dirt—the result of grass wearing away—were most commonly seen under playground equipment. Rubber mats soon became popular and were used in some settings; however, they were found to be too expensive for most municipalities and school systems. Sand and pea gravel were fairly inexpensive but required constant maintenance and replacement. Sand could be blown around and was tracked into schools, where it ruined the floors. Sand also attracted animals. Pea gravel could be thrown around and, if dispersed on concrete walks, could cause slip-and-fall accidents.

Not until 1986 did shock-absorbing surfaces with properties sufficient to reduce serious head injuries become the preferred playground surface. Regardless of the material chosen, however, the appropriate depth cannot be expected to prevent or reduce the severity of all injuries from falls. The term used to describe the shock-absorbing performance of a surfacing material is its "critical height."

Two basic groups of materials are acceptable for the surfacing of playgrounds: unitary and loose-fill.

1. Unitary materials are generally rubber mats or a combination of rubberlike materials held in place by a binder that may be poured in place at the playground site and cured to form a unitary shock-absorbing surface.

2. Loose-fill materials include, but are not confined to, sand, gravel, and shredded-wood products. These materials have acceptable shock-absorbing properties when installed over hard surfaces such as asphalt or concrete. Table 5.2 gives the appropriate depths of loose-fill materials and the critical heights at which the depths will be effective.

■ TABLE 5.2 ■

CRITICAL HEIGHTS (IN FEET) FOR LOOSE-FILL MATERIAL DEPTHS (IN INCHES)

Material	Uncompressed Depth		Compressed Depth	
	6 in.	9 in.	12 in.	9 in.
Wood Mulch	7 ft	10 ft	11 ft	10 ft
Double Shredded Bark Mulch	6 ft	10 ft	11 ft	7 ft
Uniform Wood Chips	6 ft	7 ft	12 ft	6 ft
Fine Sand	5 ft	5 ft	9 ft	5 ft
Coarse Sand	5 ft	5 ft	6 ft	4 ft
Fine Gravel	6 ft	7 ft	10 ft	6 ft
Medium Gravel	5 ft	5 ft	6 ft	5 ft

Source: Consumer Product Safety Commission

All playground supervisors should have a uniform method of reporting and documenting accidents that occur on the playground. Accident forms should include specific information including names and addresses of witnesses, how a particular piece of equipment was being used, and photographs of the accident site, if possible.

Play is critical to the physical and social development of children. Play apparatus alone does not make a playground a functional developmental area. For children to learn through recreation, properly planned programs with supervision—conducted specifically in a safe and healthy environment—are absolutely necessary.

SUMMARY

More Americans now are realizing the importance of recreational activities to good public health. Recreational activities help to renew the mind and body and therefore contribute to mental, physical, and social well-being. Americans make an estimated 7.8 billion one-day visits each year to a variety of recreational areas, participating in numerous activities that involve man-made apparatus and natural environmental resources. Although recreational areas and activities can help to provide a relaxing and rejuvenating environment, they also present major environmental health and safety concerns.

Unintentional injuries and the spread of disease increase as recreational areas become more densely populated. Also, problems associated uniquely with recreational areas—remote locations, seasonal operations, water-oriented activities, vector and animal problems, noxious plants and weeds, age-specific activities, and many others—increase the need for improved environmental health and safety awareness in recreational areas. Many common environmental health and safety problems can be avoided if design, maintenance, and human control measures are strictly enforced. Finally, management of recreational areas must provide adequate staff training and give top priority to the principles and practices of maintaining a safe and healthful recreational environment.

KEY TERMS

Avalanche, p. 82

Backsiphonage, p. 86

Conduction, p. 80

Convection, p. 80

Evaporation, p. 80

Frostbite, p. 80

Hypochlorous acid, p. 85

Hypothermia, p. 80

Loose-snow avalanche, p. 82

Mass gathering, p. 79

Playground, p. 92

Radiation, p. 80

Recreation, p. 80

Slab avalanche, p. 82

Snowmobile, p. 81

Undertow, p. 84

Wetlands, p. 78

Winter white-out, p. 81

REFERENCES

American Academy of Pediatrics Committee on Accident and Poison Prevention. 1988. Snowmobile statement. *Pediatrics*, vol. 82, pp. 798–799.

Berry, Dennis. 1989. *Pool Managers: Water Quality Handbook*. LaMotte Company, Chestertown, MD.

Bever, David L. 1996. *Recreational Safety*, 4th ed. Mosby-Year Book, Inc., St. Louis, MO.

Centers for Disease Control and Prevention. 1995, February 27. Injuries Associated with the Use of Snowmobiles. *Journal of the American Medical Association*, pp. 448–449.

Christiansen, Monty L. 1995. *Playground Safety*. Center for Hospitality, Tourism and Recreation Research, University Park, PA.

Forgey, William W. 1985. *Death by Exposure*. ICS, Merrillville, IN.

Gabert, Thomas. 1993, December. Recreational Injuries and Deaths in Northern Wisconsin. *Wisconsin Medical Journal*, vol. 92, no. 12, pp. 671–675.

Greenberg, A. 1989, November. How Safe is Skiing? *Skiing*, pp 56–62.

Greenberg, A. 1989, Spring. Is Skiing Overrated? *Skiing*, pp. 12–14.

Hauser, Dan. 1995, Spring. Riding on Thin Ice. *Snowmobile*, p. 5.

Johnson, Ralph L. 1994. *YMCA: Pool Operation Manual*, 2nd ed. YMCA of the USA, Champaign, IL.

Johnson, Robert J., C. D. Mote Jr., and John Zelcer. 1993. *Skiing Trauma and Safety: Ninth International Symposium*. ASTM Publications, Philadelphia.

Jucker, Karl, Clayne R. Jensen, and Gary Howard. 1983. *Skiing*. Wm C. Brown, Dubuque, IA.

Chapter 5

King, Steve, 1996. Prevent Playground Injuries with Professional Inspection. *Parks & Recreation*, vol. 31, no. 4, p. 62.

Koren, Herman, 1996. *Handbook of Environmental Health and Safety: Principles and Practices*, 3rd ed. CRC Press, Boca Raton, FL.

Koren, Herman. 1996. *Illustrated Dictionary of Environmental Health and Occupational Safety*. CCR Press, Boca Raton, FL.

Lisella, Frank S. 1994. *VNR Dictionary of Environmental Health and Safety*. Van Nostrand Reinhold, New York.

Miller, Dean F. 1995. *Safety: Principles and Issues.* Brown & Benchmark Publishers, Dubuque, IA.

Morgan, Monroe T. 1993. *Environmental Health*. Brown and Benchmark Publishers, Dubuque, IA.

Morgan, Monrtoe T. 1997. *Environmental Health*, 2nd ed. Morton Publishing Company, Englewood, CO.

Patton, Pettis L. 1996. Urban Playgrounds: An Institution of Learning for Children. *Parks & Recreation*, vol. 31, no. 4, p. 68.

Pope, James R. 1985. *Public Swimming Pool Management: A Manual on Sanitation, Filtration, and Disinfection*. Clemson University, Clemson, SC.

Rea, Phillip S, and Roger Warren. 1986. *Recreation Management of Water Resources*. Publishing Horizons, Columbus, OH.

Salvato, Joseph A. 1992. *Environmental Engineering and Sanitation*, 4th ed. John Wiley and Sons, New York.

Teague, Travis, 1992. *Playgrounds: Managing Your Risk*. Parks & Recreation, vol. 31, no. 4, p. 54.

Thygerson, Alton L. 1992. *Sports and Recreational Safety*, 2nd ed. Jones and Barlett Publishers, Boston, MA.

U.S. Public Health Service. *Environmental Health Practice in Recreational Areas*. PHS Publication No. 1195, Washington, DC.

U.S. Department of Agriculture. 1982. *Snow Avalanche: General Rules for Avoiding and Surviving Snow Avalanches.*

U.S. Department of Agriculture. 1994. *Snow Avalanches: Basic Principles for Avoiding and Surviving Snow Avalanches.*

U.S. Department of Health and Human Services. 1985. *Suggested Health and Safety Guidelines for Public Spas and Hot Tubs.*

U.S. Department of Health and Human Services. 2000. *Swimming Pools: Safety and Disease Control Through Proper Design and Operation.*

Wallach, Fran. 1996. An Update on the Playground Safety Movement. *Parks & Recreation*, vol. 31, no. 4, p. 46.

Wilkerson, James A. 1988. *Hypothermia, Frostbite, and Other Cold Injuries*. Mountaineers, Seattle.

6

WASTEWATER MANAGEMENT

- Discuss the need for wastewater disposal.
- Explain non-water-carried systems.
- Define and explain individual water-carried systems.
- Describe municipal wastewater treatment, its purpose, and its function.
- Discuss the principles of water pollution.

America is the same size as it was in 1492. Lakes, rivers, and streams are the same size or smaller than when the country was discovered. The population has grown rapidly, however, spawning thermal, noise, air, and water pollution. Today the production of "necessities" and the nation's affluence have generated pollution at the point of production via the use and disposal of the materials generated to satisfy the public's desires.

Water pollution (anything in water that is not water) comes from industry, domestic units, agriculture, and natural sources. Some sources of natural pollution are volcanic ash, dust storms, trees, decomposing vegetation, eroded soil, and excrement.

Industrial plants release waste into the air, onto the land, and into the water. The water used in many industrial processes picks up forms of industrial waste that remain in the water as it is discharged into the environment. This waste can be chemical (organic or inorganic), such as mercury; physical, such as heat; or biological, such as microbes borne by employees working in the plant.

Domestic water pollution constitutes a big portion of the water pollution. Domestic waste consists of kitchen and bathroom waste from homes, schools, hospitals, nursing homes, and other places where people live, work, and travel.

Pesticides, herbicides, and fertilizers are major sources of agricultural waste. Precipitation sometimes washes these compounds into streams, rivers, lakes, and oceans. This is difficult to control because it is **nonpoint pollution**. Another example of nonpoint agricultural waste is livestock drinking, urinating, and defecating in ponds, lakes, and streams. In trying to reduce agricultural waste, we can reduce the required food supply if we make mistakes.

Natural sources of pollution include, among others, volcanic ash, dust storms, decomposing

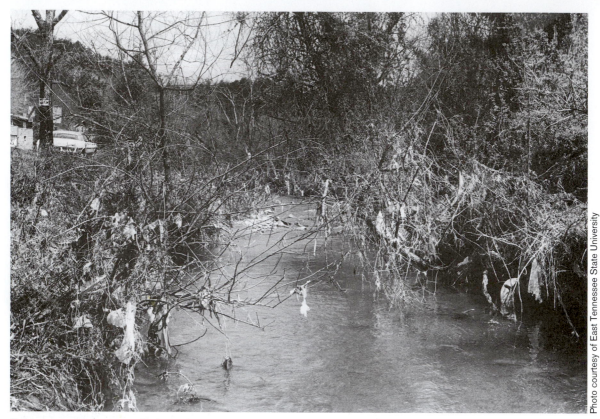

Solid waste adds to water pollution and aesthetic degradation of the environment.

Photo courtesy of East Tennessee State University

vegetation, and eroded soil. Efforts to reduce industrial and domestic water pollution concentrate on minimizing the use of materials that escape to the atmosphere and end up in water. These efforts are exerted mainly through industrial and domestic (city) wastewater treatment plants. In these plants much of the material (waste) that is not water is removed. Much research is being done throughout the world to improve the technology for wastewater treatment.

The principle of wastewater treatment can be explained by simile. Assume that we run wastewater through a large pipe that has a filter in it, and assume that the filter excludes everything except the water (Figure 6.1). If that were possible, only pure water would flow out of the pipe after being filtered. Purification would be accomplished quickly and painlessly.

Human waste products are harmful to humans. In this chapter we will focus on some techniques of disposing of human urine and feces that are capable of spreading disease. Our concern is mainly the biological causative agents of disease.

Water is a natural resource that too often is taken for granted in human culture. Unlike many other consumer goods, water contaminated by human waste cannot be simply thrown away. Water containing human waste—termed **sewage** or **wastewater**—generally contains more than 99.9% water. The remaining less than 0.1% consists of the waste we remove from the water.

Every state in the United States has a law stating that human excrement must be disposed of in a sanitary manner. Reasons for sanitary disposal of wastewaters are to prevent the pollution of surface waters, the pollution of groundwater, and hook-

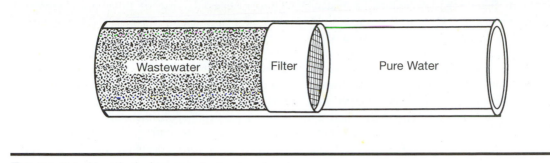

Wastewater | Filter | Pure Water

FIGURE 6.1 Hypothetical wastewater treatment system.

worm infestation by refraining from using human excrement as a fertilizer on vegetables and other foods. Further, wastewater should be disposed in a sanitary manner to prevent waste from being accessible to insects capable of transmitting disease, and for many other reasons.

Excreta disposal can be divided into two main types: non–water-carried and water-carried. We also can discuss wastewater disposal according to individual and municipal systems.

NON-WATER-CARRIED SYSTEMS

In many underdeveloped nations and in parts of the United States, dwellings are not equipped with indoor plumbing. If no water is entering the dwelling, no water is available to flush human waste away toward treatment. When these conditions are present, the best solution may be to install a **pit privy**, or pit latrine. An example is pictured.

The objective for pit construction, as it is for all disposal systems, is to construct an underground area where urine and feces can be deposited and retained in a sanitary manner. This means that the pit area is sufficiently above any water table, provides a self-closing door, and screens any openings, such as vents, which would allow access to flies or other vermin capable of spreading disease. Thereafter, the waste is deposited directly into the pit. If and when the pit becomes full, the building housing it can be relocated to a new pit. The old pit must be covered with at least 18 inches of earth.

Another type of non-water-carried sewage system is the **box and can**. These systems may be found on buses, trains, airplanes, and construction sites, or any areas where people's waste must be contained until it can be removed for treatment.

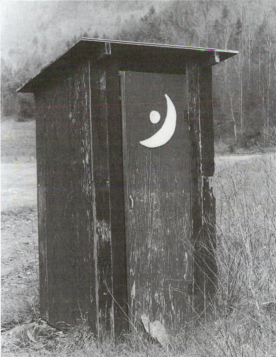

A pit privy.

Photo courtesy of East Tennessee State University

The box and can disposal system is found virtually anywhere people gather without a water-carried sewage system. The units, often termed "portable toilets" or "port-a-john," have a self-contained, above-ground chamber to collect urine and feces. A liquid chemical often is added to the chamber to reduce odors, break down the waste, and serve as a disinfectant. The box and can system must be maintained by pumping the contents of the storage chamber as necessary and transporting the waste to an approved wastewater treatment facility.

....

INDIVIDUAL WATER-CARRIED SYSTEMS

Before purchasing a tract of land, numerous factors must be considered, the most important of which could be the capability of the soil to absorb water. If potable water is available for use within the dwelling, this water must undergo treatment after its use. In this case, no central sewage disposal system is provided; therefore, the property must be evaluated for an on-site, water-carried subsurface sewage disposal system—specifically a septic tank and drainfield system. In subdivisions, the system should be an interim expedient device until a central sewerage system is constructed. In many areas, however, a central sewer, or public sewer, may not be available for decades.

The function of a **septic tank and drainfield system** is to remove as many solids as possible from wastewater and filter this waste through the soil. In many cases, plants draw the wastewater from the soil by transpiration or the soil's capillary action pulls it to the surface in order that evaporation may occur, called **evapotranspiration**.

Soil Evaluation

A critical concern that must be considered prior to construction of any subsurface sewage disposal system is the soil's capacity to absorb the wastewater. Not all soils are capable of absorbing enough water to allow construction of a subsurface system. The health department environmentalist/ sanitarian or a soil scientist evaluates the soil for appropriateness by use of (a) a percolation test, (b) soil maps, and/or (c) soil color and texture evaluation.

A percolation test involves digging a hole of a specified diameter to a typical depth of approximately 36 inches (90 cm). The hole is filled with water and allowed to presoak or saturate for a time dependent upon the soil type, generally overnight. After saturation of the soil, the hole is filled with water to a designated level. The depth of the water in the hole is measured at regular time intervals to determine how many minutes are required for 1 inch of water to exit the hole. As a result, a percolation rate, in minutes per inch, is established.

For example, if it took 1 hour for the water to lower an inch, the percolation rate would be 60 minutes/inch (24 min./cm). If the level of water in the hole lowered 1 inch (2.5 cm) in 10 minutes, the percolation rate would be 10 minutes/inch (10 minutes/25 cm). The faster the percolation rate—the less time (minutes) required to drop an inch of water in the percolation hole—the better is the percolation rate. Generally speaking, soils with a percolation rate of 60 minutes per inch (2.5 cm) or greater are not acceptable for constructing a conventional drainfield system. The percolation rate also is a factor in determining the size of the drainfield. The smaller the percolation rate, the less drainfield required. Absorption-area requirements for private residences with a disposal and washing machine are given in Table 6.1.

Soil maps also can be helpful when determining percolation rates. Upon knowing the exact location of the tract of land in question, the evaluator may refer to soil maps that tell specific soil types, textures, and applications for the area. These maps provide a general indication of the area considered for a drainfield. A more thorough evaluation may be accomplished by conducting a soil color, structure, and texture evaluation in the exact area of the drainfield.

For a soil evaluation, an evaluator bores holes with a soil auger and observes the color, structure, and texture of the soil to a desired depth. Gener-

ABSORPTION-AREA REQUIREMENTS FOR PRIVATE RESIDENCES (PROVIDES FOR GARBAGE-GRINDER AND AUTOMATIC-SEQUENCE WASHING MACHINES)

Percolation rate (time required for water to fall 1 inch, in minutes)	Required absorption area, in square feet per bedroom[1], standard trench[2], and seepage pits[3]	Percolation rate (time required for water to fall 1 inch, in minutes)	Required absorption area, in square feet per bedroom[1], standard trench[2], and seepage pits[3]
1 or less	70	10	165
2	85	15	190
3	100	30[4]	250
4	115	45[4]	300
5	125	60[4,5]	330

1. In every case, sufficient area should be provided for at least two bedrooms.
2. Absorption area for standard trenches is figured as trench-bottom area.
3. Absorption area for seepage pits is figured as effective side-wall area beneath the inlet.
4. Unsuitable for seepage pits if over 30.
5. Unsuitable for leaching systems if over 60.

Source: Manual of Septic Tank Practice, U.S. Public Health Service

ally speaking, brighter colored soils, as well as soils with greater amounts of sand or loam, tend to be better drained. Through knowledge of soils, an environmentalist/sanitarian or soil scientist can often estimate a percolation rate. Of the three types of evaluations, the percolation test is most accurate.

Before installing a subsurface sewage system, additional factors must be considered. The area must be evaluated to locate any natural drainageways, because it is not desirable to have surface water flowing over the absorption field area. The drainfield area should be located at an adequate distance (generally 100 feet) from bodies of water, water supplies, dwellings, property lines, underground utility lines, and the like. The amount of water used within a day's time must be considered before designing and installing the system. A dwelling with eight people certainly will use more water than a dwelling with two people. Therefore, the dwelling with eight would require a larger drainfield area to absorb the excess water used.

The sanitarian/environmentalist designs the on-site wastewater disposal system according to the specific properties of the evaluation. In most areas the city issues a permit before any construction can begin. The permit specifies the disposal system design. Once installed, the sanitarian/environmentalist inspects the system before the septic tank and absorption trenches are backfilled. The inspection ensures quality control and determines if the installation has been done in accordance with applicable regulations (as specified by the health department).

Septic Tank System

Now let's trace a drop of water from the dwelling through a typical septic tank and drainfield system (Figure 6.2). From a plumbing fixture such as the kitchen sink, water drains through a U-trap (often called a P-trap). The U-trap's function is to collect water, forming a barrier against gases backing up into the house from the sewer system.

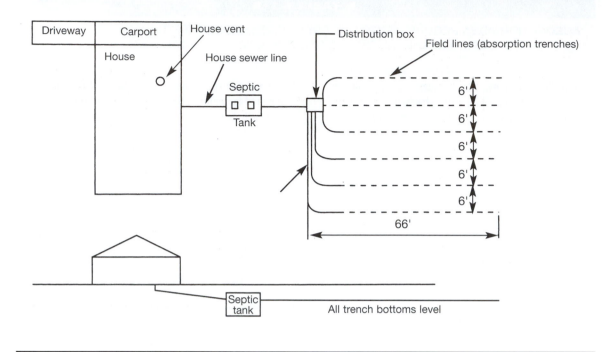

FIGURE 6.2 Layout of septic tank system.

From the U-trap the flow continues through a pipe out of the house and into the house sewer line.

The house sewer line must have sufficient diameter and slope to allow an unrestricted flow of sewage. From this point the flow continues directly into the underground septic tank. As the water enters the septic tank, the influent is diverted downward by an inlet tee. The inlet tee serves two functions: (a) it diverts the solids in the wastewater toward the bottom of the septic tank, and (b) it allows gases to back up into the household sewer line and exit through a vent. The vent, located on the house's roof, helps the wastewater to flow freely through the plumbing. It also vents into the atmosphere gases produced in the septic tank and avoids loss of water seals by siphoning.

The septic tank itself is a large chamber that is generally rectangular in shape. The tank's length is usually twice the width. The volume of individual septic tanks varies, but the tank itself should be large enough to allow the wastewater a retention time of at least 24 hours.

The septic tank (see Figure 6.3) serves three main functions:

1. It is a settling basin for removal of solids as sludge.

2. It stores the settled sludge and scum until the waste can be removed mechanically.

3. It provides a chamber for biological decomposition.

The biological activity is anaerobic, producing the gases carbon dioxide (CO_2), hydrogen sulfide (H_2S), and methane CH_4), as well as water (H_2O). The gases rise from the septic tank back into the household sewer line and out the vent. The heavier materials—those denser than water—settle to the bottom of the septic tank and produce a sludge. The solid materials—less dense than water—float to

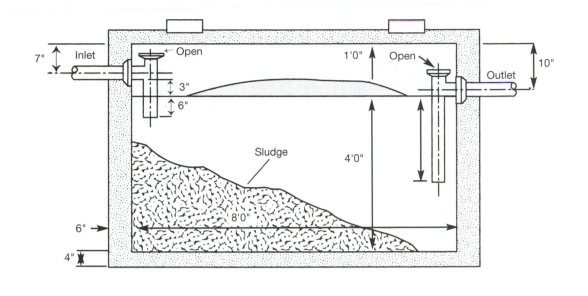

FIGURE 6.3 Septic tank.

the top of the wastewater, producing a scum layer. The objective is to allow water to flow from the septic tank with as many solids removed as possible, and with the scum also removed.

The effluent from the septic tank usually flows through a header line and into the distribution box, if present. The function of a distribution box is to collect the wastewater and distribute it evenly into each of the absorption trenches. Many current designs do not use distribution boxes. If no distribution box is used, the water simply flows directly through header lines into the drainfield or the absorption trench. This is accomplished by the old maxim of water seeking its own level.

If the distribution box is used, the water flows through the sealed lines directly into the absorption trenches. Header lines to the absorption trenches are adjusted to the height of the water in the distribution box, thereby producing an equal flow to each trench (see Figure 6.2). Once the water reaches the trenches, it is evenly distributed by way of drainage tile or percolation pipe (drainfield pipe). In some areas drainfield tile is required.

Other areas require a plastic pipe that comes in 10 feet (3.04 m) or greater lengths, or may even be continuous. This pipe is constructed with holes to allow the wastewater to flow out of the pipe and into the absorption trenches.

Absorption trenches are dug to a predetermined depth, generally about 36 inches, to absorb the wastewater. The tile, or percolation pipe, is placed over 6 inches of gravel below, and 2 inches of gravel are placed above (Figure 6.4). Generally, this (including the 5″ pipe) should total approximately 13 inches (32.5 cm) of gravel. The gravel should be clean and free of any fine particles because its void spaces serve as a storage reservoir for excess wastewater until it is absorbed into the ground (see Figure 6.5). Most of the wastewater in a traditional system will be absorbed by the soil in the absorption trenches; the rest evapotranspires.

Let us consider the possible fates of a pathogenic organism as it is transported through such a system. It may settle with the sludge in the septic tank and become food for other microorganisms. If a pathogen is not destroyed by microorganisms or

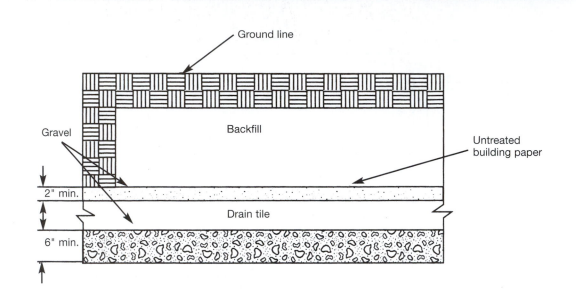

FIGURE 6.4 Lateral view through trench.

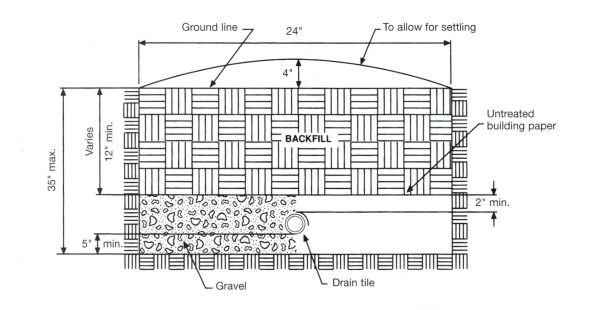

FIGURE 6.5 In-view of a drainfield line.

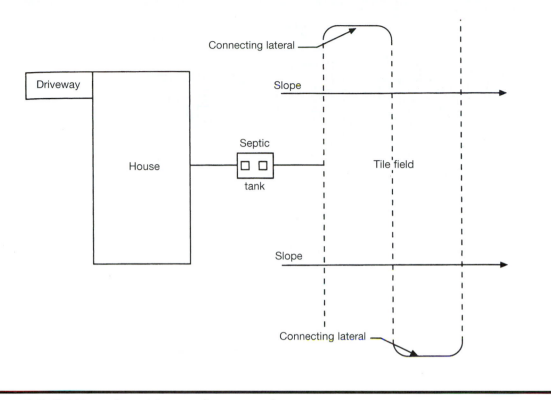

FIGURE 6.6 Field layout for serial system (home system).

the anaerobic environment in the septic tank, however, it may be passed to the absorption trenches. In the trenches, the soil should have the capability to trap any pathogens as the wastewater percolates through. Subsurface wastewater systems should not be installed in areas of fractured rock. Unlike soil, this rock does not have the capability to filter pathogens from the wastewater, thereby contributing to groundwater contamination.

Some drainfield systems are constructed without distribution boxes. An example is the serial (or hump) system shown in Figures 6.6 and 6.7. In this system all of the wastewater initially flows into the first trench. The water rises in the trench continually until it reaches the level of a preinstalled "crow over" pipe. This pipe collects the water and carries it to another trench, where the water is ab-

sorbed. The backfill in the trenches pulls the water toward the surface by capillary action. As the wastewater gets closer to the ground's surface, plants consume it and the sun evaporates it. Thus, evapotranspiration plays an important role in the serial system.

Seepage pits are used in some areas. They are deep, possibly 10 feet (3.04 m) or more, and are designed to go down until reaching the good soil. A seepage pit typically is 10 feet (3.04 m) wide, 10 feet (3.04 m) long, and 10 feet (3.04 m) deep, with 8 feet (2.40 m) of gravel in it. The void spaces in the gravel hold the wastewater during times of high use for later percolation into the ground. Seepage pits include a septic tank and possibly a distribution box. Various states have several approved types of individual sewage disposal systems.

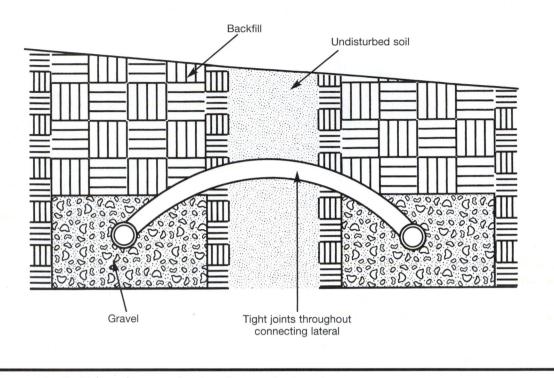

Backfill

Undisturbed soil

Gravel

Tight joints throughout
connecting lateral

FIGURE 6.7 Serial (hump) system: Section of connecting lateral.

MUNICIPAL WASTEWATER TREATMENT

Physical, chemical, and biological treatment processes all have been used in wastewater treatment, although modern treatment of municipal wastewater usually involves biological processes. Essentially, the wastewater treatment plant provides a controlled environment that enhances the growth of certain microorganisms that absorb and metabolize constituents of the waste. General requirements for the growth of microorganisms are described in Chapter 2.

Wastewater treatment processes are either aerobic or anaerobic. The aerobic process is used most frequently. The widely used activated sludge process exemplifies modern aerobic wastewater treatment. Sufficient air has to be forced into liquid in the aeration tank to maintain treatment effectiveness and prevent the unpleas-

ant odors generated by the aerobic processes. Various other conditions—including pH and temperature—must be maintained at levels suitable for microorganisms.

Here we will describe biological filtration, generally in trickling filters or biological towers. Although used less than in the past, biological filtration lends itself well to an introductory discussion of wastewater treatment.

The Process

Wastewater can be collected and treated on a large scale by municipal wastewater treatment facilities. The flow through a conventional wastewater treatment plant looks like this:

Sanitary Sewer⟶Bar Screen⟶Grit Basin ⟶Grinder⟶Primary Clarifier⟶Activated Sludge or Trickling Filter⟶Secondary Clarifier⟶Chlorine Basin⟶Stream

The wastewater exits a dwelling just as it does with the septic tank system, through the house sewer line. From the house sewer, the wastewater flows into a domestic or sanitary sewer. The sanitary sewer system consists of a series of pipes that collect the wastewater. This collection system transports the wastewater to a wastewater treatment plant.

Another type of sewer, the **storm sewer**, can be found in many areas. Unlike the sanitary sewer, the storm sewer collects surface runoff only from rainwater; it does not collect domestic waste. The storm sewer water should not flow into a wastewater treatment plant, nor should it be connected to the sanitary sewer at any point.

As the wastewater enters the treatment plant via sanitary sewer, it flows to a mechanically cleaned bar screen with a manually cleaned bypass **bar screen**. The screen is designed to remove sticks, rocks, plastics, and stringy material from the flow. The individual bars are located about 2 inches (5.1 cm) apart to remove floating sticks and other large objects. The bar screen can be cleaned and waste taken to a landfill.

From the bar screen the flow continues into an aerated grit basin or chamber. Until now water has flowed rapidly through the pipe. As the wastewater enters the **grit chamber**, however, the rate of flow slows as the water is spread over a large area. The purpose of the grit chamber is to slow down the water just enough to allow time for heavy particles, such as grit, sand, and quickly settling organic material, to be removed. The settled material is picked up by a submersible grit pump and placed in a hopper. Grease is also removed and discharged to a hopper. Both grit and grease are then taken to a landfill for disposal.

The flow may proceed through a measuring device such as Parshall flume or **venturi meter** to a **primary clarifier**, which removes most of the settable solids. This clarifier, also called a **settling basin**, allows materials to settle out. In a circular tank, the water enters through the center of the clarifier and moves outward slowly, exiting by overflowing around the rim of the unit.

The water moves slowly enough through the clarifier to allow a large amount of suspended solids to accumulate on the bottom, producing **sludge.** Machines scrape this sludge from the bottom of the clarifier and pump it away. A scum layer forms on top of the clarifier. As with sludge, a machine scrapes the scum off, feeds it into a hopper, and pumps it to a sludge treatment processor or digester.

The effluent from the primary clarifier enters activated sludge process or trickling filter. Trickling filters are large and have a medium of rocks about the side of a fist, or a synthetic material, with a depth of about 7 feet (2.1 m). The water enters the trickling filter through large arms that spray and distribute the wastewater evenly over the surface of the filter. Numerous biological organisms grow on these rocks. As the wastewater flows down through the rocks, the organisms on the rocks metabolize many of the suspended solids that were not settled in the primary clarifier. This process is much more effective if the rocks are kept wet at all times. Hence, the water is recycled in periods of low wastewater flow to create a high-rate trickling filter.

Materials continue to build up on these rocks and eventually slough off. The trickling filter is not actually a physical filter but, rather, an area of biological decomposition. The activated sludge tank serves the same purpose as the trickling filter—to remove waste from the wastewater.

The water collected at the bottom of the trickling filter flows into a secondary clarifier, moving just as it does through the primary clarifier. The secondary clarifier settles any remaining suspended solids. These solids are collected and pumped into the digester.

The activated sludge process is a biological wastewater treatment process that uses microorganisms to speed up decomposition of waste. The microorganisms feed and grow on waste particles in the wastewater; therefore, as more organisms grow and reproduce, the more waste is removed, leaving the wastewater partially cleaned. The success and operational efficiency of the activated sludge process depends on a balance of solids concentration, food, and oxygen. The activated sludge effluent flows to the secondary clarifier for water—solids separation. The solids are returned to the activated sludge process or the digester. The secondary clarifier effluent travels to the process of disinfection before the water enters the stream.

Disinfection is the process designed to kill or inactivate pathogenic organisms. The settling and biological processes remove a great number of organisms from the wastewater flow; there remain many thousands of bacteria leaving the secondary clarifier. Treatment processes available for disinfection include chlorine gas and ultraviolet systems. These systems reduce fecal coliform levels from 0–200 colonies/100ml before discharging into a stream. The flow from the disinfection process is often aerated before entering the stream.

The Digester

Recall that all of the sludge and scum collected in the clarifiers and trickling filter is pumped into a digester. The **digester** can be designed to operate as an aerobic or anaerobic. The anaerobic digester is a large sealed unit where anaerobic decomposition takes place. The sludge and scum provide food for the decomposition. Metabolization of these organic materials produces methane (CH_4), hydrogen sulfide (H_2S), and carbon dioxide (CO_2). Water (H_2O) is also a product of this metabolism.

The gases are collected and processed to produce a gas that can be readily burned. The gas, mainly methane, then can be used to heat the digesters, as well as buildings at the wastewater treatment plant and even homes and businesses. During periods of the year when heating is not required, the gas can be bottled and stored for later usage.

The sludge is stored in the digester and subjected to anaerobic decomposition for a specified time. After sufficient decomposition, the sludge is pumped out of the digester and into sludge-drying beds. The drying beds, composed of sand, are flooded with approximately 6 inches (15 cm) of wet sludge. The sludge is mainly liquid at this point. The sun evaporates the water, leaving behind a quantity of material that dries, cracks, and rolls up. You may have seen dried mud after a flash flood, where it cracks and rolls up. The sludge appears similar to that. The sludge generally takes two or three weeks to dry. Once dried, it is collected and transported to fill in eroded fields and pastures or composted.

The aerobic digestion consists of continuously aerating the sludge without the addition of food, so the sludge is always in the endogenous region. Aer-

ation continues until the volatile solids are reduced where the sludge does not create an odor, and will readily de-water. When the aerobic process achieves a required volatile solid reduction the solids can be processed and returned to the environment in a variety of ways: land application, composting, burning, chemical stabilization, drying, and pelletization.

Quality Control

Recall that 70% to 80% of all pathogens are aerobic. This sludge has just spent approximately 60 days in the anaerobic environment of the digester. Pathogenic aerobes cannot survive such stressful conditions, and they die off. As a result, the sludge is improved in sanitary quality but it still is not fully safe. It should not be applied to areas where the public gathers, such as playgrounds, football fields, and the like, or to soil growing vegetables that will be eaten raw.

Many other wastewater treatment processes—activated sludge, rotating biological contactors, contact aeration—are used in municipal and package treatment plants. Activated sludge has become more common than trickling filters in new construction. No matter what the complexity of the chemistry of physics, the objective is the same: to remove the less than 0.1% of waste dissolved in the more than 99.9% aqueous medium.

Now the question may arise: Is the effluent leaving the wastewater treatment plant and entering a river or stream free of pathogens? Some pathogens may settle out in the grit basin or in the primary clarifier, either by settling to the bottom as sludge or by floating to the surface as scum. In these cases the pathogens are transported to the digester and subjected to an anaerobic environment. Other pathogens may be passed over in the primary clarifier and trapped in the trickling filter, where they become food for other microorganisms. If some pathogens manage to escape the trickling filter, they may settle out in the secondary clarifier, where they will be subjected to the fate of the anaerobic digester. If pathogens manage to survive all of these processes, they will be passed on to the chlorine basin. In this basin, chlorine destroys the hazardous micoorganism. Sulfur dioxide is often used to de-chlorinate the effluent to reduce the toxicity of the stream. At this point the treated effluent from the wastewater plant is microbiologically safe to discharge into a river or stream.

Wastewater treatment plants have a quality control laboratory, in which tests are run on the effluent. Some tests run on wastewater are the dissolved oxygen (DO), biological oxygen demand (BOD), settable solids, chlorine residual, pH, fecal coliform, biomonitoring, nutrients, and chemical oxygen demand (COD).

A permit system under **NPDES** (National Pollutant Discharge Eliminations Systems) was established to control wastewater discharges. Publicly owned utilities and industries both are required to obtain permits to discharge pollutants to surface waters. The purpose is to ensure that existing treatment plants comply with effluent limitations and performance standards, and that new plants have the best available technology and operating methods. The program also includes requirements for monitoring and reporting discharges and requires adequate funding and staffing with qualified personnel. NPDES permits are issued for a determined time and upon expiration the permit is available for public comments. Monitoring requirements and effluent limits are subject to change during renewal.

Effluent quality rules and regulations of the Environmental Protection Agency describe the minimum level of effluent quality that secondary treatment must attain under the NPDES. Acceptable secondary effluent is commonly defined in terms of BOD, suspended solids, fecal coliform bacteria, and pH. For BOD, the arithmetic mean of the values for effluent samples collected in a period of 30 consecutive days must not exceed 30 milligrams per liter, and the arithmetic mean of values in any period of seven consecutive days must not exceed 45 milligrams per liter.

Dissolved Oxygen (DO)

In liquid wastes, **dissolved oxygen (DO)** is the factor that determines whether the biological changes are brought about by aerobic or by anaerobic organisms. Aerobic action is associated with desirable conditions and anaerobic action as being undesirable because of the foul odors it produces, such as hydrogen sulfide. Both types of organisms are everywhere in nature, so conditions favorable to the aerobic action (aerobic conditions) must be maintained; otherwise the anaerobic organisms will take over and nuisance conditions will develop. Thus, dissolved-oxygen measurements are important for maintaining aerobic conditions in natural waters that receive potentially polluting materials and in aerobic treatment processes intended to purify domestic and industrial wastewaters.

One of the most important single tests, dissolved-oxygen determination, is used for a wide variety of purposes. For example, dissolved oxygen is necessary to support normal populations of fish and other aquatic organisms. This requires the presence of dissolved-oxygen levels that support the desired aquatic life in healthy condition at all times.

Determinations of dissolved oxygen serve as the basis of the BOD test. Thus, they are the foundation of the most important determination used to evaluate the pollutional strength of domestic and industrial waste. The rate of biochemical oxidation is measured by determining residual dissolved-oxygen in a stream at various time intervals.

Biochemical Oxygen Demand (BOD)

Biochemical oxygen demand (BOD) usually is defined as the amount of oxygen microorganisms require while stabilizing decomposable organic matter under aerobic conditions. The term "decomposable" means that the organic matter serves as food for bacteria, and energy is derived from the oxidation process. The test is one of the most important in stream pollution control activities. The BOD test is essentially a bioassay procedure that measures oxygen consumed by living organisms (mainly bacteria) while utilizing the organic matter present in a waste, under conditions as similar as possible to those that occur in nature. Care must be taken in running the BOD test because, for example, if additional air is introduced, the results will not be correct. If the temperature is not 20°C—which is, more or less, a medium value as far as natural bodies of water are concerned—the test will not be correct. The organisms used to break down organic matter and the organisms in this test utilizing the oxygen are native to the soil. Generally, a 5-day BOD test is used in environmental monitoring.

Chemical Oxygen Demand (COD)

The **chemical oxygen demand (COD)** test is used widely as a means of measuring the pollutional strength of domestic and industrial waste. This test allows measurement of waste in terms of the total quantity of oxygen required for oxidation to carbon and water. It is based upon the fact that all organic compounds, with a few exceptions, can be oxidized by the acts of a strong oxidizing agent under acid conditions. During the determination of the COD, organic matter is converted to carbon dioxide and water regardless of the biological assimilability of the substances.

COD values are greater than BOD values—and may be much greater when significant amounts of biologically resistant organic matter is present. Hence, when running the BOD and COD on a sample, COD results are expected to be higher. The COD test is limited in that it is unable to differentiate biologically oxidizable and biologically inert organic matter. In addition, it does not provide any evidence of the rate at which the biologically active materials would be stabilized under conditions that exist in nature. An advantage of the COD test over the biochemical oxygen demand (BOD) test is that you do not have to wait five days for the results. The results of the dissolved oxygen test, BOD test, and COD test are all reported in milligrams per liter.

Wastewater Stabilization Ponds

Many small communities simply cannot afford the initial construction, continuous maintenance, and operation of a conventional wastewater treatment plant. In these areas the wastewater may be produced primarily in homes and small businesses and thereby are void of any significant industrial waste. Circumstances such as this usually are ideal for the installation of a wastewater stabilization pond.

A **wastewater stabilization pond** is engineered to utilize biological decomposition as a means of wastewater disposal. A wastewater stabilization pond looks similar to a large pond or a small lake. The wastewater stabilization pond is generally rectangular or oval in shape, the banks dropping sharply into the water. The size of the ponds varies. Those designed to treat large volumes of water are generally larger than those designed to treat smaller vol-

umes. The depth of the pond often is around 4 feet and should be constant over the entire area.

Once the pond is filled and in operation, microbiological decomposition of the waste occurs. The wastewater is simply piped into the pond at a location and depth where water movement through the pond causes breakup of floating solids. This condition creates an extended detention time of the wastewater, allowing many solids to settle to the bottom of the pond. These organic solids serve as food for microorganisms. There is often a large volume of these solids on the bottom, which results in an accelerated rate of microbial decomposition. As the microbes feed rapidly on this matter, they reproduce continuously, eventually depleting the oxygen supply at the bottom of the pond. This creates an anaerobic environment. This anaerobic environment is limited to only the bottom half of the pond. At the top half an aerobic environment still exists.

Because the majority of the solids have settled to the bottom of the pond, there is not as much organic matter available for decomposition in the upper half. Therefore, the microbes in the upper half do not have to work as hard metabolizing the waste and do not require as much oxygen—although abundant oxygen is introduced from the atmosphere by diffusion, and from small plants and algae by photosynthesis. On the bottom, waste products from the anaerobic microbes will be released. These include carbon dioxide (CO_2), hydrogen sulfide (H_2S), and methane (CH_4). As these gases rise from the bottom toward the surface, the aerobic organisms use them in the upper half of the pond.

The waste entering a stabilization pond should be limited to only those materials that can be degraded—those that provide food for microorganisms. Toxic materials with the capacity to kill the microorganisms should not be discharged to this type of sewage treatment facility.

The wastewater in the pond is subjected to evaporation as well as percolation (usually minimal) into the soil beneath. The remaining water exits the pond via an effluent pipe that controls the maximum water level. The maximum volume of the pond is set, and introducing new wastewater may cause the pond to overflow into the effluent pipe. Though it has a high chlorine demand, this effluent may be chlorinated, then discharged into a moving surface water supply.

Wastewater stabilization ponds should be maintained continuously by controlling excessive plant and algae growth. This keeps the areas around the banks well groomed and monitors the effluent to assure adequate disinfection.

SUMMARY

To protect the health of the public, every state requires that human waste (urine and feces) be disposed of in an approved sanitary manner. Water pollution from excreta is of particular concern because it provides a favorable environment for disease-causing organisms. Knowing the point of origin is helpful. More difficult is nonpoint pollution, such as that introduced by pesticides, herbicides, and fertilizers from agricultural waste.

Human waste disposal systems can be classified as non–water-carried and water-carried. The former are exemplified by the pit privy and the box and can. Individual water-carried systems generally consist of a septic tank and drainfield.

The location of a subsurface sewage disposal system must be predicated on a soil evaluation, a percolation test, soil maps, and evaluation of soil color and texture. Modern municipal wastewater treatment plants usually use biological processes, which encourage the growth of microorganisms that render waste constituents harmless. Wastewater treatment is either aerobic or anaerobic, of which the former is used most often, particularly an activated sludge process and biological filtration.

KEY TERMS

Aeration, p. 110

Bar screen, p. 109

Biochemical oxygen demand (BOD), p. 111

Box and can, p. 101

Chemical oxygen demand (COD), p. 112

Digester, p. 110

Dissolved oxygen (DO), p. 111

Evapotranspiration, p. 102

Grit chamber, p. 109

Nonpoint pollution, p. 99

NPDES, p. 111

Pit privy, p. 101

Primary clarifier, p. 109

Septic tank and drainfield system, p. 102

Settling basin, p. 109

Sewage, p. 100

Sludge, p. 109

Storm sewer, p. 109

Venturi meter, p. 109

Wastewater, p. 100

Wastewater stabilization pond, p. 112

REFERENCES

Hammer, Mark. 1986. *Water and Wastewater Technology*, 2nd ed. John Wiley and Sons, New York.

Issac-Renton, Judith. "Longitudinal Studies of Giardia Contamination in Two Community Drinking Water Supplies: Cyst Levels, Parasite Viability, and Health Impact." *Applied and Environmental Microbiology*. Jan 1996. v. 62 n. 1. p. 47.

National Environmental Health Association. 1979. *On-Site Wastewater Management*. Denver.

Rhyner, Charles R., et al. 1995. *Waste Management and Resource Recovery*. CRC, Boca Raton, FL.

Saluate, Joseph A., Jr. 1972. *Environmental Engineering and Sanitation*, 2nd ed. John Wiley and Sons, New York.

Sawyer, Clair N., and Perry L. McCarty. 1994. *Chemistry for Environmental Engineering*, 3rd ed. McGraw-Hill Book Company, New York.

Silverstein, Kenneth. "Everything in the Kitchen Sink (nonpoint pollution threatens city water supplies)." *American City & County*. March 1994. v. 109 n. 3. p. 26.

U.S. Public Health Service. 1967. *Manual of Septic Tank Practice*. U.S. Government Printing Office. Washington, DC.

Vesilind, Arne. 1996. *Environmental Engineering*. PWS Publishing, Boston, MA.

7

SOLID AND HAZARDOUS WASTE MANAGEMENT

Burton R. Ogle, Ph.D.

Western Carolina University

OBJECTIVES

- Identify the classifications of solid waste.
- Explain the storage of waste.
- Describe the collection of solid waste.
- Discuss the history of solid waste management and evaluate the various methods.
- Discuss the need for recycling.
- Explain the transportation of hazardous waste.
- Identify and explain hazardous waste disposal.

Ecosystems are sustainable because they dispose of waste and replenish nutrients by recycling all elements. Cavemen and early civilizations did not have a problem with waste because it consisted mainly of organic waste and the decomposers converted it into useful materials. Also, there were few people, and they generated little waste. The problem became large with more people generating more and a variety of waste—chemical, liquid, solid, nuclear, and hazardous. Little of this waste is food for the decomposers. Thus, a variety of methods must be used to manage the waste.

Until relatively recently, solid waste was dumped, buried, or burned, and some of the garbage was fed to animals. The public was not aware of the links of refuse to rats, flies, roaches, mosquitoes, fleas, land pollution, and water pollution. People did not know that the solid waste in open dumps and backyard incinerators supported vectors of diseases including typhoid fever, endemic typhus fever, yellow fever, dengue fever, malaria, cholera, and others. Thus, the cheapest, quickest, and most convenient means of disposing of the waste were used. Rural areas and small towns utilized the open dump or backyard incinerator. Larger towns and cities used municipal incinerators. Later, landfilling became the method of choice for disposing of solid waste.

As society became more affluent and demanded greater convenience, the "single-service era" began. With it came a drastic increase in the amount of waste generated. The increase in waste per person, plus more and more people—with these same people needing the land for homes, shopping centers, roads, parking lots, and so on—led to a shortage of land suitable for landfills. New York City sent a large load of "garbage" on a "cruise." New York sent a boxcar of garbage to Kansas City and, later, Wisconsin, where these areas refused to dispose of it at any price.

In the 1950s, solid waste could be buried in a sanitary landfill for 75¢ per ton. Now costs start at $25 per ton in small towns and more than $100 per ton in densely populated areas such as New Jersey. With more people and more waste, the problem has reached a critical point in many areas of the United States.

We would not be in this mess if in the past solid waste had been viewed as a resource rather than something of no value. Future generations may look at the old landfills as "resource centers." Now, as we approach the 21st century, we realize our past mistakes and are taking a new look at "garbage." Contrary to the practices of open dumping, burning, or burying waste, solid waste "disposal" methods must change.

CLASSIFICATION OF SOLID WASTE

The United States has been called a "throwaway society." We use many materials for a short time and then dispose of them. Think about the last time you visited a fast-food restaurant. Your hamburger was wrapped in paper or boxed in a container. After the meal, you likely threw away these wrappings along with your paper cup and napkins. The car you drove home from the restaurant will wear out eventually and it will be thrown away also. These are typical examples of the increasing amount of solid waste that humans generate. Americans now generate more than 230 million tons of municipal solid waste a year. That is approximately 4.6 pounds of waste per person per day, up from 2.7 pounds per person per day in 1960.

The solid waste products generated by humans can be divided into two general categories: **refuse** and larger items (such as old cars, trains, and refrigerators) that are not disposed of easily. Refuse is composed of garbage, rubbish, and ashes. **Garbage** is the organic putrescible matter from scraps of food, not only from the table but also during the growth and harvest of food on the farm and its transportation and storage.

When you buy sealed and packaged food from the grocery store and remove the food from its packages and prepare it, you produce two types of refuse. One is garbage, or food scraps, and the other is rubbish from the container. **Rubbish** is the combustible and noncombustible solid waste generated from people's activities. It includes waste such as paper, plastic bags, beverage cans, yardwork trimmings, and many other materials. Most of the municipal solid waste generated in the United States is in the form of rubbish.

Ashes, another form of refuse, are combusted materials that someone has burned to total breakdown. A person often can dump these relatively inert ashes onto the surface of the ground with few problems. Other forms of refuse may not be handled and disposed of as conveniently. Solid waste that is handled improperly can provide a breeding ground for insects and rodents. These pests can become annoying, frightening, and, most important, may spread disease to humans.

A comprehensive solid waste management program encompasses the storage, collection, and disposal of solid waste. Proper management in these three areas helps greatly in controlling insects and rodents.

STORAGE OF SOLID WASTE

A home may contain several types of solid waste receptacles. People put small wastepaper baskets in bathrooms and bedrooms. They put larger, covered containers in the kitchen to collect the garbage and rubbish from food preparation. Some people equip their homes with mechanical devices that compact waste into a storage receptacle. Others use still larger solid waste receptacles outside the dwelling to serve as a central storage point. Most homes use 20- or 30-gallon garbage cans that must be fly-tight and noncorrosive and are of sufficient number to store all of the solid waste generated until it is collected. Where recycling is practiced, receptacles are changed to accommodate recycling.

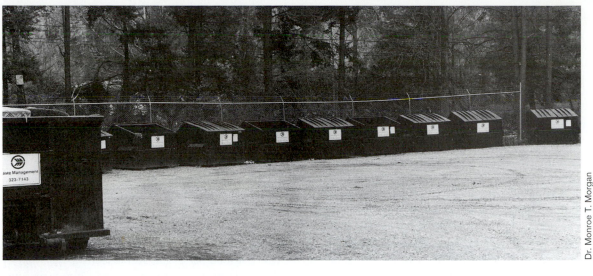

A rural community refuse collection center may look like this.

COLLECTION OF SOLID WASTE

Larger facilities such as multi-dwelling units, businesses and industries may use large-volume, noncompacting, bulk receptacles, commonly termed "dumpsters." Many rural areas use these centrally located, large-volume receptacles as a temporary means of storage. The residents in these areas simply bring their waste to the large receptacles, the contents of which are later transported to a disposal area.

Solid waste should be collected a minimum of once per week, and preferably twice per week. The collection frequency is based on the life cycle of the house fly. Under ideal conditions, a house fly develops from an egg into an adult in 8 days. These flies breed in refuse. Collecting and disposing of the solid waste within 8 days, interrupts the flies' life cycle. By collecting refuse in a timely manner, people can control fly populations to a large extent. Waste also provides food and harborage for other insects, as well as rodents capable of transmitting diseases to humans. Combustible materials, too, may build up and increase the chances of fire.

Home collection of solid waste generally is done by a private collector or a local government-owned and financed operation. Private collectors usually charge a fee to each individual homeowner, or a government contract will pay the fees. The government contract enables solid waste collection in a uniform, sanitary manner. Without such a contract, some individuals may be reluctant to pay the collector for the service and the refuse may go uncollected.

Many cities and towns require homeowners to use certain types of receptacles. Collectors usually pick up at the curb in front of the dwelling. In some neighborhoods the collectors pick up the receptacles in the backyard, as the people who live there consider receptacles too bulky to handle and unsightly in front of the dwelling.

The solid waste collection vehicle should be covered and able to compact the refuse collected. It may load from the rear, side, or top. The storage areas in these vehicles should be kept relatively clean and watertight.

Some hog-feeding operations collect only garbage. The collectors often heat garbage to 212°F for 30 minutes to kill any infectious microorganisms before farmers feed it to their livestock. If farmers feed uncooked garbage to their hogs, trichinosis is one disease that may result.

SOLID WASTE MANAGEMENT

In the past, common practice in the United States was to designate an area for solid waste disposal and simply dump this waste on top of the ground. In such an operation, old cans, tires, and other objects retained water, producing a breeding ground for mosquitoes. Further, rats, roaches, flies, and other vectors used this readily accessible garbage as food. In short, these open dumps provided an area for a variety of pests to live and breed.

People often visited these dumps in search of valuable items that others may have discarded. This created a danger from broken glass, old medicine that children may ingest, dangerous chemical compounds, and many other hazards. Open dumps also caused surrounding property to depreciate and produced noxious odors. In addition to polluting groundwater, surface water runoff from the areas often carried waste into adjacent lakes and streams, increasing water pollution. The combustible materials in these areas often caused fires. Open dumps are undesirable, and these facilities now are illegal in the United States.

Some coastal areas formerly disposed of their solid waste at sea. Workers loaded the waste into barges and transported it away from the city. Today, this practice is illegal because it produces water pollution. Another means of disposal that is now illegal is "backyard" **incineration**. Incinerators burned refuse collected in the home and produced excessive amounts of air pollution. Still used today in some areas are large municipal incinerators; however, many are converting waste-to-energy plants. The required pollution control equipment ensures that the emissions do not exceed pollution standards. The open dump, disposal at sea, and backyard incineration still are used in many countries of the world.

The EPA has recommended that solid waste management be emphasized in the following order of preference:

1. Source reduction
2. Recycle–reuse
3. Waste heat recovery—waste to energy (WTE)
4. Burying (landfill)

SOURCE REDUCTION

Years ago, children looked forward to opening new jars of peanut butter and jelly. After the contents were eaten, the jars became new drinking glasses. Bakers in the family bought new sacks of flour. The flour was eaten, and the flour sacks were transformed into clothing. Many of the food containers were reusable. Milk was picked up at the store or delivered to the doorstep in returnable bottles.

Later we entered the disposable era. Soft drink bottles and milk bottles were "nonreturnable." Salt, sugar, pepper, and catsup containers were replaced by individually wrapped packages that came to be known as "single-service" items. In restaurants, cafes, and fast-food places the dishwasher was replaced by paper, plastic, and styrofoam plates. Thus, the amount of refuse generated per person to satisfy our desire for convenience grew in alarming proportions.

The practice of single service, together with more people, 70% of whom were living in towns and large cities, led to a solid waste crisis. The problem was caused by more people creating more waste in congested areas with limited disposal sites. It was complicated by little regard for the environment or means of managing effluent from an affluent society. Now managing effluent has become big business as some have realized "there are dollars in that waste."

Although solid waste management has become big business, we still should emphasize source reduction. Probably the best way to illustrate source reduction is by the example of the old kerosene oil can. From the 1920s to the 1940s, oil was used to illuminate homes by oil lamp, and oil was used to start fires in the fireplace. Families had their own galvanized metal oil can, which they took with them to the store, where the can was filled with oil and returned to the home. These cans were not found in fields, on creek banks, or in rivers. They were reusable. A single oil can usually lasted a family a lifetime.

We've all seen plastic gallon milk jugs in creeks, rivers, fields, and lots. Could we not develop a multi-use milk container that could last a family a lifetime? This certainly would keep much waste out of landfills. Further, we could develop containers for soft drinks, beer, cooking oil, and so forth, that would reduce waste at the source with many far-reaching advantages. This could be done while meeting environmental and public health standards.

Some other ways to reduce sources of waste are as follows:

- Use fewer materials. American Indians, for example, generated little waste.
- Package things such as toothpaste in tubes instead of pump-type dispensers.
- Use cloth napkins instead of paper napkins.

- Use cloth grocery bags that go to and from the store with you again and again.
- Legislate the use of only returnable bottles.
- Use bulk sugar dispensers instead of individually wrapped packages.
- Use stainless steel instead of plastic when possible.
- Use cloth diapers instead of disposable diapers.

These measures can be reality if the public will demand them through its purchasing power.

· · · · · · · · · · · · · · ·

RECYCLE–REUSE

Recycling is one solution to the solid waste problem. Vanishing natural resources, limited amounts of land suitable and available for landfills, and economic reward are reasons that recycling is a feasible and popular method of waste disposal.

In less-developed countries, solid waste is not a problem because people use almost all of it. For example, they burn the wood, paper, and plastic products and reuse many of the glass and metal containers for food storage and even as drinking cups. In the United States, by contrast, there is a need to recycle and in some areas recycling plants are highly successful. Home recycling and resource recovery plants should replace landfills as the major means of disposing of solid waste. Recycling of materials helps alleviate the shortage of resources, greatly reduces pollution, and cuts energy demands. Rather than burying them, wastes should be returned to factories, melted down, and reshaped for reuse. Figure 7.1 summarizes the estimated savings that can be accrued by recycling.

Recycling saves energy. Fossil fuel consumption in the United States continues to soar, along with costs associated with those fuels. Through recycling, many products, particularly aluminum, plastic, and steel, have added value in that they save significant amounts of energy resources over virgin manufacturing. Figure 7.2 shows the savings that can be realized through product recovery.

Recycling creates jobs. Efforts to recycle have provided another benefit that had not been foreseen. Jobs directly associated with recycling efforts are plentiful and robust. Occupations ranging from

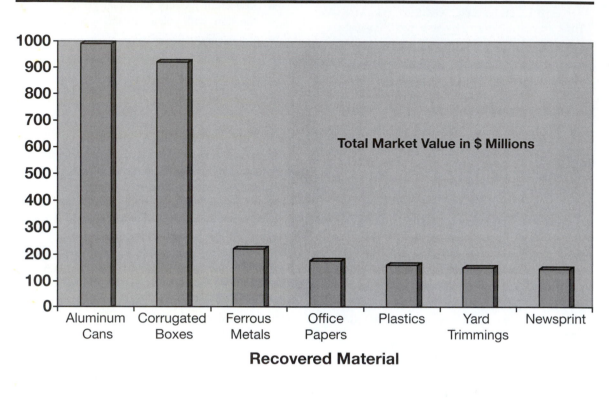

FIGURE 7.1 Estimated market value of major municipal solid waste materials.

Source: Tellus Institute, 1997

high-tech engineering careers to steady, manual labor have arisen from the recycling industry. Figure 7.3 depicts the number of jobs created in the northeast United States directly from recycling efforts.

The Benefits of Recycling

- Recycling protects and expands U.S. manufacturing jobs and increases U.S. competitiveness.
- Recycling reduces the need for landfilling and incineration
- Recycling prevents pollution caused by the manufacturing of products from virgin materials.
- Recycling saves energy.

- Recycling decreases emissions of greenhouse gases that contribute to global climate change.
- Recycling conserves natural resources such as timber, water, and minerals.
- Recycling helps sustain the environment for future generations.[1]

How Recycling Stacks Up

Buying recycled office paper—and recycling it—has never been easier. Even actions this simple can make a real difference in a product's environmental impacts. When compared to manufacturing and dis-

---

[1]*Source:* The United States Environmental Protection Agency, 1998

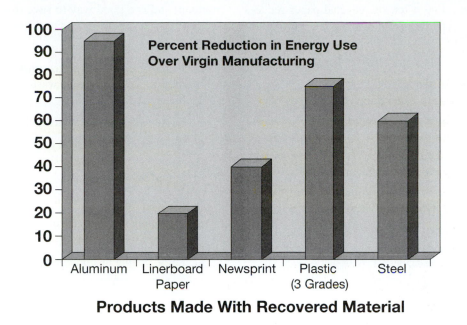

Products Made With Recovered Material

Source: Tellus Institute, 1992

FIGURE 7.2 Energy savings of products made with recovered materials.

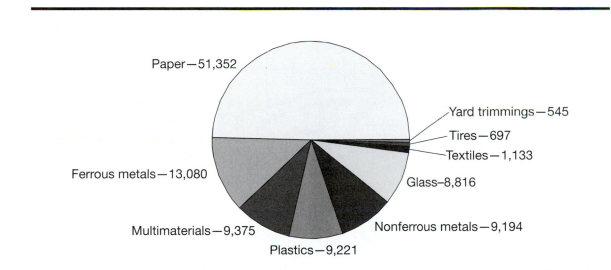

Source: Roy F. Weston, 1994

FIGURE 7.3 Summary of recycling jobs in the Northeast, by material.

posing of a ton of virgin office paper, manufacturing and recycling a ton of recycled paper reduces solid waste, energy use, pollution, and greenhouse gas emissions. Specifically, manufacturing and recycling a ton of recycled office paper:

- Reduces solid waste by 49%.
- Reduces total energy consumption by 43%.
- Reduces net greenhouse gas emissions by 70% of carbon dioxide equivalents.
- Reduces hazardous air pollutant emissions by 90% and particulate emissions by 40%.
- Reduces absorbable organic halogen emissions to water by 100% and suspended solids by 30%.[2]

---

[2]*Source:* Environmental Defense Fund, 1995

Even though recycling is good for the environment and is a good way to save resources, it is not utilized as much as it should be. Some reasons are:

- People have become accustomed to convenience, and separating waste is an inconvenience.
- People are used to throwing things away.
- The market for waste is not sufficient. Locating a recycling store beside the grocery store would help.
- Stronger laws are needed to require recycling.
- Recycling programs lack sufficient funding for research and start-up demonstrations.
- Some people just do not care.

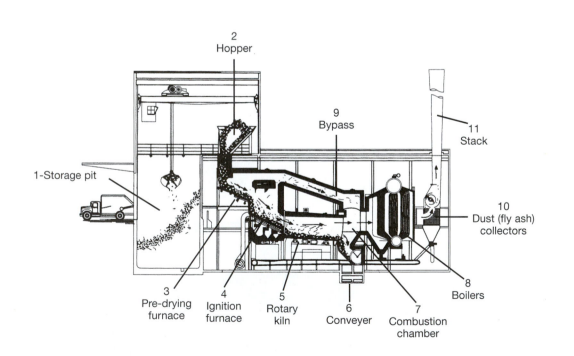

2
Hopper

9
Bypass

11
Stack

1-Storage pit

10
Dust (fly ash) collectors

3
Pre-drying furnace

4
Ignition furnace

5
Rotary kiln

6
Conveyer

7
Combustion chamber

8
Boilers

Source: Solid Waste Management, Environmental Protection Agency

FIGURE 7.4 One type of municipal refuse incinerator.

Chapter 7

Scientists have done research to find ways to recycle various materials, thereby reducing the cost of solid waste management and overloads on landfill space. We still need to find ways to recycle more plastics, cloth, asphalt, glass, leather, wood, and other materials. Industry also is encouraged to recycle its solid and liquid waste. In addition, laws should be passed to require reduction in the generation of solid waste.

WASTE TO ENERGY AND INCINERATION

The municipal incinerator (Figure 7.4) is a means of solid waste treatment. These incinerators can be centrally located close to the sources of the solid waste prior to processing. The temperatures within the incinerator must be very high (1800°F) to prevent air pollution. These incinerators often are expensive to construct and they must include a site location to dispose of the ashes. Burning refuse to generate electricity is another possibility, and selling the electricity or steam helps offset the cost of the incinerators. This technology commonly is called **energy recovery** or **waste-to-energy (WTE)** because the heat derived from incinerating refuse is a useful resource. Burning refuse can produce steam used directly for heating buildings or generating electricity. Internationally, well over 1,000 waste-to-energy plants are operating in Brazil, Japan, Russia, and Europe. In the United States, more than 110 waste incinerators burn over 45,000 tons of refuse daily. Some are simple incinerators, and others produce energy. Figure 7.5 portrays the waste-to-energy incinerator.

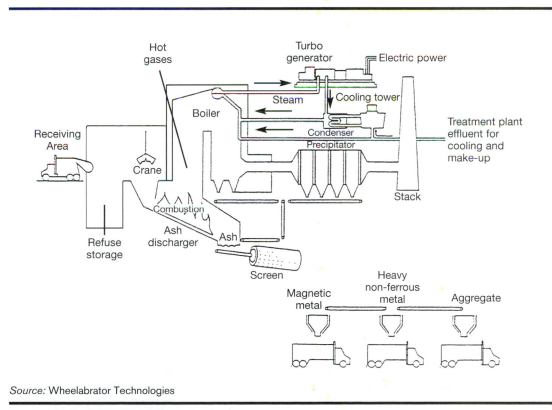

Source: Wheelabrator Technologies

FIGURE 7.5 Waste-to-energy incinerator.

SANITARY LANDFILL

One of the most widely used means of solid waste disposal is the **sanitary landfill**. Briefly, in a sanitary landfill, the solid waste is buried in sections and covered with soil. If the landfill is operated properly, it can be located near populated areas. A landfill should not be located in areas with high groundwater tables, and preferably where the soil is a sandy loam. Roads leading into the landfill should be constructed to handle traffic from heavy collection vehicles.

A properly operated sanitary landfill eliminates insects, rodents, safety hazards, fire hazards, and other problems that exist in open dumping. Figure 7.6 gives an example of regulations for sanitary landfills. This one closely resembles federal guidelines.

Buffer zone standards for siting new landfills apply to Class I disposal facilities. A Class I disposal facility is a sanitary landfill that serves a municipal, institutional, or rural population to be used for disposal of domestic, commercial, institutional, municipal, demolition/construction, farming wastes, discarded automotive tires, and dead animals. According to the standards, Class I facilities must be located, designed, constructed, operated, and maintained such that the fill areas are a minimum of:

- 100 feet from all property lines
- 500 feet from all residences
- 500 feet from all wells determined to be downgradient and used as a source of drinking water by humans or livestock
- 200 feet from normal boundaries of springs, lakes, and other bodies of water

Landfills also must operate under leachate migration control standards. The facility must have a liner designed to last the estimated life of the site as well as the post-closure care period. The facility also should be designed, constructed, and installed to prevent any leaching of waste or waste constituent from the facility into adjacent subsurface soil, groundwater, or surface water. This waste migration must not occur at any time during the use of the facility or during the post-closure period.

The facility's liner must be constructed of materials that have the appropriate chemical properties and sufficient strength and thickness to prevent failure. Failure of the liner may result from pressure gradients, physical contact with the waste or leachate to which it is exposed, climactic conditions, stress of installation, and stress of daily operation.

The liner must be placed on a foundation or base capable of providing support. The foundation also must provide resistance to pressure gradients both above and below the liner. This prevents failure of the liner from settlement, compression, or uplift.

Any surrounding earth likely to be in contact with the waste leachate must be covered by the liner. The liner also must be designed to meet a minimum performance standard of 3 feet of recompacted soil; this achieves a maximum hydraulic conductivity of 1×10^{-7} cm/sec.

A geologic buffer must be located directly beneath the liner. It shall measure not less than 5 feet from the bottom of the liner to the seasonal high water table of the uppermost unconfined aquifer or the top of the formation of a confined aquifer.

If compacted earth liners are used, the minimum allowable thickness shall be 3 feet unless otherwise approved. If geomembrane liners are used, they must be used in conjunction with a compacted earth liner that must be at least 3 feet thick. Together the two liners also must achieve a maximum hydraulic conductivity of 3 feet or 1×10^{-6} soil. The compacted earth liner used with the geomembrane liner also shall be free of sharp objects, and compatible with supporting soils and with leachate expected to be generated. The geomembrane liner also shall have sufficient strength and durability to function for the life of the facility plus the post closure care period.

A leachate collection and removal system is required immediately above the liner. It is designed, constructed, maintained, and operated to collect and remove leachate from the facility. This system must be constructed of materials that are chemically resistant to the waste managed in the facility and the leachates expected to be generated. The materials also must be of sufficient strength and thickness to prevent collapse under the pressures exerted by overlying wastes, waste cover materials,

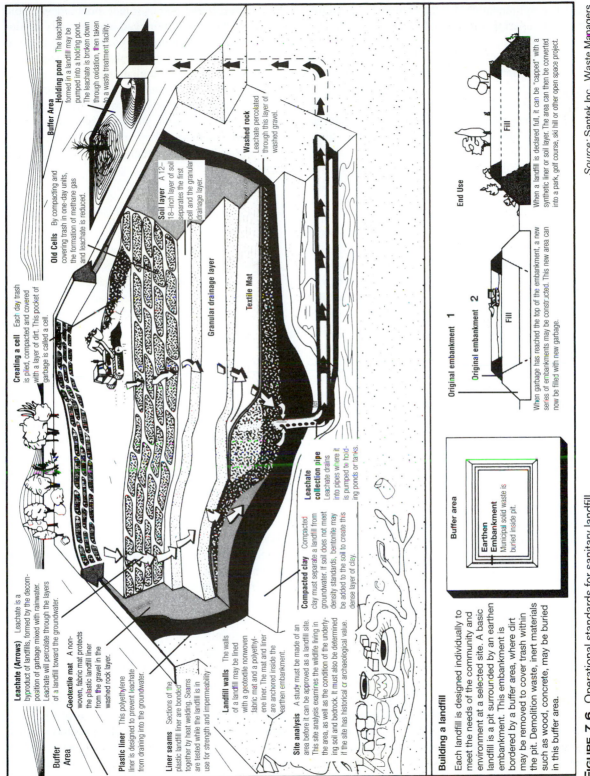

Buffer Area

Leachate (Arrows) Leachate is a byproduct of landfills, formed by the decomposition of garbage mixed with rainwater. Leachate will percolate through the layers of a landfill toward the groundwater.

Geotextile mat A nonwoven, fabric mat protects the plastic landfill liner from the gravel in the washed rock layer.

Plastic liner This polyethylene liner is designed to prevent leachate from draining into the groundwater.

Liner seams Sections of the plastic landfill liner are bonded together by heat welding. Seams are tested while the landfill is in use for strength and impermeability.

Landfill walls The walls of a landfill may be lined with a geotextile nonwoven fabric mat and a polyethylene liner. The mat and liner are anchored inside the earthen embankment.

Site analysis A study must be made of an area before it can be approved as a landfill site. This site analysis examines the wildlife living in the area, as well as the condition of the underlying soil and bedrock. It must also be determined if the site has historical or archaeological value.

Compacted clay Compacted clay must separate a landfill from groundwater. If soil does not meet density standards, bentonite may be added to the soil to create this dense layer of clay.

Leachate collection pipe Leachate drains into pipes where it is pumped to holding ponds or tanks.

Creating a cell Each day trash is piled, compacted and covered with a layer of dirt. This pocket of garbage is called a cell.

Old Cells By compacting and covering trash in one-day units, the formation of methane gas and leachate is reduced.

Soil layer A 12–18-inch layer of soil separates the first cell and the granular drainage layer.

Washed rock Leachate percolated through this layer of washed gravel.

Granular drainage layer

Textile Mat

Buffer Area

Holding pond The leachate may be formed in a landfill into a holding pond. The leachate is pumped down through oxidation, then taken in a waste treatment facility.

Building a landfill

Each landfill is designed individually to meet the needs of the community and environment at a selected site. A basic landfill is a pit surrounded by an earthen embankment. This embankment is bordered by a buffer area, where dirt may be removed to cover trash within the pit. Demolition waste, inert materials such as wood, concrete, may be buried in this buffer area.

Buffer area

Earthen Embankment Municipal solid waste is buried inside pit.

Original embankment **1**

Original embankment **2**

Fill

When garbage has reached the top of the embankment, a new series of embankments may be constructed. This new area can now be filled with new garbage.

End Use

Fill

When a landfill is declared full, it can be "capped" with a synthetic liner or soil layer. The area can then be converted into a park, golf course, ski hill or other open space project.

Source: Santek Inc., Waste Managers

FIGURE 7.6 Operational standards for sanitary landfill.

and any equipment used at the facility. Other equivalent or superior protection may be substituted for this buffer. The leachate collection and removal system must be protected, by design or operational features, or both, from equipment mishandling that might reasonably be expected during operation.

These landfill facilities must be designed, constructed, operated, and maintained such that the final cover includes a cap that will provide long-term minimization of migration of liquids through the closed facility, function with minimum maintenance, promote drainage, accommodate settling and subsidence so the cap's integrity is maintained, and meet specific closure requirements.

Further, the leachate collection reservoirs shall be constructed (e.g., lined) such that collected leachate is contained. The reservoir also must have sufficient capacity to store the volume of leachate expected to be generated in 30 days. The facility must have a reliable and convenient means of detecting the level of collected leachate in the reservoir and sampling the leachate.

During construction or installation, liners and cover systems (e.g., membranes, sheets, or coatings) must be inspected for uniformity, damage, and imperfections (e.g., holes, cracks, thin spots, foreign materials) immediately after construction or installation. For example, geomembrane liners and covers must be inspected to ensure tight seams and joints and the absence of tears, punctures, or blisters. Further, soil-based and admixed liners and covers must be inspected for imperfections including lenses, cracks, channels, root holes, and other structural nonuniformities that may cause an increase in the permeability of the liner or cover.

....

COMPOSTING

Composting is an effective method of solid waste disposal. In **composting**, biodegradable materials break down through natural processes and produce humus. The metabolism of microorganisms is what breaks down the waste aerobically or anaerobically.

Materials that are nonbiodegradable must be separated from the degradable materials and disposed of in some other manner. Some common nonbiodegradable materials are glass, plastics, rubber products, and metals. Once nonbiodegradable materials have been removed and a totally biodegradable waste has been established, it is brought to a grinder. Grinding increases the surface area of the waste and enhances biological degradation.

Aerobic composting involves decomposition in the presence of air (free oxygen). Anaerobic implies decomposition in the absence of the atmospheric oxygen. Most modern compost systems are aerobic rather than anaerobic for several reasons.

1. Aerobic processes are not accompanied by the foul stench present at an unsealed anaerobic composting operation.

2. In crop production industries, composting is safer because temperatures do not reach pasteurization temperatures that exceed the thermal death point of most plants, animals, and parasites.

3. Aerobic composting is more rapid than anaerobic composting.

An aerobic compost operation ideally is an optimal environment for the growth of aerobic organisms. The material to be composted is the food. Therefore the "food" should have a C/N* ratio favorable for decomposition. The microbes desire a C/N of 25:1 to 30:1. If the C/N is too low (l20:1), the ammonium compounds will volatilize into the air, causing an unpleasant odor. Various groups of organisms have different optimum temperatures (some prefer 25°C, some 37°C, and others 55°C), though the optimal temperature for a process as a whole integrates the optimums of the various microbes. The pH of aerobic composting varies depending on the organisms' need for oxygen. Aeration is important and is provided by turning the compost mechanically to expose it to oxygen to speed decomposition. Microbes must have moisture, and such is the case in composting. The amount of moisture needed varies, as does the composition of the material being composted. The moisture content should be approximately 45% to 50%. If the moisture is too low, microbial activity slows, and biological activity ceases at a moisture content of about 12%. If the moisture content is too high, it reduces the amount of free oxygen present and slows the process so that it may become anaerobic. Many times sludge is added to waste for composting to provide microbial food and trace elements.

The three main types of composting are windrow, static pile, and in-vessel.

1. *Windrow.* A sludge/refuse mixture configured in long rows (windrows) that are aerated by convection air movement and diffusion or by turning periodically through mechanical means to expose the organic matter to ambient oxygen.

2. *Static pile.* A stationary mixture is aerated by a forced aeration system installed under the pile.

3. *In-vessel composting.* Composting takes place in enclosed containers in which environmental conditions can be controlled. The waste decomposes into a harmless organic material that can be used as a soil conditioner and enhancer for agricultural applications.

What Are the Benefits of Using Compost?

Soil Enrichment:

- Adds organic bulk and humus to regenerate poor soils.
- Helps suppress plant diseases and pests.
- Increases soil nutrient content and water retention in both clay and sandy soils.
- Restores soil structure after reduction of natural soil microbes by chemical fertilizer.
- Reduces or eliminates the need for fertilizer.
- Combats specific soil, water, and air problems.

Pollution Remediation:

- Absorbs odors and degrades volatile organic compound.
- Binds heavy metals and prevents them from migrating to water resources or being absorbed by plants.
- Degrades, and in some cases, completely eliminates wood preservatives, petroleum products, pesticides, and both chlorinated and non-chlorinated hydrocarbons in contaminated soils.

Pollution Prevention:

- Avoids methane production and leachate formation in landfills by diverting organics for composting.
- Prevents pollutants in stormwater runoff from reaching water resources.
- Prevents erosion and silting on embankments parallel to creeks, lakes, and rivers.
- Prevents erosion and turf loss on roadsides, hillsides, playing fields, and golf courses.

Economic Benefits:

- Results in significant cost savings by reducing the need for water, fertilizers, and pesticides.
- Produces a marketable commodity and a low-cost alternative to standard landfill cover and artificial soil amendments.
- Extends municipal landfill life by diverting organic materials from the waste stream.
- Provides a less costly alternative to conventional bioremediation techniques.[3]

STOP

••••••••••••••

MEDICAL WASTE DISPOSAL: METHODS AND PROBLEMS

Because of great concern about the spread of infectious diseases through contact with blood-borne pathogens, one of the major challenges facing the health-care industry is the safe handling and disposal of medical waste. According to the American Hospital Association (AHA), the average hospital generates about 25 pounds of waste per day per patient bed. Infectious waste accounts for about 20% of that total. Hospitals and other generators of medical waste are at financial as well as legal risk for the safe and timely disposal of infectious waste.

The Environmental Protection Agency (EPA) and Centers for Disease Control and Prevention (CDC) recognize as medical infectious waste: contaminated sharps (such as needles), objects, blood

---

[3]*Source:* U.S. Environmental Protection Agency, 1997

and blood products, pathological wastes (anatomical waste and tissue samples), and laboratory waste capable of producing disease. Thus, consideration of several factors is necessary, including the presence of a pathogen of sufficient virulence, dose, portal of entry, and resistance of host. For a medical waste to be infectious, it has to contain pathogens with sufficient virulence and of sufficient quantity so that exposure to the waste by a susceptible host would result in an infectious disease. In 1987 the CDC indicated that, though any items that have had contact with blood, exudes, or secretions are potentially infective, to treat all waste as infective is not usually practical or necessary. Differentiating infectious and medical waste is difficult, as the terms often are interchanged.

Health Concerns

From a safety standpoint, a twofold problem exists when handling medical waste.

1. Health-care workers, waste haulers, and the public must be protected from the risks that medical waste poses to their health.

2. Government and industry must minimize the amount of medically related waste released into the environment.

The health problems are primarily occupational, as the greatest concerns are the health and well-being of health-care workers and waste haulers. Cases of public exposure to wastes generated by health facilities are rare and isolated. Far more common are occupational illnesses, resulting from exposure to infectious materials. Therefore, efforts should be focused on educating and training workers, managing waste on- and off-site, and diminishing the demand for disposable medical materials.

The American Hospital Association (AHA) established perhaps the most meaningful interpretation of medical waste by offering the following classes of waste materials:

1. Cultures and stacks

2. Pathological waste

3. Human blood and blood products

4. Used sharps

5. Animal waste

6. Waste from patients with highly virulent diseases

7. Unused sharps

Methods of Disposal

Several treatment technologies are available to dispose of medical waste. The most commonly encountered methods are steam sterilization, shredding/chlorinating, microwave disinfection, incineration, and other combustion technology.

STEAM STERILIZATION

The advantages of steam sterilization, or **autoclaving**, are low capital investment and operating costs, relatively small space requirements, and simplicity of operation. Disadvantages include limited capacity, the requirement of special waste packaging and handling, and odor and drainage problems. Autoclaving is not recommended for pathological wastes, waste with high liquid content, and waste contaminated with volatile chemicals. After autoclaving, the appearance of waste remains unchanged. Although needles, syringes, blood bags, and the like are sterile, they also are recognizable. This has the effect of making much of this waste unacceptable for disposal in a landfill or other disposal setting. Also, compacting autoclaved waste tends to break open waste bags and other containers, exposing and spilling their contents. Consequently, waste haulers and landfill operators may not be willing to accept autoclaved waste in spite of its sterile condition.

SHREDDING/CHLORINATING TECHNOLOGY

In the past few years, a technology has been promoted featuring a combination of shredding and chemical sterilization. Currently two models are available. One size treats small, limited quantities of laboratory wastes and sharps. The other model is a relatively large-capacity system that treats almost all infectious waste a hospital generates. With the large-capacity system, waste is loaded manually onto an inclined conveyor belt, which feeds into a high-torque, low-speed shredder. Waste is discharged from the bottom of this shredder into a high-speed hammermill that granulates the waste. During both shredding stages, waste is sprayed continually with a sodium hypochlorite solution. An inclined, perforated conveyor at the hammermill's discharge separates the granular waste from the excess liquid (slurry). The slurry is collected in a basin and piped to a sewer drain. The solids are discharged into a cart, where they are retained for off-site disposal. The shredding rate is adjusted so the sodium hypochlorite contact time is sufficient for complete sterilization.

The principal advantages of shredding/chlorination systems are simplicity, substantial reduction in volume, alteration of appearance, and wide range of use. Disadvantages are their relatively high costs, limited throughput capacities, and potential slurry contamination. Noise levels and chlorine concentrations also are high. The slurry discharged to the sewer may have concentrations of heavy metals, organics, and other contaminates requiring a discharge permit. In addition, special precautions may be needed to ensure compliance with workplace standards.

MICROWAVE DISINFECTION

Microwave technology represents an innovative alternative to common waste disposal systems in that it offers waste treatment and volume reduction without introducing undesirable treatment by-products into the environment (air, ground, or water). Briefly, the medical waste is transported mechanically to a closed chamber, where it is injected with steam under pressure and then shredded. The waste then is conveyed through chambers where a series of 12 microwave units maintain a constant high temperature (greater that 200°F) for 45 to 60 minutes depending on load density. Final shredding at the discharge point further reduces the volume and renders the waste completely unrecognizable. This process can accommodate large quantities of waste, making it acceptable for large, multisystem operations and commercial establishments. Disadvantages are the high initial cost and the need to provide alternative means for disposing of certain medical wastes, primarily chemotherapy waste.

INCINERATOR TECHNOLOGY

Incineration uses controlled, high-temperature combustion to destroy organics in waste materials. Modern incineration systems are well-engineered, high-technology processes designed to maximize combustion efficiency and completeness with a minimum of emissions. Three basic hospital/institutional technologies currently in use are multiple-chamber, rotary kiln, and controlled air incinerators.

1. *Multiple-chamber incinerators.* Also referred to as Incinerator Institute of America (IIA) technology, the multiple-chamber incinerator was developed in the mid-1950s and was virtually the only system installed in hospitals through the mid-1960s. Multiple-chamber incinerator processes are designed for pumping air in excess levels, and they use settling chambers to control combustion and limit emissions. Despite this emission-limiting function, most of these devices require emission control systems to comply with standard emission regulations. Further, they cannot meet the current performance and operating requirements of many states without substantial upgrading and the addition of state-of-the-art combustion control equipment.

2. *Rotary kiln incineration.* Rotary kiln incineration features a cylindrical, refractory, lined combustion chamber. The chamber rotates on a slightly inclined horizontal axis. Waste is loaded at the elevated end of the kiln. The rotary action moves the waste through the system. The kiln rotation promotes good burnout and superior ash quality. These systems require secondary combustion chambers and air pollution control equipment to ensure compliance with emission regulations.

3. *Controlled air incinerators.* Also called modular combustion and starved-air incineration, controlled air incineration is basically a two-stage combustion process. In the first-stage chamber, solid waste is burned in a starved air (reducing) environment. In the second-stage chamber, combustion products and volatile gases are burned under excess air conditions. The first controlled air

incinerators were installed in the United States around 1962. This technology was popular initially because of its relatively low cost. Its popularity grew quickly because most of these systems could comply with air pollution control regulations readily without having to add costly air pollution control equipment. More than 95% of all hospital/infectious waste incinerators installed during the past 20 years have been of this type. Soon, however, this type of incineration will not be in compliance with stringent emission control regulations being legislated in many states. Installation of pollution control equipment will be required on a great many of these systems.

THERMAL PLASMA TECHNOLOGY

Thermal plasma treatment represents an innovative departure from the more conventional incineration technology. Invented by Vance IDS of Florida and known commercially as Incandescently Heated Bio-Hazardous Waste Disposal, this process exposes medical waste to intense incandescent heat, electrically generated in an inert (argon gas) plasma ion cloud and controlled atmosphere. Chamber temperatures reach approximately 20,000°F, which literally vaporize materials introduced into the chamber to their basic molecular components. Because of near complete ionization, temperatures outside the chamber do not exceed 90°F.

This process yields pure carbon black, which is a marketable by-product and can be used in road construction. The process has a greater than 99% waste reduction factor. Argon gas is reclaimed and returned to the system, and the balance of the residue, a nonleaching aggregate cinder, is pulverized and can be released safely into the sewer system or accumulated indefinitely on-site, available for sale to concrete manufacturers as a hardener. The cleaned by-product gases, consisting of oxygen and carbon monoxide, are vented out through the sewer trap and pipe vent. Temperature, time, pressures, waste weight, and generation location are recorded and saved so a complete report can be generated.

While exceedingly promising, this technology is largely unproved and is expensive. Its greatest

potential at this time exists where large regional waste processing and disposal facilities are feasible. Many states currently mandate that infectious waste be treated on-site. They also restrict off-site transport of the waste or prohibit it from being landfilled, or both. Many additional states are planning similar restrictive legislative measures. At present, incineration is the only method the EPA recommends for disposing of virtually all types of infectious wastes. Offset disposal difficulties and limitations probably are the greatest incentives for hospitals and other institutions to select a type of on-site treatment. Many hospitals that are unable to utilize on-site treatment may be required to ship their waste across the country to the disposal facilities. These services typically are costly, and at times prohibitively expensive.

This method has several advantages, however, as off-site disposal is simple and requires relatively short implementation time. It avoids problems with locating and permitting on-site treatment systems. Also, building space and associated support systems are not required. These benefits usually are not enough, however, to make an off-site facility the most attractive alternative. The Medical Waste Tracking System of 1988 and comparable state legislation have imposed additional difficulties with this treatment option. Packaging, manifesting, and tracking requirements, with their accompanying severe penalties, for noncompliance, provide the most recent major deterrent to off-site waste disposal.

Health-care providers face several sets of new and complex requirements. Federal and state laws have extended a facility's liability for waste handling beyond the walls of the hospital itself. The insurance industry labels this increasing exposure to liability as "environmental impairment risks." If current trends continue, legal regulations faced by generators and disposers of medical waste will only get tougher and more complicated. Commercial insurers currently are limiting liability coverage for the transportation and disposal of medical waste. These factors have increased the need for hospitals to protect themselves from a dangerous liability situation. The plethora of new regulations coming from different directions warrants care in determining which regulations take precedence.

In the 21st century, the disposal of medical waste will become more complex and problematic. It is a serious problem now, and all indications point to a future full of legal and insurance fights, dangerous and deliberate violations, and vast room for improvement. For these reasons, health-care providers not only must become more responsive to changing regulations but also more proactive and responsible in dealing with the overall medical waste issue.

START ················

HAZARDOUS WASTE

As the nation becomes increasingly industrialized and more technologically advanced, more wastes are generated. Some of the waste is hazardous. The Resource Conservation and Recovery Act (RCRA), which was enacted by Congress in 1976 to address the management of waste in the United States, identifies hazardous waste as follows:

1. *Toxicity*. **Toxic** means potentially poisonous to humans. Toxicity is determined by a toxicity characteristics leeching procedure (TCLP). Technicians expose a waste to laboratory-created landfill conditions and allow it to equilibrate. After 24 hours, water samples are tested for levels of substances high enough to be hazardous.

2. *Ignitability*. **Ignitable** compounds are liquids with a flashpoint below 60°C or nonliquids liable to cause fire via friction, moisture absorption, or spontaneous chemical change. Organic solvents, oils, plastics, and paints are ignitable compounds.

3. *Corrosivity*. **Corrosive** wastes, those with a pH below 2 or above 12.5, can eat away living tissues or corrode materials through chemical reaction. These corrosive materials, such as acids, alkaline substances, cleaning agents, and battery residues, present a threat to people who come into bodily contact with leaky containers.

4. *Reactivity*. **Reactive** wastes include obsolete munitions and certain chemical wastes that react vigorously with air or water. They may explode and generate toxic gases. An example is the waste from the firecracker industry.

In 1999, over 20,000 hazardous waste generators produced over 40 million tons of hazardous waste regulated by RCRA.

An example of a hazardous waste problem (though not regulated under hazardous waste law) is the former use of polychlorinated biphenyls (PCBs). These are organochloride chemicals structurally similar to the pesticide DDT. Because PCBs have excellent insulating properties, they were used widely in transformers and other electrical components. They also had a wide range of use in soap, paint, glue, waxes, brake lining, caulking compounds, and epoxy resins. In 1968 in Japan, cooking oil was contaminated accidentally with PCBs, and several thousand people suffered subsequently from enlarged liver, disorders of the intestinal tract and lymphatic systems, and loss of hair. In the early 1970s, PCBs were found in cow's milk, inland and deep-sea fish, meats, and humans. Tests have indicated that PCBs interfere with reproduction in fish, rodents, and many species of birds and monkeys. PCBs are suspected of being carcinogenic. Moreover, PCBs are not easily biodegradable—which raises concern where even small quantities have been spilled in the environment. Compounding the problem is that when PCBs decompose, their products are even more poisonous than the original material. Production of PCBs stopped in the United States in 1977. Decades more will have to go by for the compounds to be removed from the environment.

Sometimes workers must dispose of a batch of chemicals because of overheating or some other problem. Many of these wastes are toxic, and some are deadly. Thus, they should not be mixed with domestic waste or pumped into streams, lakes, or oceans. In the past, the easiest way to dispose of the wastes was to pack them in 55-gallon steel drums (the "garbage cans" of the chemical industry) and store them elsewhere. As the drums accumulated, often in the thousands, they created new toxic waste sites. Some examples of hazardous waste incidents are as follows.

- In the early 1940s, Hooker Chemical Company of Niagara Falls, New York, dumped approximately 19,000 tons of waste into a canal site. In 1953, the company covered the dump site with dirt and sold the land to the

Board of Education of Niagara for $1. The deed of the sale indicated that the site contained "waste products resulting from the manufacturing of chemicals." The deed further stated that Hooker would not be responsible for the condition of the land. The site later was used for an elementary school and playground, with housing also in the area.

The steel drums eventually rusted, corroded, and leaked. The contents seeped into the soil and groundwater and eventually entered the lakes, rivers, and streams. Heavy rain during the spring of 1977 raised the level of the groundwater and turned the area into a muddy swamp. Many of the school children and people living in the neighborhood suffered serious illnesses. The citizens reported skin sores, epilepsy, rectal bleeding, liver malfunctioning, miscarriages, severe headaches, and birth defects.

An environmental survey revealed that the drums were leaking and that several other dumps contaminated with hazardous waste were scattered around the city. Almost overnight, a new and serious environmental concern was brought to the attention of the public. The dump site was evacuated, families were relocated at a cost of $37 million to the State of New York, and cleanup began (and may never really end). The hazardous waste era had arrived.

An estimated 1000 kg of wastes containing dioxin had been buried in that area. Dioxin is a highly toxic substance—one of the deadliest known. Through this unfortunate incident, it was found that dioxin could enter drinking water supplies and cause severe problems.

- At a rural site 25 miles south of Louisville, Kentucky, 6,000 drums full of toxic chemicals and 11,000 more partly full were found. The corroding drums oozed hazardous chemicals into the soil. An investigation found that the deceased owner of the land had pocketed money that was supposed to be used for proper disposal of the waste.

- Iberville Parish, Louisiana, was the site of a truck driver's death. The driver had dumped a load of hazardous chemicals into a waste pit. The dumped chemicals reacted with chemicals already in the pit, producing a cloud of hydrogen sulfide gas that paralyzed the driver's respiration. Investigators noticed later that the disposal site was operating without proper permits.

- Montaque, Michigan, was a site of water contamination. Illegal dumping of carbon tetrachloride and chloroform, as well as tetrachloride othylene, poisoned well water in the area. This accident was uncovered in 1977, when a former employee of Hooker Chemical complained to Michigan authorities about the hazardous wastes. Investigators also discovered a secret dump site and many drums that had been allowed to drain onto the property. Hooker subsequently had to pay to provide local residents with a proper waterline or take water to them. As a result of the legal action, Hooker was forced to construct a huge clay-lined vault to contain its wastes and begin efforts to decontaminate the groundwater.

- Residents of Seymour, Indiana, were evacuated from their homes in March 1980 when hydrogen gas reacted with solvents from more than 60,000 containers of hazardous wastes that a company had dumped improperly in the nearby area. The EPA declared a water emergency at Seymour. The cost of complete removal of the waste was estimated at $12 million.

Federal officials believe there may be as many as 50,000 dangerous chemical dumps in the United States.

Transportation of Hazardous Waste

Railroads, trucks, and barges transport hazardous waste in the United States. The transportation of hazardous wastes can pose a threat to the public. To promote safety and protect the public's health, companies follow four basic control measures for the movement of hazardous waste from a generator to disposal.

1. *Hazardous waste manifest.* The concept of a cradle-to-grave tracking system is considered a key to proper management of hazardous waste. Manifest copies accompany each barrel of waste that leaves the site where it is generated and are signed and mailed to the receiving sites to indicate the transfer of waste from one location to another.

2. *Labeling and placarding.* Each container is labeled and marked. The transporting vehicle is placarded before a waste is transported from the generating site. Companies post warning labels such as: explosive, strong oxidizer, compressed gas, flammable liquid, corrosive material, and poisonous/ toxic substances.

3. *Haulers.* Because of the dangers involved, haulers of hazardous waste are subject to operator training, insurance coverage, and special registration of vehicles transporting hazardous waste. Handling precautions include restrictive use of the transport trucks and the use of gloves, face masks, and coveralls for the workers' protection.

4. *Incident and accident reporting.* Accidents involving hazardous waste must be reported immediately to the state regulatory agency, as well as local health departments. Necessary information that will help responders contain the material should be made available.

Hazardous Waste Disposal

When choosing a hazardous waste disposal site, evaluators must consider many factors. These include hydrology, geology, climatology, ecology, and public and environmental health. Some disposal options include the so-called secure landfill; chemical, physical, and biological treatment processes; incineration; and deep-well injection.

SECURE LANDFILL

In the past, the **secure landfill** was one of the more frequently used methods of disposing of hazardous waste. Regulations now drastically limit their use.

A secure landfill consists of ground excavation and some sort of insulation to prevent waste from escaping into air, water, and land. This is accomplished by locating the landfill away from aquifers that are used for drinking water supplies. The operated area is lined with concrete or some approved impermeable liner. Compacted earth (preferably clay) is placed over the liner, then another liner is poured. The barrels, many times specially lined, coated with concrete, and so on, are placed in the area and covered with earth. Secure landfills now are covered by the "land ban," which specifies treatment methods for wastes before they can be placed into or on the ground. Treatment methods are designed to ensure that contaminants do not migrate from the disposal area.

Builders design each level of the landfill so workers can monitor leachate. Preferably, surface waters are diverted away to reduce the chance of water entering, covering the barrels, and causing rust.

CHEMICAL, PHYSICAL, AND BIOLOGICAL TREATMENTS

The goal for chemically, physically, and biologically oriented treatment processes is to reduce the volume of waste and the hazardous characteristics of the waste. Chemical methods include neutralization, precipitation, solidification, and oxidation reduction. Physical processes include evaporation and compaction of some material. Biological techniques depend largely upon microorganisms to decompose toxic organic compounds. These treatment methods greatly reduce the volume of waste to be landfilled or incinerated and avoid migration of hazardous components from the disposal area.

INCINERATION

Incineration, burning at high temperatures, is a significant means of handling hazardous waste. Combustion is intended to convert waste to a less bulky, less toxic, and less noxious material. The products of combustion are mainly carbon dioxide, water, and ash. Some products of incomplete combustion (PICs) are harmful. If the water or gaseous products of combustion contain undesirable compounds, further treatment is necessary. This treatment usually consists of scrubbing for the gaseous material and wastewater treatment for the water. The residue is disposed of in secure landfills. Incineration reduces the volume of landfilled hazardous waste, thus saving landfill space. Incinerators are expensive, however, and the waste, ash, gases, and water must be controlled to prevent damage to the environment and the public's health.

Remediation

DEEP-WELL INJECTION

In hazardous waste management, as with radiological health, emphasis should be placed on reducing the amount at the source of generation. Sometimes this can be accomplished by reusing and recycling the waste and by modifying the industrial process to eliminate or reduce the waste generated. Presently, waste minimization is the preferred method of hazardous waste management. All facility permits issued effective September 1, 1985, and thereafter specify that a waste minimization program must be in place. Further, all generators, upon completing a manifest, must specify that they have such a program. In 1980, the U.S. Congress passed **CERCLA** (the Comprehensive Environmental Response, Compensation and Liability Act), known as the **Superfund** program, to clean up contaminated waste sites. In 1984, Congress added amendments to the 1976 Resource Conservation and Recovery Act, to better manage hazardous waste. The Superfund Amendments and Reauthorization Act was passed in 1986. These acts are summarized in Chapter 14.

SUMMARY

Responsible, effective, solid waste management begins by reducing the volume at the point of generation and by recycling. The remaining waste may be treated, for example, by incineration or disposed in a sanitary landfill. Requirements for landfills have been strengthened and now include liners, leachate collection and treatment, management of gases produced by decomposition, and more. Composting has again become a popular and effective method for reducing the solid waste burden in the United States. Effective and cost efficient measures for

managing infectious waste are continually being explored.

Hazardous waste programs have developed over the last 30 years. The hazardous waste manifest system provides a mechanism to track transfers of hazardous waste from cradle to grave. Efforts to minimize the production of hazardous waste offer a greater degree of safety and cost savings. Recycling of materials that we typically disposed of 20 years ago has shown to save money on raw materials, reduce energy consumption, and create new jobs. Simple disposal of municipal solid waste on land has been replaced largely by burial of treated waste. Remediation of contaminated sites is increasing, as necessary specialized technology is developed.

KEY TERMS

Ashes, p. 116	Reactive, p. 131
Autoclaving, p. 128	Refuse, p. 116
CERCLA, p. 134	Rubbish, p. 116
Composting, p. 134	Sanitary landfill, p. 124
Corrosive, p. 131	Secure landfill, p. 133
Energy recovery, p. 123	Superfund, p. 134
Garbage, p. 116	Toxic, p. 131
Ignitable, p. 131	Waste-to-energy (WTE), p. 123
Incineration, p. 118	

REFERENCES

American Public Works Association. 1970. *Municipal Refuse Disposal*. Public Administration Service, Chicago.

Blackman, William C., Jr. 1995. *Basic Hazardous Waste Management*, 2nd ed. Lewis Publishers.

Doucet, Lawrence G. 1990. Infectious Waste Treatment and Disposal Alternatives. Peekskill, NY: *Professional Development Series #057005*.

Environmental Protection Agency. 1997. *Innovative Uses of Compost Erosion Control, Turf Remediation, and Landscaping*. U.S. Government Printing Office, Washington, D.C.

Environmental Protection Agency. 1998. *RCRA, Superfund & EPCRA Hotline*. U.S. Government Printing Office, Washington, D.C.

Griffin, Roger D. 1989. *Principles of Hazardous Materials Management*, 2nd ed. Lewis Publishers.

LaGrega, Michael D., P. L. Buckingham, J. C. Evans, and Environmental Resources Management Group. 1994. *Hazardous Waste Management*. McGraw-Hill, New York.

Miller, Tyler. 1988. *Living In the Environment*, 5th ed. Wadsworth Publishing, Belmont, CA.

Martin, William F., John F. Martin, and Timothy G. Prothero. 1987. *Hazardous Waste Handbook for Health and Safety*. Butterworth-Heinemann, Boston, MA.

Pfeffer, John T. 1992. *Solid Waste Management Engineering*. Prentice Hall, Englewood Cliffs, NJ.

Public Health Service. 1982. *Sanitation in the Control of Insects and Rodents of Public Health Importance*. U.S. Government Printing Office, Washington, DC.

Rhyner, Charles R., Leander J. Schwartz, Robert Wenger, and Maty Kohrell. 1995. *Waste Management and Resource Recovery*. CRC, Boca Raton, FL.

Roy F. Weston, Inc. 1994. Value added to recyclable materials in the northeast. Prepared for the Northeast Recycling Council, Brattleboro, VT.

Slavik, Nelson S. 1988. OSHA/EPA Handling and Disposal of Hazardous Materials. *Technical Document Series #055970.*

Tellus Institute. 1997. Estimated value of MSW materials recycled in 1995. Prepared for U.S. EPA, Washington, D.C.

Tellus Institute. 1992. Energy implications of integrated solid waste management systems. Prepared for New York State Energy Research and Development Authority, Boston, MA.

United States Council for Automotive Research. 2001. *Passenger cars, the most recycled products on earth.* http://www.uscar.org.

Vesiland, Anne. 1996. *Environmental Engineering*. PWS Publishing Company, Boston.

Vesiland, P. A. 1983. *Environmental Pollution and Control*, 2nd ed. Ann Arbor Science, Michigan.

VECTORS AND THEIR CONTROL

Darryl Barnett, Dr. P.H.

Eastern Kentucky University

OBJECTIVES

- Identify the rodent that is of greatest public health interest.
- Identify the arthropods of greatest public health interest.
- Name the most prominent disease agents.
- Describe the transmission route from the vector.
- Discuss the habitat of public health-related rodents and arthropods.
- Discuss the most important control methods for the vectors.

Vector-borne diseases are a major problem worldwide and are becoming an increasing problem in the United States due to humanity's encroachment into new areas, the compression of the world by ease of travel, by illegal importation of animals that can serve as reservoirs, and possibly by increased immigration from areas endemic with previously unseen causative agents in the United-States. A **vector** is any organism that transmits a pathogen, or disease-causing agent. Among vector-borne diseases are murine typhus, bubonic plague, leptospirosis, salmonellosis, rat bite fever, rickettsialpox, trichinosis, lymphocytic choriomeningitis, toxoplasmosis, and listeriosis. Two types of vectors that are most problematic are discussed in this chapter: rodents (mainly rats) and insects of the arthropod class. Money spent on managing solid wastes to control these vectors pays off because it reduces the need for spending on vector control programs and vector-borne diseases.

RODENTS

Commensal Rodents

Rodents are undesirable for several reasons. They destroy property, frighten people, spread disease, and compete with humans for food. Improperly managed solid waste creates an ideal habitat for insects and rodents.

Rats plague many store owners and farmers. Rodents are undesirable in feed and seed stores because they destroy the seed, corn, and other supplies. Rats also are undesirable in poultry houses and bird farms. They destroy and contaminate structures, as well as harm young birds and chicks. In some areas of the world, rats destroy as much as one-third of the entire harvest.

Because rats gnaw and burrow, they can cause structural damage to buildings. They have been known to gnaw insulation off wiring, which has started fires in buildings. Norway rats *(Rattus norvegicus)* prefer to burrow and live below the ground. Therefore, they have been known to burrow and weaken the foundation bulkhead of dams and thus create the condition for flooding and other forms of destruction. We wish to control rodents to protect our property and enhance our health. If we are going to control them, we must know something about their biological characteristics and habits.

Biological Characteristics

Domestic rodents include the previously mentioned Norway rats, plus roof rats *(Rattus rattus)* and house mice *(Mus musculus)*. They are members of the order *Rodentia*, family *Muridae*. These rodents are "commensal," which means they live at people's expense. They eat their food, live in their houses, and share with them their diseases—without contributing anything beneficial to the relationship.

Rodents are characterized by a single pair of incisor teeth on each jaw and by the absence of canine teeth. They usually have a tail with fine scales and few hairs, although many American rodents, such as field mice, wood rats, squirrels, and chipmunks, have hair and a bushy tail.

The Norway rat (Figure 8.1) is predominantly a burrowing rodent. The most common and largest of the domestic rats, it is found throughout the temperate regions of the world including the United States. Some common names of this species are: brown rat, house rat, barn rat, sewer rat, and wharf rat. The Norway rat has a heavy, stocky body and averages 7 to 18 ounces in weight and between 7 to 10 inches in length. A distinguishing characteristic of the Norway rat is that the combined head and body are longer than the tail. The total length of Norway rats (tail plus body and head) is between 13 and 18 inches. The Norway rat has coarse fur, usually brownish or reddish gray, a blunt nose, and small, close-set ears that appear to be half buried in

fur. The eyes are small compared with those of other rats. The gestation period for the Norway rat averages 22 days with the rats reaching sexual maturity in 3 to 5 months after birth. Norway rats have from four to seven litters per year, with the average female weaning 20 rats per year. The rats' life expectancy is about one year. Preferable food is garbage, meat, fish, vegetables, fruits, and cereal. The Norway rat needs only 0.5 to one ounce of water per day.

The *roof rat (Rattus rattus)* is smaller than the Norway rat (see Figure 8.1) and is a more agile climber. In the United States, the roof rat is found mainly in the South, across the entire nation to the Pacific coast. It is found in Hawaii as well as colder regions of the world. The roof rat's body is slender and graceful. It weighs 4 to 12 ounces and is 6 to 8 inches long. A distinguishing factor of the roof rat is that the tail is longer than the combined body and head. Tail length is from 7 to 10 inches, and total length of the roof rat is from 14 to 18 inches. The roof rat has a pointed nose, large ears, and large eyes. The average gestation period of the female roof rat is 22 days; the young reach sexual maturity in 3 to 5 months. Females average four to six litters per year, with an average of six to eight offspring per litter. The roof rat prefers to live above ground, indoors, in attics, between floors, in walls, in enclosed spaces, or outdoors in trees and dense vine growth. The roof rat's preferred foods are vegetables, fruits, and cereal grains. It also competes with people for other foods.

The *house mouse (Mus musculus)* is abundant throughout the United States, as well as the rest of the world. It has a long, slender, graceful body (see Figure 8.1), with an average weight of 0.5 to 0.75 ounces. Its tail is 3 to 4 inches long, which is a little longer than the head plus the body. It has a pointed nose, large ears, and large eyes. The house mouse reaches sexual maturity in 1.50 to two months after birth. The gestation period is 19 days, and the mother has an average of eight litters per year. The offspring range from five to six per litter. Longevity for a house mouse is usually less than one year. These mice prefer convenient indoor spaces between walls and cabinets, in furniture, or in stored goods. Outdoors they live in weeds, rubbish, and grasslands. The preferred food is cereal grains, but

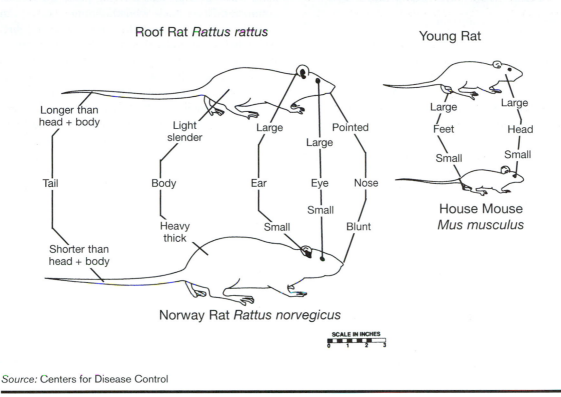

Roof Rat *Rattus rattus*

Young Rat

Longer than head + body	Light slender	Large	Pointed
Tail	Body	Ear	Large	Eye	Nose
	Heavy thick	Small	Small	Blunt
Shorter than head + body			

Large Feet — Small

Large Head — Small

House Mouse
Mus musculus

Norway Rat *Rattus norvegicus*

SCALE IN INCHES
0 1 2 3

Source: Centers for Disease Control

FIGURE 8.1 Field identification of three domestic rodents.

they will eat most types of the other edible food that people consume.

Rodents are sensitive to touch. They have guard hairs (vibrissae) all over their bodies, which serve as feelers or sensitive whiskers. Hence, rats and mice prefer to run along walls and between objects where they can keep their sensitive whiskers in contact with vertical or side surfaces. This compensates for their poor vision; and they also are believed to be color-blind. Having an extremely keen sense of smell, rodents can readily detect the odors of most foods that humans consume. Rodents also have a well-developed sense of taste and will eat most foods that humans eat, preferring fresh food to spoiled food. Rats tend to associate sickness caused by poison bait with the bait and will not take the poison again, thus becoming bait-shy.

While the Norway rat prefers to burrow and live below the ground and the roof rat prefers to live above the ground, the house mouse, as its name suggests, prefers living in human quarters. The rodents' burrows seldom are far from a source of food and water.

It was once believed that rodents must gnaw to wear off the average growth of 4 to 6 inches per year on their incisors. However, this is false since the opposing pair of incisors serve as a chisel to keep both worn down. However, rats do gnaw to gain entrance and to obtain food. In so doing, they are destructive to human belongings.

Some signs that indicate the presence of rodents are observing live or dead rats, hearing rats, and seeing rodent droppings, runways, burrows, nests, and signs of gnawing. Further evidence is seeing feeding stations, or spots where rats have pulled food scraps and left them after eating what they wanted. Additional signs are urine, rat hair, and rat body odors.

Four Rodent Control Measures

Rodent control management is divided into four distinct areas:

1. Eliminating sources of food.
2. Eliminating breeding and nesting places.
3. Rat-proofing buildings and other structures.
4. Killing them.

A good job of solid waste management goes a long way toward creating an unfavorable environment for rodents. Storing, collecting, and disposing of refuse in a sanitary manner does much to deprive the rodents of their requirement for survival: food.

Rats prefer to consume people's food while it is in the pantry, grocery store, or on shelves. If they cannot get to this food supply before people do, however, they will survive easily on people's garbage. Therefore, garbage storage, collection, and disposal are vital to eliminating rodents. Another situation in which rats obtain food is the feeding of pets. Sometimes owners overfeed cats or dogs and after dark the rodents come in and eat the food. Interestingly, rats can live for a long time by eating apples. Hence, apple trees in a community can serve as a food supply for rodents if other basic requirements for survival, such as harborage, are provided. Because rats prefer to live close to people's food supply, people must be careful to make the food unavailable for them. This includes food in the home, restaurants, grocery stores, schools, and other places where humans live, work, travel, and recreate.

Elimination of breeding and nesting places is another way to control rodents. The rubbish in an open dump provides a home, or harborage, for the rodents, and their food source is readily available. Some communities require that all lumber, fire wood, and the like be stored at least 6 inches above the ground. At this height, the materials do not provide a home for rats, which prefer dark, moist places in which to burrow. For this reason, wood should not be piled directly on the ground, and trash and other rubbish should be removed from the premises periodically to prevent nesting. Old appliances such as washing machines, televisions sets, and refrigerators, as well as cars, trucks, and other

solid waste also provide a living place for rats. A common mistake made while building a house is to pour the patio and steps before the ground (fill dirt) has settled adequately. When the dirt finally settles, it leaves a space under the patio and other areas that is suitable for rat harborage.

If the rats cannot be starved to death and, for some reason, their breeding and nesting places cannot be removed, we must concentrate on building them out (Figure 8.2). Most modern homes are rat-proofed. The crawl space under the house usually has ventilators, each having a grid with a screen behind it to prevent rodents from entering. Likewise, attics typically have ventilators with screens on them. Because the Norway rat prefers to burrow, the footings on houses are poured in an L-shape with the boot (the toe of the L) on the outside. The rats will burrow down, encounter the concrete, and not burrow further. This prevents them from entering buildings where food is stored. Other means of rat-proofing include placing metal strips on doors where rats may gnaw to gain entrance and putting hardware cloth (rat wire) over windows. All potential entrances to buildings such as openings around pipes, cracks in walls, and other places where a rat could gain entrance should be sealed with concrete. In sum, one has to do everything possible to build out dwelling places and businesses so rodents cannot gain entrance.

The final measure to control rodents is to kill them. If a killing program is necessary, we have failed in the first three endeavors: starving them to death, denying them a home, and building them out. Extermination then becomes necessary. The preferred method is by natural means. Traditionally, this meant the household cat. No chemicals are added to the environment and the cat becomes part of the family. While cats may have an impact on a house mouse population, they are typically not effective against rat infestation. Cats are also not recommended for restaurants, grocery stores, and other food establishments.

Rodenticides are available on the market, but many are toxic to humans. When selecting rodenticides and making them available to rats, extreme care is recommended. Two rodenticides recommended for use by laypersons are red squill and warfarin.

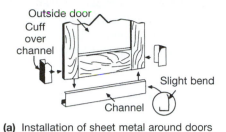

Outside door
Cuff over channel

Slight bend

Channel

(a) Installation of sheet metal around doors

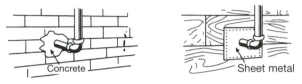

Bend-Over

1½"
1½"

Rivet

(b) Use of hardware cloth screens

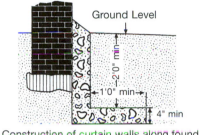

Concrete

Sheet metal

(c) Sealing openings through walls

Ground Level

2'0" min

1'0" min

4" min

(d) Construction of curtain walls along foundations

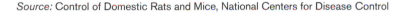

Source: Control of Domestic Rats and Mice, National Centers for Disease Control

FIGURE 8.2 Common measures to build out rats.

Red squill generally comes wrapped in paper similar to candy or gum. It is a one-time rodenticide. A sufficient amount of red squill must be made available to the rats to kill them the first time, because they tend to become bait-shy. If rats eat enough of the red squill, they will be killed by paralysis of the heart muscles. Because red squill is an emetic, humans who consume red squill will regurgitate the poison immediately. Rats cannot regurgitate, thus once ingested, the red squill will kill them.

The second recommended rodenticide group is called *anticoagulants*, of which the most common is warfarin. Warfarin generally is put in corn meal. The rats feed continuously during the night and eat the poisoned corn meal. The warfarin reduces the clotting ability of the blood and increases the permeability of the capillaries. Eventually they begin hemorrhaging and the blood seeps through the blood vessels, weakening the rats until they eventually die. Warfarin is considered safe around children (unless they live in a famine area) because they do not often eat dry corn meal. If a person ingests warfarin, vitamin K in the form of phytonadione is given orally to protect against the anticoagulant effect. Foods high in Vitamin K include leafy vegetables. Warfarin should be made available to rats in adequate quantities until the rat population is completely killed. This is a good choice, as rats do not tend to become bait-shy to warfarin as they do with red squill and some other rodenticides. However, some rats have been reported to develop a resistance to warfarin.

A patch test may be used to determine if a poisoning program is effective in killing all the rats. This consists of spreading flour on the floor and around the walls. If the next morning five- and four-toed footprints and tail marks are seen in the flour, the rats have not been killed and the program must continue.

Another common way to kill rats is by traps. Mousetraps have been used for many years. They are placed along walls, near runways, burrows, and other areas where rodents will likely encounter them. The traps have bait, such as peanut butter or cheese, which attracts the rodents to the trap. Subsequently, the rats are attracted to the traps, trigger them, and are caught. Rats do tend to become trap-shy. If the rat is caught squealing and suffering in the trap, other rats tend to associate this and stay clear of this strange object in their environment.

The most desirable, most economical ways to control rats are to try to starve them to death and to deny them a place to live. These measures also create a clean environment for humans.

Sylvatic Rodents

Sylvatic rodents do not typically live close to people, thus they are normally found in the wild. However, on occasion people do encounter various sylvatic rodents and their parasites while participating in outdoor work or recreational activities. These rodents and parasites can serve as either reservoirs or modes of transmission for several well-known diseases. These diseases are plague, Lyme disease, and hantavirus pulmonary syndrome.

PLAGUE

Plague is a historical disease that visited devastation upon Europe in the middle ages. In its history it has most often been associated with commensal rodents. However, sylvan rodents are capable of carrying and harboring the oriental rat flea (*Xenopsylla cheopis*), which is a capable vector of human plague. A few of the sylvan rodents associated with plague include prairie dogs (*Cynomys sp*), california ground squirrels (*spermophilus beecheyi*) and chipmunks (*tamias sp*).

LYME DISEASE

Lyme disease can be a serious debilitating chronic disease in humans. The transmission of lyme disease is most often associated with the deer tick (*Ixodes scapularis*) or the western blacklegged tick (*I. pacificus*). However, a sylvan rodent, the white-footed mouse (*Permyscus leucopus*) plays an important role in this disease. This mouse serves as one of the natural reservoirs for the causative agent of lyme disease (*Borrelia burgdorferi*). When a larval or nymphal stage tick feeds on the mouse it acquires the causative agent and is able to transmit the agent to a human when it feeds in the nymphal or adult stage.

HANTAVIRUS PULMONARY SYNDROME

The hantavirus pulmonary syndrome (HPS) first came to note in 1993 during an outbreak in the Four Corners area of the southwestern United States. In quoting the Centers For Disease Control, it could be considered "an old disease that has been newly recognized." Extensive research indicated that it can have a commensal linkage, but the rodent vectors are normally considered to be sylvan in nature. HPS is described as a pan-American zoonosis, which has several different viral causative agents, related to distinct rodent hosts. The original Four Corners outbreak found the causative agent to be a virus, since named Sin Nombre, and the reservoir to be the deer mouse (*P. maniculatus*). Since the 1993 outbreak three additional viruses with different rodent hosts have been identified.

The Black Creek Canal virus has been linked in Florida to the cotton rat (*Sigmodon hispidus*); in Louisiana and Texas the bayou virus has been associated with the rice rat (*Oryzomys palustris*); and in the northeastern United States cases of HPS have been linked to New York-1 virus. This latter virus has been connected to both *P. leucopus* and *P. maniculatus*. Exposure to the causative agent is related to disturbing rodent urine, droppings, or nests, particularly in confined spaces. If disturbed, the viral particles can become airborne and subsequently can be inhaled. Transmission can also occur due to particle exposure via broken skin, mucous membranes, ingestion, and from rodent bites.

Regardless of whether the rodent population is "commensal" or "sylvan," control efforts must be focused on denying harborage and food sources to the population. As part of a total program, trapping and rodenticides must be utilized to provide final control. In situations where fleas and ticks provide transmission from a rodent reservoir, prevention and control measures must be taken in conjunction to control the ectoparasites and reduce exposure to the population.

· · · · · · · · · · · · · ·

ARTHROPODS

Arthropods are animals belonging to the phylum *Arthropoda*, meaning "jointed foot." Insects, the largest class of arthropods, typically have three pairs of legs, a segmented body with a head, thorax, and abdomen, plus mouthparts consisting of palpi and a **proboscis**. The proboscis is utilized by mosquitoes, fleas, lice, cockroaches, and flies to pierce the skin and to take a blood meal. In the case of some flies, a sponging mouthpart is used to feed. This type of mouthpart uses saliva to break down the food in order for the fly to feed. The sponging mouthpart contributes to the spread of organisms by contamination and from the fly saliva. Insects generally are acknowledged as the arthropods of greatest public health significance.

The second most prominent class of arthropods of public health significance is the **arachnids**, which include ticks and mites. Arachnids typically have the head, thorax, and abdomen unified into one body region. As adults, they have four pairs of legs and no antennae. Mouthparts consist of a cutting organ called the *chelicerae*, which enables insertion of the hypostome. This anchors the arachnid and allows blood feeding from the host. The tick is among the most efficient of the arthropod vectors.

Insects

MOSQUITOES

Mosquitoes, a member of class *Insecta*, are a formidable public health problem because they are responsible for spreading disease organisms to millions of people each year. These pathogens include arboviruses, which are responsible for yellow fever; various encephalitides; dengue and its hemorrhagic fever; the protozoans, which cause the various forms of malaria; and the nematodes, which cause filariasis.

Mosquitoes have a complete **metamorphosis**, a four-stage life cycle, as shown in Figure 8.3. The first three stages occur in water. The *Anopheles* and *Culex* genuses lay their eggs on water, while the eggs of the *Aedes* genus mosquito, of primary public health interest, are found on the sides of containers or in tree holes just above water level. This knowledge is valuable when determining the proper strategy for eliminating egg-laying areas for specific mosquitoes. The next two stages, larva and pupa, known in the mosquito, as the **wriggler** and the **tumbler**, must have access to air. This necessity enables a means of killing them by spraying larvacides on the surface of water. The adult mosquito, both male and female, is an active flyer, varying in both range and preference for meal sources. Mosquitoes typically are active in the evening and night and during the day while resting in shaded areas. Most prefer temperatures in the 80° to 90°F range. The male feeds on plant juices, and the female feeds upon the blood of warm-blooded or cold-blooded animals.

Thus, the female is responsible for transmitting disease organisms. Most female mosquitoes require a blood meal before they are able to lay each batch of fertile eggs. Only one mating is required, however, to fertilize egg production for a lifetime.

The mosquito transmits the disease agent primarily with its salivary glands and proboscis or piercing part which is designed for piercing the skin and sucking blood. While the mosquito is taking blood, salivary secretions from the gland are injected as an anticoagulant. The disease-causing agent, which normally has migrated from the intestinal system, is injected with the salivary secretion. It is in this manner that mosquitoes spread disease organisms.

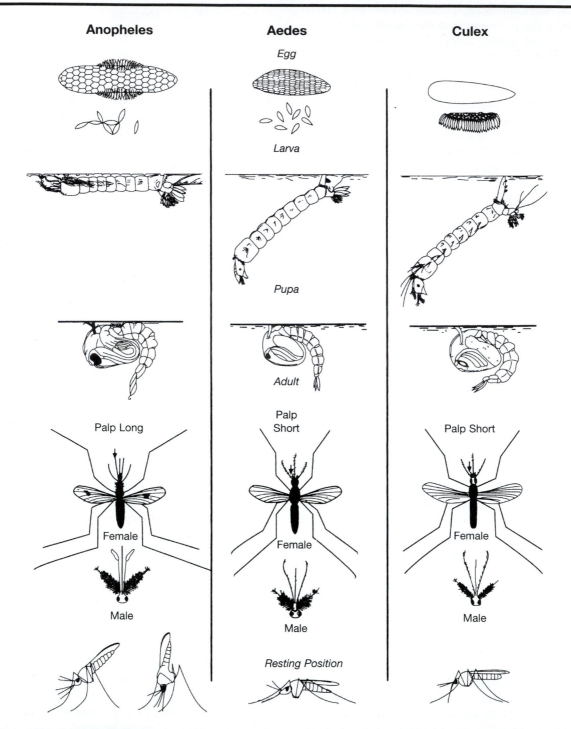

FIGURE 8.3 Stages in life cycle of mosquitoes.

Chapter 8

Mosquito control is founded on an integrated approach, including the use of the following:

- chemicals such as insecticides and larvacides
- biological control such as the *Gambusia affinis*, a predatory fish, and parasites such as the nematode *Ronomermis culicivorax*
- sanitation efforts

The latter includes good solid waste control, eliminating the artificial containers favored by *Aedes aegypti*, and vehicle tires, which are favored breeding spots for *Aedes albopictus*. Sanitation also includes other types of habitat elimination such as draining transient water pools (for example, ditches and canals), which are ideal habitats for *Culex tarsalis*. Proper storage, collection, and disposal of solid waste results in the elimination of breeding areas and ultimately can save money and time in the control of arthropods.

While the historically endemic mosquito borne diseases in the United States continue to be of concern, a new encephaltide arbovirus arrived in the United States in 1999. This is the West Nile virus, a flavivirus closely related to the St. Louis encephalitis virus. This virus initially affected people in the New York City area with 62 severe disease cases and seven deaths. It is currently unknown how the virus entered the country, but it is suspected to have been present at least from the spring of 1999. This arbovirus is vectored primarily in the United States by mosquitoes of the *Culex sp*. Birds serve as the primary reservoir with the mosquito feeding upon the amplified bird host. The mosquito can then feed upon humans and domestic animals. Both can develop clinical illness but are normally considered to be incidental or dead end hosts from which a susceptible mosquito cannot obtain the virus. Most recent reports indicate that the virus has been identified as far south as Florida and as far west as Ohio and Kentucky.

Prevention and control efforts have included surveillance for cases and the use of sentinel flocks with serum sampling. Larvaciding and adulticiding efforts have been used to reduce mosquito populations and to reduce contact with adult mosquitoes.

FLIES

Flies, like mosquitoes, belong to the class *Insecta* and have a complete metamorphosis. While we are familiar with the adult stage, the egg and pupa stages are rarely seen. The larval stage, also known as a **maggot**, is viewed with disgust. When the eggs are laid in the flesh of mammals, the resulting larvae invade the surrounding living tissue, resulting in a condition known as **myiasis**. Medical researchers, however, recently have found the larval stage of the blowfly, a family that includes common greenbottles and bluebottles, can be used beneficially to devour dead tissue around infected wounds. Myiasis may occur in a different form known as "obligate" myiasis. This occurs when the fly larva must spend part of its developmental stage in living tissue. Documented cases in the United States have been related to travelers exposed to the human botfly (*Dermatobia hominis*) in the tropics and on rare occasion to botflies, which normally deposit their eggs in animals. Examples of these include *Wohlfahrtia vigil*, *Cuterebra sp,* and *Cordylobia anthropophaga*. These flies create a painful boil-like or furuncular lesion, which contains the developing larva. These types of flies are of concern in areas such as institutions, which contain elderly or helpless individuals.

Society has historically viewed flies as carriers of disease-causing agents and as destroyers of food. From a public health viewpoint, flies can be classified as *biting flies* (sand flies, horseflies, deerflies) or *nonbiting flies* (houseflies, bottleflies, screw worm flies). The latter also are called **synanthropic** flies, referring to their close association with humans (Figure 8.4). Today, the presence of flies is viewed as a gauge or sentinel that sanitation efforts are not being carried out properly. Flies are sources of annoyance, painful bites, and disease transmission. Thus, they currently are considered one of the greatest public health hazards facing humans.

In the southern United States, the most abundant synanthropic fly is the housefly (*Musca domestica*). In the northern part of the country, the most common is the blowfly. The former is considered to be the greater threat to human health. The housefly and the blowfly do not bite but have "sponge-like" mouthparts. A fly with this type of mouthpart can devour only liquids. It constantly

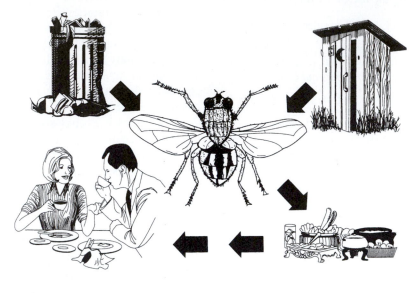

Source: U.S. Public Health Service

FIGURE 8.4 Mechanical transmission of disease-causing organisms by flies.

tests for food sources by excreting saliva, which dissolves the food. This is evidenced by the light brown spots left on areas that have been visited by large numbers of flies.

Domestic flies spread the causative agents of disease in the following ways:

1. On their mouthparts
2. Through their vomitus
3. On their body and leg hairs
4. On the sticky pads of their feet
5. Through the intestinal tract by means of fly feces

These are the mechanical transmission methods that spread the causative agent of the diseases and conditions including typhoid fever, paratyphoid, dysentery, and diarrhea.

In addition to being annoying, the biting flies also contribute to the spread of disease. The stable fly (*Stomoxys calcitrans*), black fly (*Simulium venustrum*), and tsetse (*Glossinia palpalis*) are examples of vicious biters. Enormous numbers of black flies have been known to attack cattle and kill them. Deerflies, horseflies, sand flies, and other biting flies attack humans, causing great discomfort. These flies require a blood meal to produce eggs and they typically transmit the disease agent from the salivary gland while feeding. Diseases spread by these flies are categorized as biologically transmitted diseases of the **cyclo-propagative** type. This means that the causative agent undergoes a change in its form and additionally proliferates within the fly. Diseases transmitted in this manner include African sleeping sickness, onchocerciasis, loiasis, and many others, causing suffering and death to millions of people the world over. Thus, control of these flies is essential to the control of many serious and widespread diseases.

Controlling the fly is based upon an understanding of the fly's life cycle and other biological factors. Eliminating breeding media, such as horse manure, cow manure, privies, and garbage, is necessary for effective fly control. Thus, good solid waste management is basic to denying breeding areas and food sources for adult flies.

COCKROACHES

The cockroach, a member of the class *Insecta*, has a three-stage life cycle consisting of the egg, nymph, and adult. The three-stage life cycle is known as incomplete metamorphosis. Cockroaches have become well adjusted to living with and near humans. The hardiness of the cockroach is well known. They have been found to withstand radiation doses 50 times that which can kill a human. In addition, immunologists have found that cockroaches have an immune system comparable to that of mammals. Cockroaches also are purported to be the source of allergens to many people living in inner-city crowded conditions. They harbor in cracks and crevices in and around human habitats. Like many other household pests, they travel between sources of disease pathogens (privies, sewers, garbage) and food intended for human consumption. However, little evidence supports the outbreak of specific diseases as a result of cockroaches. Because their activity is well known and they have been shown to carry *Salmonella typhimurium*, *Entamoeba histolytica*, and the virus for poliomyelitis, they are assumed to be a threat to human health. They carry the organisms on their feet, body hairs, and mouthparts, and in their intestines.

Cockroaches eat almost anything from fingernails to steak. They are fond of starchy items such as cereals, bakery products, and bookbindings. These roaches also will feed upon beer, cheese, leather, wallpaper, and dead animals. They discharge a nauseating liquid from the mouth and thoracic glands, which imparts an unsavory odor and taste into infested food. They regurgitate partly digested food from their mouths and defecate while feeding, both of which are loaded with microorganisms.

Roaches do not fly but can move by a gliding motion. Most cockroaches are nocturnal, appearing during daylight only if disturbed or very hungry. They prefer to live in warm, moist areas such as cracks and crevices near stoves, refrigerators, hot water heaters, coffee urns, and warm water pipes.

Of the several species of cockroaches, the three most common are discussed here.

1. The American cockroach, *Periplaneta americana*, is believed to have originated in Central Africa but now is found worldwide. The nymphs are white but soon turn a grayish brown and eventually become dark brown in color. This roach has a particular appetite for beer and sweets and often is called the "water bug."

2. The German cockroach, *Blattella germanica*, is native to Europe. It is the pest found most commonly in restaurants and homes. It can enter homes from infested establishments (grocery stores) by means of bottled drinks, packaging, potatoes, onions, other foods, and used furniture. This roach is a pale, yellowish brown and is easily identified by two, dark brown stripes on the pronotum (head). German cockroaches are prolific reproducers. The female carries the eggs in an egg pouch or **ootheca**, protruding from the abdomen until one day before they hatch. These roaches also are known as "Croton bugs."

3. The Oriental cockroach, *Blatta orientalis*, is a dark brown or black species believed to be the third most common cockroach in the United States. It is less domesticated than most species. The habitat includes sewers, damp basements, outbuildings, and the like. This roach has a strong, repulsive odor. It has the longest life cycle of the three discussed here, and it tends to favor colder climates.

FLEAS

Fleas have complete metamorphosis and are members of class *Insecta*. Their effect on people varies from a red spot at the site of the bite to an intense generalized rash. Flea bite sensitization also may occur. The most severe effect is the transmission of disease organisms to people. Although fleas tend to have a preferred host, they will freely utilize another in the absence of their normal host.

Normal flea hosts range from avians to rats to people. The flea normally lays its eggs in the host's hair or feathers. The eggs fall from the host, with the larval stage feeding on organic debris and the pupa stage being spent in a cocoon. Within 24 hours of emergence from the cocoon, adult fleas, both male and female, are ready to feed. Similar to the mosquito, the flea needs the blood meal in order to lay eggs. Fleas are characterized as capillary feeders, using stylets to penetrate the skin and to form a tube to transmit the blood. This enables them to transmit disease pathogens through regurgitation or salivary contamination. They also may transmit disease through fecal contamination. The most noted flea-related diseases are typhus fever and plague. The most notable flea in these diseases is probably the *Xenopsylla cheopis*, also known as the oriental rat flea. This flea is especially vulnerable to blockage of the **proventriculus** by the plague organism *Yersinia pestis*, which causes the flea to regurgitate into a bite wound, thus transmitting the organism to the host.

Control of the flea centers on repressing the flea both on the host and premise areas such as pet bedding. Treatment with pesticides to eliminate the flea in yards and lawns is central to their control. In addition, control of the hosts, such as rats, is paramount in eliminating disease outbreaks.

LICE

The final member of the class *Insecta* of public health importance is the louse. Louse-borne conditions and diseases historically have been associated with people living in crowded or wartime conditions when bathing and clothes-washing facilities have not been available. Louse hosts are as diverse as that of fleas and, similar to fleas, they are not exclusively selective to that host. The three lice of public health interest are the similar-appearing body louse (*Pediculus humanus humanus*) and head louse (*Pediculus humanus capitis*), plus the infamous crab louse (*Pthiris pubis*). These species are known as sucking lice because they take blood meals, and they are found only on mammals.

They undergo incomplete metamorphosis, beginning as an egg (nit) either attached to a hair (head and pubic louse) or attached to clothing (body louse). Heat from the head or body incubates and hatches the eggs into the nymph stage. The adult is similar to the nymph, but larger. The adult is equipped with mouthparts comparable to that of the flea for puncturing and pumping blood, as the louse depends upon blood for sustenance. All three types are responsible for **pediculosis**, heavy infestations of lice characterized by hardened, scarred, pigmented skin and secondary infections, usually a result of intense scratching.

Only the body louse is associated with diseases of public health interest such as louse-borne typhus (*Rickettsia prowazeki*), trench fever (*Rickettsia quin-*

tana), and relapsing fever (*Borrelia recurrentis*). Although these lice are blood feeders, transmission of the causative organism in these diseases typically does not occur from the bite of the louse. It normally occurs through contamination of the bite site from scratching. Fecal material enters these wounds directly or from the louse being crushed and spilling intestinal contents into the wound.

The control of lice focuses on treatment of the host and the host's clothing. Common laundering of clothing with hot water or dry cleaning is satisfactory. Approved insecticides may be used for dusting the host or for treating nonclothing items. Emulsifiable concentrates in the form of a head and body shampoo also are available for elimination of all three types of lice. Prevention is the best tool for eliminating louse outbreaks. Proper hygienic habits, especially teaching children not to share clothing, hats, combs, and brushes with peers, is the most effective means of eradicating pediculosis.

Arachnids

Ticks and mites are of high public health concern. They are of the order *Acarina,* specified by its members' nonsegmented bodies. They belong to the class *Arachnida*, along with mites, spiders, and scorpions.

TICKS

The effect of ticks on humans varies from tick bite paralysis, caused by neurotoxic salivary secretions, to the transmission of disease organisms including protozoa, rickettsia, viruses, and bacteria. Some species of tick can transmit pathogenic organisms from the adult stage to the egg stage through a process known as **transovarian transmission**, and from one developmental stage to another, call **transstadial transmission**.

Ticks are divided into two main groups:

1. Hard ticks (*Ixodidae*)
2. Soft ticks (*Argasidae*)

Hard ticks and soft ticks are easily differentiated by the location of the head (capitulum), presence of the scutum, and body shape. Ticks have a four-stage life cycle. Adults mate on the host and the female lays eggs when she drops to the ground. The larvae, also called "seed ticks," develop and attach to a vertebrate host, which leads to the nymph stage. The nymph then finds another host for feeding, and molts to the adult. Depending on the species, the life cycle varies by the number of hosts necessary for development to an adult; these ticks are known as "one host," "two-host," "three-host," or "plural-host."

The method of transmitting disease pathogens varies with the pathogen and with the tick. Some pathogens, such as *Rickettsia rickettsii* (Rocky Mountain spotted fever) and *Borrelia burgdorferi* (Lyme disease), are transmitted by tick bite and by contamination of an open wound by crushed tick tissue or feces. These are related to the hard ticks *Dermacentor andersoni*, *D. variablis*, and *Amblyomma americanum*. The soft tick genus *Ornithodoros* transmits the pathogen for tick-borne relapsing fever (Borrelia sp) by salivary secretions and also by infectious fluids from the coxal glands on the body.

Because the tick is such a significant public health vector of disease, prevention and control is of great importance in disease reduction. Strategies for individuals include tucking trouser legs into sock tops, keeping clothing buttoned, inspecting the body during and after possible exposure to the tick, and using tick repellents such as Deet (N, N-diethyl-meta-toluamide) prior to potential exposure. Additional efforts in residential areas include keeping lawns and yards closely cut. This helps control both the tick and the small rodent hosts. Larger vegetated areas can be sprayed with the appropriate insecticide. Control efforts, too, must focus on hosts such as domestic animals, including the use of tick/flea collars, plus the dipping, spraying, and dusting of animals. Buildings, kennels, homes, and bedding areas must be treated simultaneously with the host to ensure proper control and elimination. Recent research in Lyme disease prevention has demonstrated a reduction in tick numbers in certain areas by feeding the deer population vermectin-treated corn.

MITES

The final group of arthropods of public health importance is the mite. Like ticks, mites belong to order *Acarina* and have four life stages. Mites may be found in vegetation, on various hosts such as mice, rats, and birds, on organic material such as straw and wood, and living on people. They are responsible for transmitting to humans dermatitis, scabies, allergies, and, most importantly, disease pathogens. Dust mites, ubiquitous to many homes, have been implicated as the cause of many allergic responses. Mites have also been implicated in the transmission of diseases such as scrub typhus (*Rickettsia akamushi*) and rickettsialpox (*Rickettsia akari*).

The life cycle of the mite is important in its effects on people.

Scabies, a mite infestation of people causing itching and irritation, often leads to secondary infections induced by scratching. Scabies is caused by the female (*Sarcoptes scabiei var. hominis*) burrowing, after mating, into the epidermal stratum corneum, where she feeds on lymph. There she lays the eggs and leaves scybala (fecal material).

The larva of the chigger (redbug) causes the intense itching of **dermatitis**. It also feeds on lymph and the lyses of tissue. The reaction to the saliva contributes to the itching and general reaction.

The scrub typhus agent is passed by a chigger mite (*Leptrotrombidium akamusi*) transstadially to its larva stage, which feeds on a person, thus passing the disease agent to a new host. The adult does not feed on vertebrate hosts. The agent for rickettsialpox is passed similarly, by the bite of the house mouse mite (*Liponyssoides sanguineus*), which carries the agent in its saliva.

Management of mites depends upon the type of mite. Those that are host-related can be reduced by controlling the host (birds, rats, house mice) by modifying buildings, trapping, and poisoning. Those that live on vegetation are best approached by keeping lawns cut short, eliminating tall weeds, and removing vegetation from near buildings. Pesticides also are used for outdoor residual treatment, fumigation, and by personal treatment after exposure. Pre-exposure repellents also are recommended. Personal hygiene is paramount, as scabies is passed from person to person in many ways. Hot water and soap are recommended after exposure.

SUMMARY

Throughout history, insects and rodents have plagued humans. These pests have destroyed human food supplies and spread disease-causing agents to humans. Thus, vector-borne diseases, one of the four classifications of disease, have caused much suffering and death. An example occurred during the 1340s when one-fourth of the world's population died of bubonic plague, a disease spread by rats and fleas. Vectors still are prominent in spreading some vector-borne diseases, particularly in developing countries. Thus, efforts to prevent these diseases are aimed at preventing and controlling the vectors.

Control measures, in order of desirability, first should utilize natural measures such as removing the food or breeding places. The second most preferred method is biological control, such as having a cat around to hunt mice or fish to eat the larvae of mosquitoes. Third, and least desirable, is to kill the adults, such as poisoning or spraying chemicals to kill mosquitoes.

KEY TERMS

REFERENCES

Control of Domestic Rats and Mice. 1986. U.S. Public Health Service, Government Printing Office, Washington, DC.

Fleas of Public Health Importance and Their Control. 1988. Centers for Disease Control, Atlanta, GA.

Flies of Public Health Importance and Their Control. 1988. Centers for Disease Control, Atlanta, GA.

Household and Stored-Food Insects of Public Health Importance and Their Control. 1988. Centers for Disease Control, Atlanta, GA.

James, M. T., and Robert F. Howard. 1969. *Herms's Medical Entomology.* 6th ed. Macmillan, New York.

Lice of Public Health Importance and Their Control. 1988. Centers for Disease Control, Atlanta, GA.

Mites of Public Health Importance and Their Control. 1988. Centers for Disease Control, Atlanta, GA.

Mosquitoes of Public Health Importance and Their Control. 1988. Centers for Disease Control, Atlanta, GA.

Recognition and Management of Pesticide Poisoning. 4th ed. 1989. U.S. Environmental Protection Agency, Washington, D.C.

Sanitation in the Control of Insects and Rodents of Public Health Importance. 1982. Centers for Disease Control, Atlanta, GA.

Ticks of Public Health Importance and Their Control. 1989. Centers for Disease Control, Atlanta, GA.

Ware, George W. 1989. *The Pesticide Book.* Thomson Publications, Fresno, CA.

9

TOXICOLOGY

Maurice Knuckles, Ph.D.

Environmental Health Administration, Washington, DC

Welford C. Roberts, Ph.D.

The Uniformed Services University of the Health Sciences

OBJECTIVES

- Understand that there are various types of and facets to toxicology.
- Acquire an understanding of elementary general toxicology concepts.
- Define and explain selected toxicological terms.
- Discuss the factors that should be considered when assessing the toxicology of a xenobiotic agent.
- Know where to find additional resources and information concerning chemical toxicity.

INTRODUCTION

What Is Toxicology?

Traditionally, toxicology has been characterized as the study of poisons. However, that definition is not useful in view of the admonition by Paracelsus (physician; 1493–1541) that "all substances are poisons . . . ; the right dose distinguishes a poison from a remedy poison." Today, toxicology may be defined as the study of how **xenobiotics** (substances foreign to the body) affect biological systems. Those foreign substances may be beneficial therapeutic agents (pharmaceuticals) or harmful environmental agents such as lead, pesticides, or industrial solvents.

The role of the general toxicologist is to determine the adverse effects of xenobiotics on human health using a variety of study types. Other areas include environmental toxicology, which focuses on the adverse effects of pollutants on ecological systems; regulatory toxicology, which utilizes data from various types of toxicology studies to set exposure standards; and forensic toxicology, which deals with the harmful effects of chemicals from a medico-legal perspective. Let's explore the significance of the field of toxicology by examining a simple scenario.

A Scenario—Baltimore, Maryland, July 2001

A train accident involving the release and burning of several toxic chemicals occurred in Baltimore, Maryland, in mid-July 2001 (Moske and Ruane, 2001; Gallo, 2001). The 4,000-ton freight train was traveling from Richmond, Virginia, to Philadelphia, Pennsylvania. As it passed through downtown Baltimore, it entered an old, 1.5 mile long, uphill tunnel that was constructed in the late 1800s, where it derailed. It carried a cargo of industrial solvents, acids, and other corrosive chemicals. A fire developed and hydrochloric acid leaked from one tank car. Chemicals such as petroleum distillates, tripropylene, acetone, and wood and paper products were burning. Smoke clouds exited the tunnel into the downtown area and acid leaked into the city's Inner Harbor. All of this continued over a four-day period. This area of the city attracts tourists and conventions, and has numerous hotels, merchant shops, restaurants, and other businesses. There is a convention center in the area and it is the site of the Camden Yards major league baseball stadium. There was traffic congestion in the area on the day of the derailment, and the first game of a baseball doubleheader was in progress.

Given this scenario—the chemicals involved, fire and spillage, the potential exposure to an extremely large number of people, leakage to the environment—there are a number of things that emergency responders must consider to prevent or minimize harm to the people and the environment. One of the first and major considerations is the potential or actual hazard posed by the chemicals. The toxicology of the chemicals of concern is a key element in this determination. Some questions that may be presented to emergency responders in such a situation may include: Should people be concerned about their health? Are the chemicals toxic? What are the immediate and long-term health effects? How will the chemicals affect the environment and associated wildlife? Are they going to be around a long time or just a short period of time? Toxicology can help provide answers to these and similar questions and serve as a tool to estimate risk and mitigate the actual or potential hazards.

Baltimore's downtown area was disrupted for several days. The second game of the baseball doubleheader was postponed because the stadium was evacuated (Gallo, 2001). However, fortunately, firefighters were able to control the mishap successfully and there were no major injuries or fatalities to the general public or the emergency responders themselves. The hydrochloric acid that leaked into the harbor reportedly produced abnormal acidity for approximately 2 hours with no reported adverse effect (Roig-Franzia, 2001a,b).

THE ENVIRONMENTAL HEALTH PARADIGM

In order for a toxic substance to affect people, it must come in contact with them and enter their body. The **Environmental Health Paradigm** (Figure 9.1) illustrates how xenobiotic chemicals, such as toxic substances, may be emitted by a polluting source and move through the environment to come into contact with people (Miller and Roberts, 2001). When contaminants are released into the environment, they can enter the air, water, or soil. These are called **exposure pathways**, and when more than one is involved collectively they are identified as **multiple pathways**. All of these pathways can contaminate food sources. Also, as contaminants move through the environment they can affect the fauna and flora within ecosystems.

Contaminants can only affect people's health when they contact and enter the body through an **entry route**. The typical entry routes include intake through the lungs by breathing (**inhalation**), passage through the skin (**absorption**), or entry by the mouth (**ingestion**). Substances also may be injected into the body (**parenteral**), for example, accidental needle sticks by health care professionals. People may receive contaminants into the body through multiple entry routes.

Even when contaminants do come into contact with people, they may or may not cause an adverse effect. This is due to how **susceptible** people are to the agent. Susceptibility may vary between groups of people or individuals. Factors such as genetics, general health, and others may influence susceptibility. The less susceptible people are, the more **resistant** they are to chemical toxicity.

The Environmental Health Paradigm also implies that if contaminants do not enter environmental compartments (i.e., air, water, soil), or if they do not contact or enter the body, then they would not cause adverse human health effects. If a person is not susceptible (i.e., is resistant) to the effects of a contaminant, then disease would not occur. In order to prevent contaminants from harming people or the environment, controls may be established at key places along the paradigm. For example, pollution can be prevented by using nontoxic substances at

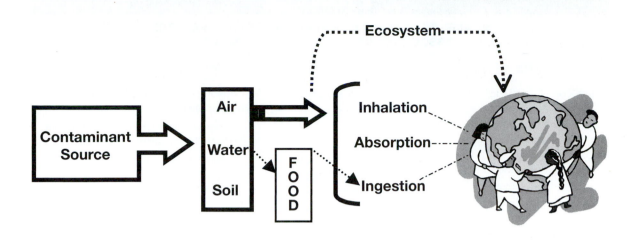

FIGURE 9.1 Environmental health paradigm.

the source. If the source does generate toxic contaminants, they can be contained, recycled, or modified so that pollutants do not enter the environment.

Exposure and Route of Entry

Before any adverse human health effects will take place, exposure must occur. Figure 9.1 shows that people may be exposed to contaminants through the air, water, food, and soil, and they may enter the body by inhalation, absorption, or ingestion. Exposure to substances that may induce toxic effects usually occur by accident, intentional ingestion, occupational contact, or environmental exposures. However, it is important to understand that all exposures do not lead to a toxic manifestation due to a number of factors. A sufficient concentration of the chemical agent or a **metabolite** (breakdown product) must reach and persist at an organ or tissue where the toxic effect is elicited (target organ). Key factors influencing whether a toxic effect will be manifested includes the route of exposure and the duration and frequency of exposure. Each of these factors influence the magnitude of the dose received.

The toxicity of an agent may be altered depending upon its route of exposure. A volatile agent inhaled is likely to be more toxic than the same agent exposure via skin contact. For example, an industrial solvent inhaled may put large quantities of the chemical agent directly into systemic circulation whereas absorption through the skin may be significantly less. The duration of exposure (short term or long term) and how often one is exposed will influence the magnitude of the absorbed dose and whether a toxic effect will be manifested.

When contaminants reach a person's entry site, they may cause local or **point of entry effects** and/or they may be absorbed and distributed to other places in the body. Table 9.1 presents examples of point of entry effects and factors associated with systemic distribution.

Typically, when contaminants are measured in an environmental media they are reported as concentrations, for example, milligrams per liter (mg/L) (water, air), milligrams per cubic meter (mg/m^3) (air), and milligrams per kilogram (mg/kg) (soil, food). Also, the concentrations may be reported as parts-per-million (ppm), parts-per-billion (ppb), or parts-per-trillion (ppt).[1] These concentrations may

---

[1]**part-per-million (ppm)**: that is, one part contaminant per million parts of the environmental medium (e.g., one part contaminant per million parts of air); **part-per-billion (ppb)**: that is, one part contaminant per billion parts of the environmental medium: **part-per-trillion (ppt)**: that is, one part contaminant per trillion parts of the environmental medium.

EXAMPLES OF POINT OF ENTRY EFFECTS AND FACTORS ASSOCIATED WITH SYSTEMIC DISTRIBUTION

Mechanism and Site of Entry		Point of Entry Effects	Systemic Distribution
Absorption	Skin	Irritation, sensitization, defatting	Absorption, entry into circulatory system, distribution
Ingestion	Mouth/Stomach	Irritation	Absorption into circulatory system via biliary-hepatic system, distribution
Inhalation	Lungs	Irritation, particulate entrapment (e.g., phygocytosis)	Enter alveolar space, pass through capillaries, enter circulatory system (gases, vapors)

be thought of as measures of exposure. When chemicals enter and pass through air, water, or soil, they may change chemically due to physical, chemical, or biological processes in the environment or they may remain unchanged. When changes do occur, the modified chemical may be either more or less toxic.

Disposition of Toxicants

Once an exposure occurs, all or a portion of the agent will be absorbed into the blood or be eliminated in expired air or feces (Figure 9.2). The absorbed dose is distributed via the blood to various organs and tissues, and a portion of the absorbed dose may be bound to plasma proteins or distributed to a storage site in the body. For example, absorbed lead will be distributed to the bone storage site. Once bound to a plasma protein such as albumin or deposited into a **storage** site, the agent is no longer biologically active or able to induce a toxic manifestation. The portion still biologically active is then subjected to **biotransformation**, which occurs primarily in the liver. There are a number of reactions that together transform the agent into a metabolite that is more water soluble, the goal being to facilitate elimination of the agent from the body. Elimination of the chemical agent ends any potential toxic effects.

However, the process of biotransformation does not always result in the total elimination of the compound, nor is a less toxic metabolite (from **detoxification**) a guaranteed result. In some cases, the metabolite may become more toxic to the target organ than the parent compound and may be reabsorbed into the blood. When the parent compound or metabolite reaches its target organ in a sufficient concentration and for a sufficient time period, a toxic effect will be manifested. This is one of the conditions where susceptibility or resistance can influence a population's response to a chemical.

················

DOSE-RESPONSE RELATIONSHIP

The magnitude of the toxic effect (**response**) is dependent upon the dose of a chemical reaching the target organ; and the dose reaching the target organ is dependent upon the exposure. The relationship between the exposure characteristics and the spectrum of effects together are referred to as the dose-response relationship. Typically, the dose-response relationship for toxic chemicals is depicted by the S-shaped **sigmoid curve** (Figure 9.3). The lower portion of the curve shows no measurable response until a **threshold dose** is reached. The threshold is the dose at which a response can be measured. Once the threshold is reached, the dose-response curve becomes linear where each increase in dose is accompanied by an increase in response. In acute (high dose–short term) toxicology studies, the demonstration of a dose-response relationship is

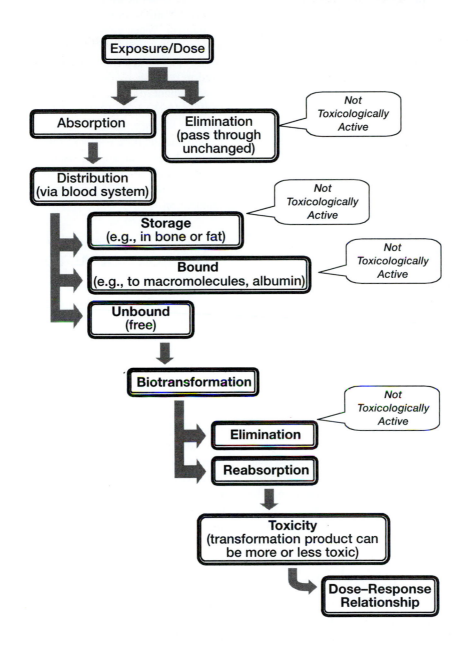

FIGURE 9.2 Possible fates of xenobiotic chemicals in exposed people.

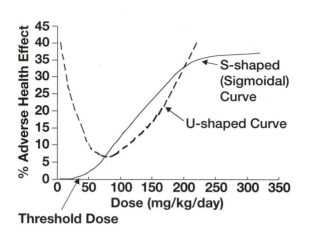

FIGURE 9.3 Examples of dose-response curves.

important in establishing the toxicity of a chemical. As the dose increases further, a maximum response is reached as indicated by the flattening of the sigmoid curve. Once the maximum response has been reached, any additional increase in dose may only prolong the effect. It is important to recognize that the sigmoid dose-response curve is not the only dose-response curve. For essential nutrients, a **U-shaped dose response curve** is typical where too little or too much of an essential nutrient may result in an adverse response or death. Exposure to single agents can produce more than one toxic response and the dose response-relationship may be different for each response.

···············

ENVIRONMENTAL HEALTH REGULATIONS AND RISK ASSESSMENT

One of the ultimate goals of toxicology is to determine the potential harmful effects of a chemical agent using a variety of study types—acute, subchronic, chronic, developmental, reproductive, carcinogenic, and so forth. Based upon these studies, the risk to human health and other biological systems can often be determined.

Since toxicology studies allow one to measure and estimate the potential for chemicals to cause adverse human health effects, it is an important discipline for environmental and health regulation development. When environmental health regulations and guidelines are developed, the goal usually is to protect public health. Toxicology is one of the tools used in the **risk assessment** process leading to the development of such regulations and guidelines (NRC, 1983; PCCRARM, 1997a,b). Toxicology helps to identify and characterize the nature of the hazard and the dose response relationship. Chapters 16 and 17 present a more detailed description and discussion about human risk assessment and the related processes of risk management and risk communication.

···············

ENVIRONMENTAL TOXICOLOGY

One of the specialized areas of toxicology places emphasis on the potential for chemicals to harm the ambient or natural environment. Thus, the area of **environmental toxicology** or **ecotoxicology** assesses and estimates the fate and effects of toxic substances on the natural environment to include its fauna and flora, and focuses on populations, communities, and ecosystems (Kendall, Bens, and Cobb, 1996). Toxic substances can alter the environment in a manner that renders it difficult to sustain healthy life and may even cause death. In addition to fauna and flora, people also can be affected. However, this section will focus on primarily the nonhuman concerns.

Chemical pollutants can impact the environment in a variety of ways. They may alter air quality. For example, chlorofluorocarbons (CFCs; the refrigerant Freon™ is an example) lead to the depletion of atmospheric ozone and allow increased levels of ultraviolet (UV) radiation to reach the earth's surface. These higher levels are associated with an increased risk in the development of skin cancer in people. Air quality issues are presented in more detail in Chapter 14.

The occurrence of acid precipitation ("acid rain") is an example of how pollution may affect multiple environmental compartments (Nadakavukaren, 1995). Automobile exhausts, discharges from fossil fuel (oil, coal) burning power plants, and other sources emit sulfur dioxide (SO_2) and nitrogen dioxide (NO_2) into the atmosphere. Interaction between these and reactive oxidizing agents in the atmospheric, for example, hydrocarbons and others, can convert SO_2 and NO_2 to sulfuric and nitric acids, respectively. The acids fall to the earth, sometimes after being transported hundreds of miles from their origin, as rain, snow, fog, or other precipitation. The acid conversions also can take place in soil on the ground. The increased acidity from the precipitation can alter vegetation and animal populations in an ecosystem. It can also affect the chemistry of soil and natural waters by causing metals to leach from minerals and rocks, which in turn can be toxic to aquatic life, vegetation, and other mammals, including people, as they are passed along the food chain.

Environmental toxicology focuses on various **environmental compartments** to include the **atmosphere** (air), **hydrosphere** (water), **lithosphere** (soil), and **biosphere** (living organisms). Environmental chemistry and chemodynamics are important tools used to assess how chemicals interact with the environment. **Chemodynamics** is the term applied to the movement and transport of xenobiotics within (**intraphase**) and between (**interphase**) environmental compartments. When one studies or assesses the impact of xenobiotics, their **environmental fate** is determined. This is a determination or estimate of how chemicals will enter and move through the environment, how they will be transformed into other chemicals, where they will accumulate, and how long they will persist. **Thermodynamic and equilibrium modeling** based upon chemical and physical properties (such as oxidation state, lipophilicity, and volatility) are used to predict transport and chemical concentrations in environmental compartments. Environmental fate studies and assessments focus on how chemicals are released into the environment, partition among environmental compartments, move and react within each compartment, partition within each compartment, and move into organisms.

Bioavailability is important in environmental toxicology because chemical, physical, and biological processes can affect the ability of toxic substances to move through the environment. The previous acid rain examples illustrated how a chemical change (decrease in pH) can leach metals and enhance their biological availability. The species of a chemical (e.g., oxidation state) or its form (e.g., organic versus inorganic) may affect its bioavailability. This is exemplified by the occurrence of "Minamata disease" caused by mercury-containing waste that was discharged from a plastics factory in Minamata, Japan between the years 1953 and 1961(Potts, 1996; Nadakavukaren, 1995). The factory discharged mercury in its inorganic metallic form. Bacteria (*Methanobacterium amelanki*) converted the inorganic mercury to the more toxic methyl mercury, which moved more rapidly through the food chain (microscopic algae » zooplankton » fish). It bioconcentrated in predator fish at levels up to 100,000 times greater than that in surrounding waters. When people consumed the contaminated fish, they developed neurotoxic conditions and fetuses had teratogenic effects.

Environmental toxicity assessment also includes measuring and assessing the impact of chemical contaminants on the health of the flora and fauna that occupy ecosystems. Kendall et al. (1996) and Menzer et al. (1994) discuss methods for both aquatic and terrestrial toxicology assessments; the reader should refer to these references for additional detail. These types of assessments generally evaluate the effect that chemicals may have on selected species that inhabit the ecosystem. Several different species may be tested to evaluate effects at different trophic levels in an ecosystem and the transfer of contaminants through trophic levels. Modeling and geographic information system (GIS) technologies are also used to estimate and predict ecosystem effects.

A tiered testing approach is used to evaluate aquatic systems, starting with short-term screening tests and advancing to more complex chronic definitive tests, as necessary. Examples of aquatic species that are tested often include algae (e.g., *Scenedesmus quadricuda*), duckweed (*Lemna minor* and *Lemna gibba*), freshwater invertebrates (e.g., the water fleas, *Daphnia magna* and *Daphnia pulex*), and fish (e.g., rainbow trout [*Salmo gairdneri*], bluegill [*Lepomis macrochirus*], fathead minnow [*Pimephales promelas*], and others). The specific species tested will vary with the nature of the ecosystem. For example, species tested for fresh-water systems will differ from those tested for salt-water systems.

Toxicology testing of terrestrial systems may employ field testing methods requiring trapping, remote sensing, and sampling, and enclosure studies (i.e., testing and maintaining specimens in outdoor, open-air facilities). These environmental toxicology evaluations may be acute, short-term, longer-term subchronic or chronic, and even lifetime studies. Some examples of the species that may be tested in terrestrial studies are presented by Menzer et al. and include birds (e.g., bobwhite quail [*Colinus virginianus*] and mallards [*Anas platyrhynchos*]), mammals (e.g., mink [*Mustelo vison*], European ferret [*Mustela purotius furo*]), insects and arthropods (e.g., honeybees [*Apis mellifera*], harvester ants [*Pogonomyrmex owyheei*], and crickets [*Acheta domesticus*]), amphibians (e.g., the frog embryo teratogenesis assay-*Xenopus* [FETAX]), earthworms (*Eisenia foetida*), and plants (e.g., lettuce [*Lactuca sativa*], soybean [*Glycine max*], and barley [*Hordeum vulgare*]).

Just as there is a risk assessment process to address the potential for toxic substances to harm humans, a separate paradigm was developed for the environment. **Ecological risk assessment** is "a qualitative and/or quantitative appraisal of actual or potential effects of" contaminants and pollutants "on plants and animals other than people or domesticated species." Details about ecological assessments can be found in the U.S. Environmental Protection Agency's environmental evaluation manual for Superfund sites (USEPA, 1989). The process consists of four interrelated activities:

1. The **problem formulation** includes a qualitative evaluation of contaminant release, migration, and fate; identification of contaminants of concern, receptors, exposure pathways, and known ecological effects of the contaminants; and selection of endpoints for further study.

2. The **exposure assessment** quantifies the contaminant release, migration, and fate; characterizes exposure pathways and receptors; and measures or estimates exposure point concentrations.

3. The **ecological effects assessment** includes literature reviews, field studies, and toxicity tests, and it links contaminant concentrations to effects on ecological receptors.

4. The **risk characterization** is a measurement or estimation of both current and future adverse effects.

······················

OTHER RESOURCES AND SUMMARY

The discipline of toxicology is quite diverse and complex. Some toxicologists are generalists, just as some medical doctors are general practitioners. Others are very specialized and may concentrate on a specific organ system (e.g., reproductive toxicology, ototoxicology, hepatotoxicology, and others), or a specific outcome (e.g., cancer, developmental/teratological effects, etc.). The nature of a toxicological outcome can vary widely with the type of chemical agent and its effect. For example, irritants (e.g., mineral acids) can affect mucous membranes (eyes, respiratory tract) and asphyxiants can deprive the body of oxygen by displacement (e.g., carbon dioxide) or metabolically (e.g., cyanide). Other effects caused by chemicals include anesthesia (e.g., organic solvents), fibrosis (e.g., asbestos), sensitization (e.g., toluene diisocyanate), cancer (e.g., benzene), and others. Generally, we are exposed to multiple chemicals; therefore, toxicologists must consider the combined effects, which may differ significantly from the effects of any single chemical.

The broad range of toxicology and its complexity cannot be presented in extensive detail in a single book chapter. We have focused on some very general aspects of toxicology, with some emphasis on regulatory toxicology (and risk assessment) and ecological toxicology. There are a variety of resources that the interested reader may consult to acquire additional and more specific detail about chemical toxicity. Examples of these include:

■ Toxicology textbooks such as those by Klaassen (1996) and Hayes (1989).

■ On-line databases like the Hazardous Substances Data Bank (HSDB), Integrated

Risk Information System (IRIS), Chemical Carcinogenesis Research Information System (CCRIS), GENE-TOX, Environmental Mutagen Information Center (EMIC), and Developmental and Reproductive Toxicology and Environmental Teratology Information Center (DART / ETIC) (NIH/NLM Online).

- ■ Publications by federal agencies that routinely assess chemical toxicity: Examples include the U.S. Environmental Protection Agency, the Occupational Safety and Health Administration, the Agency for Toxic Substances and Disease Registry, and the Food and Drug Administration.

There are numerous professional, peer-reviewed journals that report various aspects of toxicology. Some examples are: *Toxicological Sciences, The Toxicologist, Environmental Toxicology and Chemistry Journal, Regulatory Toxicology and Pharmacology, Archives of Environmental Contamination and Toxicology, Archives of Environmental Health, Bulletin of Environmental Contamination and Toxicology, Ecotoxicology, Ecotoxicology and Environmental Safety, Environmental Toxicology and Pharmacology, Environmental Toxicology and Water Quality, Environmental Toxicology, International Journal of Toxicology,* and *Toxicology and Ecotoxicology News*.

There are literally thousands of chemicals used globally by people on a daily basis. Additionally, new chemicals are being developed and used constantly. People and the environment are constantly exposed to a barrage of xenobiotics. Ideally, we should know what hazards these chemicals present to people and the environment before they enter the market and institute processes and procedures to prevent harm. For many existing chemicals that are in use the hazards are known. However, there are also many existing chemicals whose hazards are not known. Issues concerning toxicities of mixtures are not well understood. Toxicology is one of the tools that will help health, environmental, and other professionals gain an understanding about chemical hazards and develop technologies to protect people and the environment.

KEY TERMS

REFERENCES

Gallo, J. 2001. Orioles have tough day at park; Team drops first game to rangers; Second is called because of train fire. *Washington Post*, July 19, p: D1.

Hayes, A. W. (ed.). 1989. *Principles and Methods of Toxicology*, 3rd ed. New York: Raven Press.

Kendall, R. N., C. M. Bens, G. P. Cobb III, et al. 1996. *Aquatic and Terrestrial Ecotoxicology*. In: Klaassen,

C. D. (ed.). *Casarett and Doull's Toxicology, The Basic Science of Poisons*. 5th ed. New York: Mc-Graw-Hill, pp. 883, 888–898.

Menzer, R. E., M. A. Lewis, and A. Fairbrother. 1994. *Methods in Environmental Toxicology*. In: Hayes, A.W. (ed.). *Principles and Methods of Toxicology*, 3rd ed. New York: Raven Press, pp. 1389–1418.

Miller, R. D. and W. C. Roberts. 2001, In Press. *Environmental Health*. In: *Textbook of Military Medicine*. Falls Church, VA: TMM Publications.

Mosk, M., and M. E. Ruane. 2001. Fire rages in tunnel; Baltimore crews try to reach hazardous spills. *Washington Post*, July 20, p: A1.

Nadakavukaren A. 1995. *Our Global Environment, A Health Perspective*, 4th ed. Prospect Heights, IL: Waveland Press, Inc., pp. 270–272, 490.

NIH/NLM (Online). National Institutes of Health, National Library of Medicine internet site (http://toxnet.nlm.nih.gov/).

NRC (1983). National Academy of Science, National Research Council. *Risk Assessment in the Federal Government: Managing the Process*. Washington, DC: National Academy of Science.

Potts, A. M. 1996. *Toxic Responses of the Eye*. In: Klaassen, C. D. (ed.). *Casarett and Doull's Toxicology, The Basic Science of Poisons*, 5th ed. New York: McGraw-Hill, p. 607.

PCCRARM (1997a). Presidential/Congressional Commission on Risk Assessment and Risk Management. 1997. Framework for Environmental Health Risk Management; Final Report, Volume 1.

PCCRARM (1997b). Presidential/Congressional Commission on Risk Assessment and Risk Management. 1997. Framework for Environmental Health Risk Management; Final Report, Volume 2.

Roig-Franzia, M., and M. Ball. 2001a. In Baltimore, toxic scare abates. *Washington Post*, July 22: p. C1.

Roig-Franzia, M., and M. Ball. 2001b. Last toxic train car leaves tunnel; As chemical scare recedes, Baltimore returns to favorite summer pursuits. *Washington Post*, July 22: p. C1.

USEPA (1989). U.S. Environmental Protection Agency. Risk Assessment Guidance for Superfund, Volume II: Environmental Evaluation Manual (EPA/540–1-89/001).

10

RADIOLOGICAL HEALTH

Albert F. Iglar, Ph.D.

East Tennessee State University

OBJECTIVES

- List the major sources of radiation.
- Identify major forms of radioactive decay and major types of ionizing radiation.
- Describe units of measure important in radiological health.
- Identify the types of radiation-monitoring instruments and their applications.
- Discuss how to control radiation from internal and external sources.
- Describe the nuclear power cycle as a potential source of exposure to ionizing radiation.
- Describe typical disposal of radioactive wastes.

Radiological health, sometimes termed health physics, refers to the protection of humanity from hazards to health, balanced against the benefits of radiation. This means that programs of protection against radiation have not necessarily aimed at reducing exposure to radiation to zero, because benefits of radiation (such as the use of X-rays to diagnose disease) should be maintained, and because no control is practical for background radiation (from cosmic radiation, terrestrial sources, and body burden).

Radiological health also is limited to **ionizing radiation**, that which interacts with matter to form charged particles. This is defined to include certain electromagnetic radiation (x-radiation and gamma rays) and particle radiation (alpha, beta, neutron, and other radiation). Certain radiation that is ionizing under limited circumstances, such as ultraviolet, visible light, and others, is not considered in radiological health.

A distinction often is made between directly ionizing radiation, which includes only radiation composed of charged particles, and indirectly ionizing radiation, which includes neutral particles and electromagnetic radiation. Directly ionizing radiation produces relatively large numbers of ions, mainly by magnetic interaction with the orbital electrons of atoms from a distance. By contrast, indirectly ionizing radiation produces relatively small numbers of charged particles, and these produce additional ions.

SOURCES OF RADIATION

In the United States, diagnostic use of X-rays is a particularly significant source of nonoccupational exposure to ionizing radiation. Thus, state regulatory agencies typically attempt to minimize exposure by assuring that safe X-ray equipment is provided and that it is properly installed, maintained, and operated. In recent years, radon (or, to be specific, certain of its decay products) has come to be viewed as an important source of nonoccupational exposure to radiation. **Radon** is found naturally in soils, although to widely varying degrees. Various factors in the construction of buildings (such as openings that can admit gases) can increase the entry of radon. Testing of the air in homes for radon is at least recommended, and sampling can be done easily, by exposure of an activated carbon collector or by other methods. If excess levels are found, various construction measures are available to relieve the problem. The guideline for radon is 4 picocuries per liter of air.

Other sources of exposure to radiation also can be significant. Use of radionuclides (especially technetium-99m) in medicine, as well as in industry and research, represents multiple sources of exposure. The nuclear power cycle (nuclear power) generally presents little nonoccupational exposure to ionizing radiation, but there is concern for the possibility of catastrophic releases and for an increased number of sources in the future. Consumer products such as smoke detectors generally provide minimal exposure to ionizing radiation. Nuclear weapons present a concern, both from the viewpoint of testing in the atmosphere (now lessened) and from the possibility of use in war.

RADIOACTIVITY

Atomic structure is closely related to emission of radiation. Figure 10.1 shows the general structure of selected isotopes of hydrogen and uranium. Numerous nuclides (a nuclide has a particular atomic number and mass number), including both natural and man-made ones, undergo spontaneous disintegration to more simple forms. This process, which involves emission of radiation, is termed **radioac-**tivity. This disintegration of given nuclides occurs in such a way that the nuclide approaches stability. An important criterion of the stability of a nuclide is its neutron-to-proton ratio. For atoms with low atomic weight, a neutron-to-proton ratio of approximately 1 is required for stability. Higher ratios are required for stability in atoms with greater atomic weight.

Forms of decay of radioactive nuclides include:

1. *Alpha emission.* Alpha particles have a relative charge of +2 and a mass number of 4, and are identical in structure to helium nuclei. They are emitted by nuclides of relatively high atomic weight, and the loss in mass forms a product that tends toward stability. All comparable alpha particles from a given nuclide have the same energy, although a given nuclide may emit multiple alpha particles of different energy. Thus, all comparable alpha particles from a given nuclide travel the same distance in a homogeneous material. Alpha particles produce high ionization per unit length of path, although they travel relatively short distances comparatively because of their high charges. Alpha emitters are of particular concern if they enter the body and become internal sources. Thus, this aspect of radiation protection means taking measures to prevent alpha emitters from entering the body. One important approach is to keep levels of radionuclides low in the workplace atmosphere, essentially by process enclosure, ventilation, and air cleaning.

2. *Beta emission.* Beta particles have a relative charge of –1 and a mass number of zero (although they have a small mass). While identical to high-speed electrons, beta particles are emitted by the nucleus. Beta emitters have neutron-to-proton ratios that are too high for stability, and the emission of a beta particle causes a neutron to be replaced by a proton, thus decreasing the neutron-to-proton ratio. Beta particles from a given nuclide have a range of energies, but characteristic mean and maximum energies. Beta particles penetrate farther than alpha particles in general (dependent on their energy), which corresponds to the lesser degree of ionization produced in

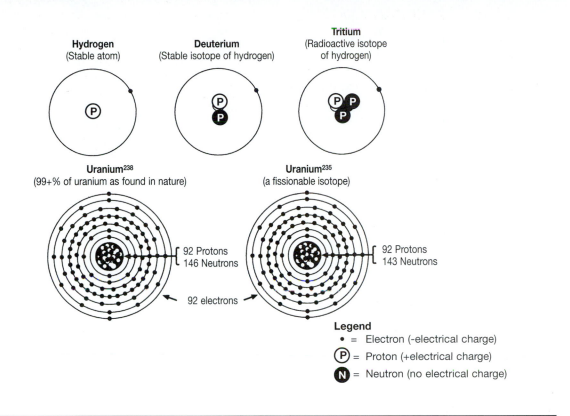

FIGURE 10.1 Atomic structure of selected isotopes of hydrogen and uranium.

matter. Beta radiation is of potential concern if from an internal source, so measures such as avoiding contamination of air or skin are required. Beta emitters also may be significant as external sources, though shielding may be relatively simple (such as with plastic).

3. *Positron emission.* Positron particles have the same mass as beta particles, but the opposite relative charge, +1. They are emitted by the nuclei of atoms with neutron-to-proton ratios too low for stability, and they produce a product with a higher ratio. Positron emission is a form of decay of some radionuclides, but positrons are not a radiation hazard because positrons are annihilated when they combine with orbiting electrons, the result being production of energy.

4. *X-ray and gamma ray emissions.* These are forms of electromagnetic radiation, consisting of photons traveling in waves at the speed of light. Gamma rays, however, are emitted by nuclei, typically following particle emission, whereas X-rays originate in the orbiting electron structure. An example of the emission of an X-ray photon is found in orbital electron capture, also termed k-capture, in which the nucleus captures an orbiting electron, usually from the k-shell. An electron with a higher energy level fills the vacant position, with its excess energy given off as an X-ray photon. Orbital electron capture tends to occur in nuclides that have neutron-to-proton ratios too low for stability, and this form of decay causes an increase in the ratio. X-rays and gamma rays have characteristic energies for particular nu-

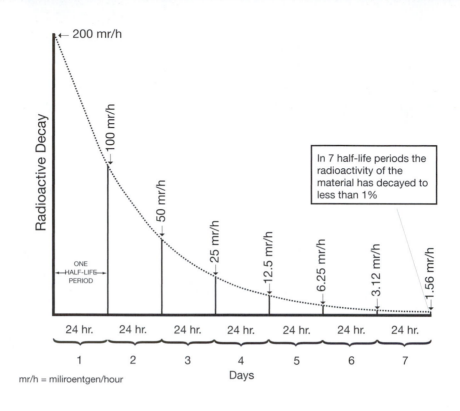

FIGURE 10.2 Decay of hypothetical substance with half-life of 24 hours.

clides. X-rays and gamma rays are highly significant if from external sources, and nuclides that emit X-rays and gamma rays also are hazardous as internal sources.

5. *Neutron emission.* Neutrons have mass numbers of 1 (though the mass is somewhat greater than that of a proton) and no net charge. They are highly penetrating, in part because they lack a great tendency to directly produce ionization. Neutron radiation can be significant from both internal and external sources and is associated especially with nuclear fission.

6. *Other forms of decay.* Various other sorts of decay include internal conversion (a gamma photon from a nucleus transfers sufficient energy to an orbiting electron to eject it from the atom) and isometric transition (a higher

energy nuclide emits a gamma photon and reaches a lower energy ground state).

All atoms of a given radionuclide decay in a defined manner. Although many nuclides have multiple modes of decay, each occurs in a definite proportion of the instances. The result of radioactive decay is, in some cases, transmutation into a new radionuclide. Three radioactive series are found in nature, one nuclide decaying to form another, until a stable nuclide is reached. These are the uranium, thorium, and neptunium series. A fourth series, the actinium series, can be generated artificially.

Radiation from a specific nuclide exhibits a given energy pattern, with energies being expressed in units of mega electron volts (MeV). Further, the decay occurs with regularity for a given radioactive species. That is, a constant fraction of the total number of atoms present decays per unit time. This fraction is unchangeable, except for certain cases involving fissionable nuclides.

Related to this is the concept of **half-life**. The half-life is a constant length of time for any radionuclide, and refers to the time required for half of the atoms of a particular radionuclide to decay. As an illustration, Figure 10.2 shows the decay of a hypothetical substance with a half-life of 24 hours.

．．．．．．．．．．．．．．

UNITS OF MEASURE IN RADIOLOGICAL HEALTH

Activity refers to the quantity of a radionuclide with regard to its rate of undergoing radioactive disintegration. The recommended unit of activity for many purposes is an SI unit, selected as an international standard; the Becquerel (Bq), defined as the quantity of any radionuclide that produces 1 disintegration per second. The customary unit of activity in the United States has been the Curie (Ci), essentially defined as that quantity of any radionuclide that produces 3.7×10^{10} disintegrations per second. This is a huge quantity of activity, so smaller units are used, including millicuries ($1 \text{ mCi} = 10 \times 10^3 \text{Ci}$), microcuries ($1 \text{ Ci} = 10^{-6}\text{Ci}$), and picocuries ($1 \text{ pCi} = 10^{-12}\text{Ci}$).

Radiation monitoring instruments—at least the ones used most commonly—measure exposure based on gas ionization, and related to a unit termed the roentgen. One roentgen is defined as the amount of X-rays or gamma radiation, that together with the associated particle radiation, produces, per standard cubic centimeter of air under standard conditions, in air, one electrostatic unit of positive ions plus one electrostatic unit of negative ions.

Other units of radiation that are especially important in estimating dose of radiation for comparison with standards are:

1. *Units of absorbed dose.* The unit customarily used in the United States has been the RAD. One RAD is defined as the dose of any form of ionizing radiation that produces energy absorption of 1×10^{-5} joules/gram in any specified material. For the SI system, the unit of absorbed dose is the **Gray** (Gy), defined such that one Gray refers to absorption of 1×10^{-3} joules/gram (1 Gy = 100 RAD).

2. *Units of dose equivalency.* The basis for this approach is that the same absorbed dose can yield very different effects depending on the type of ionizing radiation involved. The common U.S. unit of dose equivalency, the REM, is calculated as follows:

Dose Equivalency = Absorbed Dose × Quality Factor
     (in REMs)   (in RADs)

The quality factor (QF) indicates the approximate relative tendency of each type of radiation to produce a biological effect. The quality factors of x, gamma, and beta radiation are taken as 1. The quality factor for neutrons, however, depends on their energy but usually ranges from about 2 to 11, and for alpha the QF is listed as 20. Basic standards for radiation exposure may be expressed in REMs. For the SI system of units, dose equivalency is expressed in **Sieverts**, defined by a similar equation, using absorbed dose in Grays and quality factor.

．．．．．．．．．．．．．．

INSTRUMENTS FOR MEASURING RADIATION

The most familiar instruments for measuring radiation operate on the principle of gas ionization. The Geiger-Muller counter (sometimes termed **Geiger counter** or GM counter), the best known of these, mainly is used as a portable survey monitor. In this application, it provides a sensitive means of locating environmental contamination. The **proportional counter**, also a gas ionization instrument, is used particularly for differentiating radiation in field surveys. **Ionization chamber instruments**, which also utilize the gas ionization principle, are less sensitive but highly accurate. In their most common application, they are used as portable instruments to measure somewhat higher levels of radiation.

The **scintillation detector** is primarily a laboratory-based instrument, often in a system that includes a dedicated microcomputer. Liquid scintillation counters are used especially for measuring and identifying nuclides that emit beta radiation. They find application in the life sciences, most notably for detection of carbon-14 and hydrogen-3. Solid scintillation detectors are used for evaluation of gamma emitters. The semiconductor detectors used in analogous instruments, however, bring greater sensitivity and improved resolution.

The **dosimeter** indicates cumulative exposure to radiation over time. The most familiar is the nuclear emulsion monitor, more often known as the film badge. Although it provides a permanent record, like other dosimeters it is under the control of the person being monitored. Other devices that serve a similar purpose are thermoluminescent dosimeters (TLD detectors) and pocket chamber dosimeters.

CONTROL OF EXPOSURE TO RADIATION

Radiation can have effects ranging up to loss of life in acute exposure (Figure 10.3). In the case of chronic exposure to radiation, the most notable effects are cancer and hereditary defects. These are termed **stochastic effects**, meaning that the dose of radiation determines the probability that the effect will occur. In addition, the stochastic concept includes the nonthreshold basis, that no dose of radiation is so low as to avoid these effects totally, and that even low doses may produce severe effects. Under the stochastic principle, certain control of radiation exposure is required based on the ALARA (as low as reasonably achievable) principle. Radiation protection includes control of nonoccupational exposure, which involves minimizing exposure to X-rays, controlling exposure by food, air, and water, and other measures. One important distinction concerns control of exposure from external sources versus control of exposure from internal sources. Control of occupational exposure also is important as described in the following.

Control of External Sources

External sources refer to those outside the body, such as diagnostic X-ray equipment, a fission reactor, and other sources. The three major methods of control for radiation from external sources are time, distance, and shielding.

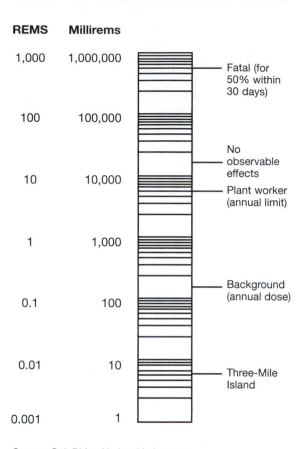

Source: Oak Ridge National Laboratory

FIGURE 10.3 Effects on humans expected at various doses of radiation.

TIME

The basis for limiting time is that dose of radiation is the product of dose rate multiplied by time. For example, consider an occupational situation where radiation exposure is 2 mREM per hour, and it is desired to limit total exposure of any worker to 10 mREM per week. The desired limit would be met if each worker were exposed for only 5 hours per week (10 mREM/week divided by 2 mREM/hour = 5 hours/week). This administrative control is relatively simple and inexpensive to implement, although it requires effective supervision (as well as the availability of alternative jobs for workers) and

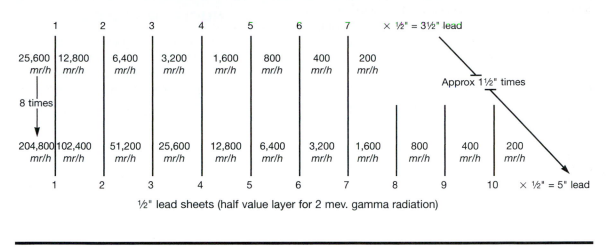

FIGURE 10.4 Typical effect of adding successive half-value layers of shielding.

probably is most applicable to low to moderate levels of exposure to occupational radiation.

DISTANCE

Distance as a means of control is predicated on an important characteristic of nonlaser electromagnetic radiation: that intensity of the radiation is inversely proportional to the square of the distance from the source. Thus, for example, if the distance from a point source of gamma radiation were doubled, the intensity would be only one-fourth as great. Similarly, if the distance from the source were tripled, the intensity would be only one-ninth as great. Because the range of alpha and beta radiation is relatively short, this concept usually is limited to X-rays and gamma radiation. The concept also is more difficult to apply to multiple sources and to sources that are too large to be approximated as points. Depending on distance for occupational radiation protection requires effective supervision.

SHIELDING

Shielding often is the preferred means of protection against external sources of radiation because it may create an environment that is inherently safe. That is, there may be no direct dependence on administrative limitation of exposure time of workers or distance from the source. An important principle of shielding

is that a constant fraction of incident radiation is lost in successive equal increments of thickness of the material. In the case of gamma rays and X-rays, the loss in energy occurs by three mechanisms: the photoelectric effect, the Compton effect, and pair production. The same effect of shielding also may be described in terms of the half-value layer, which is the thickness of a particular shielding material that will reduce the intensity of X-rays or gamma radiation of a particular energy by one-half. Although various examples of shielding could be cited, the most familiar probably is the shielding in a room where diagnostic X-rays are performed. Shielding commonly can be found in walls, doors, and floors, depending on the situation. Figure 10.4 illustrates the concept of half-value layer in shielding (though in a much different situation than x-ray rooms).

Control of Internal Sources

In the occupational context, control of exposure from internal sources requires preventing contamination of the person, the workplace air, and the workplace itself. A first measure is to enclose the processes that might spread radionuclides in the air or other parts of the workplace environment. A glove box is a simple example of an enclosure that seals radionuclides from the environment of the workplace, yet allows manipulation. With some processes, a combination of at least partial enclosure, supplemented by exhaust ventilation, can be effective in preventing the spread of contaminants into the workplace. Generally this also means that the exhausted air must be treated. For radionuclides in particulate form, this usually involves a roughing filter followed by a HEPA (high efficiency) filter.

For some occupational settings, at least minimal potential or actual contamination of the workplace apparently is likely. Standard practice is that access to these areas be limited to employees whose jobs require that they be present and who have received appropriate training. They wear protective clothing over the entire body. In some situations, workers use respirators to avoid inhaling radionuclides. Before leaving the regulated area, the usual procedure is for workers to remove clothing in a contaminated area, shower, cross carefully into a designated clean area, dress in uncontaminated clothing, and be checked for contamination by use of a radiation monitor.

NUCLEAR POWER

Nuclear power, or more precisely nuclear fission for generation of electricity, is a particular focus of public concern. Potential sources of exposure to radiation encompass the total nuclear fuel cycle (Figure 10.5), including mining, refining, enrichment, generation of power, reprocessing of spent fuel elements, management of waste, and others. The discussion here emphasizes generation of electricity.

In most nuclear power plants in the United States, uranium-235 is used as the source of energy. Nuclei of the element tend to disintegrate naturally, with the emission of neutrons and heat. In a nuclear reactor, the neutrons cause the disintegration of more atoms of uranium-235 in a controlled chain reaction. The heat generated is used to produce steam, which turns a turbine and then a generator to provide electricity.

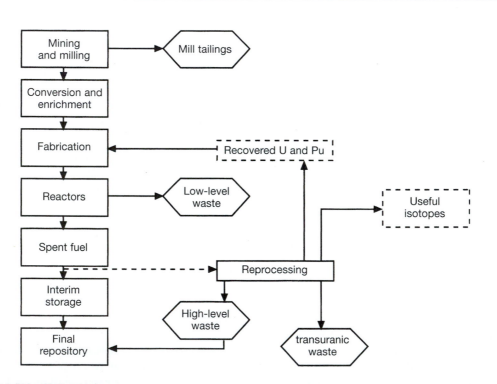

Source: Oak Ridge National Laboratory

FIGURE 10.5 Nuclear power cycle.

The intention is to design safety into the plant at a fundamental level. The fuel is limited to a maximum of a few percent of uranium-235, depending on design, and the geometry of fuel materials is such that a compact mass cannot be assembled easily. These measures make it impossible for a nuclear power plant to explode as a fission bomb. Further, the uranium fuel is in a form (often uranium dioxide) that is resistant to solution in water and is sealed inside corrosion-resistant metal tubes.

Redundancy is an important principle in the design of nuclear power plants. This means that plant features critical to safety, such as cooling systems, are represented by replicate units to assure safety under various equipment failure scenarios. In practice in the United States, reactors are enclosed in massive concrete and steel containment structures, designed to preclude disastrous release of radioactive material in the maximum credible accident. Control rods made of neutron-absorbing materials are available for insertion in the reactor.

Despite these precautions, fear of radiation and safety issues are present. Certain discharges of radioactive material are permitted to air and water, although the amounts have been judged to be safe. Further, considering the large release of radioactive material in 1986 from the nuclear power plant at Chernobyl in the Ukraine, renewed attention to safety is surely appropriate. (Note: that this release was due to a chemical explosion, not nuclear.) In the United States, future reactors are expected to be designed to be inherently safe by emphasizing negative reactivity. This means that if the fission should start to go out of control, it would have the effect of suppressing the reaction. Figure 10.6 shows one proposed design concept of a modern reactor.

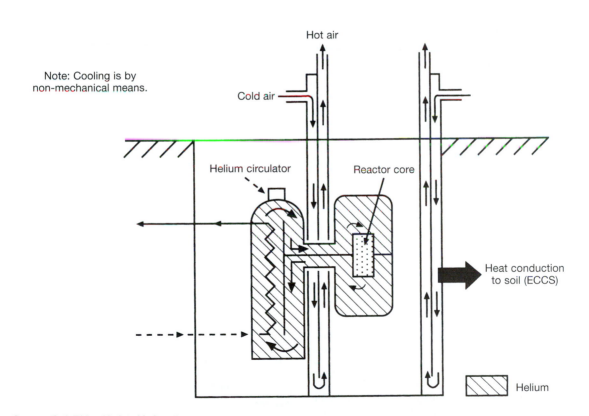

Source: Oak Ridge National Laboratory

FIGURE 10.6 High-temperature, gas-cooled reactor.

Breeder reactors represent a way to increase the supply of fissionable fuel for reactors. The basis for the most frequently discussed breeder reactors is the high concentration of uranium-238 found in natural uranium. The fissionable isotope, uranium-235 typically is only 0.71% of the total, and nearly all of the remainder is uranium-238. In fission reactors, uranium-238 can react to form plutonium-239, which is also fissionable. A breeder reactor is designed to enhance this reaction, with the result that it produces considerably more fissionable material than is destroyed. In the United States, the Clinch River Breeder Reactor plant was canceled as a result of concern about safety. (One major concern was over the safety of liquid sodium as a coolant.)

·················

RADIOACTIVE WASTE

Problems with the management of radioactive wastes have been significant. In the United States, **low-level radioactive waste** usually has been disposed of by near-surface burial. Despite precautions, this has brought such problems as subsidence of filled areas and contamination of groundwater. Now there is interest in other management methods, such as preventing contamination, compaction of waste, concentration of radioactive material (such as by absorption on activated carbon), incineration when appropriate, other waste treatment and containment or encapsulation, or other stabilization of the material. At present, high-level radioactive waste is largely stored at the nuclear power plants where generated. Quantities are somewhat larger than anticipated due to failure to develop breeder reactors or commercial nuclear fuel reprocessing in the United States. High-level radioactive waste can be sealed deep in the ground in a **mined geologic repository**. This would involve converting waste to a form that is resistant to environmental transport, sealing it in corrosion resistant containers, and burying in tunnels which are subsequently sealed.

The concept involves ability to monitor for leaks. A mined geologic repository has been under study and development at Yucca Mountain, Nevada, though this has faced opposition.

SUMMARY

Radiological health requires the control of ionizing radiation, that which interacts with matter to produce charged particles. The major types of ionizing radiation are alpha, beta, gamma, X-ray, and neutron. Major sources of exposure include radon, medical use of X-rays, occupational sources, and others.

Exposure may be external (controlled by time, distance, and shielding) and internal (controlled by preventing radionuclides from entering the body). Exposure from the nuclear power cycle and from waste management is presently low but is a subject of concern.

Radiological health is regulated at both the federal and state levels. Central are the efforts of the Nuclear Regulatory Commission, though the Environmental Protection Agency and others also have programs. Significant regulatory efforts are also found in state agencies as part of a division of responsibility with federal authorities.

KEY TERMS

Activity, p. 165

Dosimeter, p. 166

Geiger counter, p. 165

Gray, p. 165

Half-life, p. 165

Ionization chamber instruments, p. 165

Ionizing radiation, p. 161

Low-level radioactive waste, p. 170

Mined geologic repository, p. 170

Proportional counter, p. 165

Radioactivity, p. 162

Radon, p. 162

Scintillation detector, p. 165

Sievert, p. 165

Stochastic effects, p. 166

REFERENCES

Eisenbud, Merril. 1987. *Environmental Radioactivity*, 3rd ed. Academic Press, Orlando, FL.

Gershey, Edward L., Robert. C. Klein, Esmerelda Party, and Amy Wilkerson. 1990. *Low-level Radioactive Waste*. Von Nostrand Reinhold, New York.

Gammage, Richard B., Stephen V. Kaye and Vivian A. Jacobs (ed.). 1985. *Indoor Air and Human Health*. Lewis Publishers, Chelsea, MI.

International Physicians for the Prevention of Nuclear War and the Institute for Energy and Environmental Research. 1992. *Plutonium: Deadly Gold of the Nuclear Age*. International Physicians Press, Cambridge, MA.

Martin, Alan, and Samuel A. Harbison. 1986. *An Introduction to Radiation Protection*, 3rd ed. Chapman and Hall, New York.

Murray, Raymond L., and Judith A. Powell (eds.). 1994. *Understanding Radioactive Waste*. 4th ed. Battelle Press, Columbus, OH.

National Research Council. 1995. *Technical Bases for Yucca Mountain Standards*. National Academy Press, Washington, DC.

Mettler, Fred A. Jr., and Arthur C. Uptoin. 1995. *Medical Effects of Ionizing Radiation*. 2nd ed. Saunders, Philadelphia, PA.

Stannard, J. Newell. 1988. *Radioactivity and Health: A History* (Prepared for U.S. Department of Energy under contract DE-AC06–76RL0 1830). Office of Scientific and Technical Information, Washington, DC.

Stewart, Donald C. 1988. *Handling Radioactivity*. Robert E. Krieger Publishing Co., Malabar, FL.

United States Environmental Protection Agency. 1986. *Radon Reduction Techniques for Detached Houses*. Publication EPA/625/5–86/019. Center for Environmental Research Information, Cincinnati, OH.

United States Environmental Protection Agency. 1994. *A Citizen's Guide to Radon*, 2nd ed. Publication 402-K92–001. U. S. Government Printing Office, Washington, DC.

Wagner, Henry N. 1989. *Living with Radiation: The Risk, the Promise*. Johns Hopkins University Press, Baltimore, MD.

11

FOOD PROTECTION AND SAFETY

Frank C. Gomez, Dr.P.H.

Touro University International

INTRODUCTION

Food Safety and Globalization

During the last decade the importance of protecting the public from the consequences of food-borne illness and ensuring that the food supply is safe from pathogens has become a national priority. Although protection of food from **conta-**mination and **adulteration** has always been an important goal of public health, the emergence of new food-borne pathogens and the globalization of the food industry present a new set of threats to public health.

The food service industry and regulators, alike, are faced with controlling five times the number of food-borne pathogens than were commonly known only 50 years ago. Compounding the pathogen problem has been the significant shift in the manner in which food is now produced, processed, distributed, and served to consumers. Multinational corporations now provide a substantial amount of our food. Suddenly, the effects of globalization and corporate mergers have increased the risk of widespread and far-reaching outbreaks of food-borne illness affecting many more people than previously known to mankind. Managing food safety is now significantly more complicated than it was just a few years ago.

The globalization of the food service industry has also elevated the relative importance of managing food safety in multinational corporations as they understand the linkages between the food safety of their food products to the survival and profitability of the corporate entity.

Lifestyle, Food Safety, and the Emerging Food-Borne Pathogens

Although the emergence of the multinational food service corporations has definitely had an impact on food safety, lifestyle changes throughout the societies of the developed and developing countries have also contributed to an increased risk of food-borne illness. Most people consumed a greater variety of foods that originate from countries throughout the world. Additionally, the tremendous increase in the availability of fast foods has made it more convenient for families to eat meals away from home. These factors place more people at greater risk for developing food-borne illness.

The combined factors of lifestyle changes, the globalization of the food service industry, and the impact stemming from the growing importance of the multinational corporations have resulted in the need for a comprehensive food safety program throughout the United States and abroad.

The realization that globalization of the food service industry has an effect on our ability to protect the food supply under our traditional regulatory scheme was significantly challenged by three emerging pathogens and the inability of government and the food service industry to adequately

control them. These three emerging pathogens are E. coli 0157:H7, bovine spongiform encephalopathy (BSE), and foot-and-mouth disease.

Of the three diseases mentioned above, only E. coli 0157:H7 is generally recognized as a significant food-borne pathogen. However, the impact of bovine spongiform encephalopathy (BSE), which is linked to **Creutzfeldt-Jakob disease (CJD)**, and foot-and-mouth disease on the importance of a strong food safety inspection program cannot be denied. Let's examine the impact of these diseases on the food safety regulatory process and the need to manage food safety from the farm to the table.

Foot-and-mouth disease is an acute infectious viral disease that affects cattle, sheep, pigs, and goats. It also affects elephants and other wild animals. Domestic animals acquire the disease by direct or indirect contact with an affected animal, or by contact with feed or virtually any material containing the virus. It is a disease that is very difficult to control. Although the disease does not affect humans, it does have a dramatic impact on farmers and the farming community.

Bovine spongiform encephalopathy (BSE) is defined as a "progressive neurological disorder of cattle that results from infection by unconditional transmissible agent." The exact nature of the agent that is linked to a variant form of Creutzfeldt-Jakob disease (vCJD) is unknown; however, recent studies have associated vCJD with **prion protein (PrP)** from BSE-infected cattle.

BSE has not been detected in the United States, although it has been found in several European countries. There is evidence that the recent outbreak of BSE in Europe was caused by feeding rendered ruminant products to young calves. Like foot-and-mouth disease, BSE brought fear to European and American consumers, which resulted in stronger regulatory efforts to control these diseases on the farm.

Although BSE and foot-and-mouth disease focused attention on the need for reform in food safety programs for federal, state and local regulators, the consumers' confidence in the protection of the food supply from food-borne pathogens had already been severely weakened by the emergence of E. coli 0157:H7.

Escherichia coli 0157:H7 is an emerging food-borne pathogen that has been of concern since it was identified as a cause of an outbreak of food-borne illness associated with undercooked ground beef in 1982. Since this initial documented outbreak of E. coli 0157:H7 it is estimated by CDC to cause an estimated 73,000 cases of illness and 61 deaths in the United States each year.

E. coli 0157:H7 is found in the intestines of cattle. During slaughter the carcass can become contaminated and the organisms are thoroughly mixed when ground beef is processed. Known sources of E. coli 0157:H7 include raw milk, juice, fruits, vegetables, alfalfa sprouts, and sewage-contaminated water. In fact, any food or water contaminated by cattle can be a source of the organism.

Young children and the elderly are especially susceptible to E. coli 0157:H7 infections, which may cause severe bloody diarrhea and in a few cases result in hemolytic uremic syndrome (HUS), which can lead to acute kidney failure.

The impact on the food service industry from the emergence of E. coli 0157:H7, bovine spongiform encephalopathy (BSE), and foot-and-mouth disease has been dramatic. It threatens the economic survival of virtually any food service corporation responsible for a major outbreak of food-borne illness. This fact has been especially true for those businesses involved in an outbreak of E. coli 0157:H7.

It is clear that control of foot-and-mouth disease, bovine spongiform encephalopathy (BSE), and E. coli 0157:H7, as well as food-borne pathogens such as salmonella, shigella, and campylobacter, must begin at the source on the farm and continue to the dining table.

· · · · · · · · · · · · · · ·

UNDERSTANDING FOOD-BORNE ILLNESS

The Major Causes of Food-Borne Illness

Food-borne illness is caused by the ingestion of contaminated food. The terms food-borne illness and food-borne disease are used interchangeably

and mean that an illness, serious injury, or death was caused by a responsible etiologic agent and food was the mode of transmission.

Food-borne illness is a significant problem in the United States. According to CDC an estimated 76 million persons experience food-borne illnesses in the United States every year. This data is based on CDC's Emerging Infections Program Food-borne Diseases Active Surveillance Network (FoodNet) which collects data on nine food-borne diseases in selected sites. The FoodNet study also estimates that there are 325,000 hospitalizations and 5,000 deaths related to food-borne diseases in the United States each year.

Most food-borne illnesses in the United States are those caused by several specific bacteria and viruses. The bacteria are campylobacter (*Campylobacter jejuni*), salmonella (*S. typhi, S. enteritidis*), *Listeria monocytogenes*, and E. coli O157:H7. The most commonly implicated virus is known as the Norwalk or Norwalk-like viruses.

Classification of Food-Borne Illness

Although the Centers of Disease Control and Prevention (CDC) tracks only nine food-borne diseases as being the most important to control to protect the public's health, there are over 250 different food-borne illnesses which have been identified and classified as follows:

- Pathogenic bacteria
- Viruses
- Parasites
- Natural toxins
- Prions

Food-borne illnesses are also classified as **infection**, **intoxication**, or **toxin-mediated infection**. A food-borne infection occurs when the food-borne pathogen is the cause of the infection. An example of a food-borne infection is *Salmonellosis*.

A food-borne intoxication occurs when the food-borne pathogen produces a toxin in the food before consumption. If the levels of the toxin produced is sufficiently high, the consumer will become ill. Intoxication may also occur if a person consumes food that has become contaminated with toxic chemicals or pesticides from sources other than bacteria. Examples of bacteria which cause intoxications are *Staphylococcus aureus* and *Clostridium botulinum*.[1]

A toxin-mediated infection is a disease caused by toxin formation during infection, such as *Clostridium perfringens*, instead of before infection occurs as with an intoxication.

Conditions for Bacterial Growth In Food

Pathogenic bacteria are by far the most common cause of food-borne illness. Understanding how bacteria cause food-borne illness will allow you to understand the rationale for the various laws and regulations that control the food service industry, and why various food handling methods are used when preparing food for transporting, storage, preparation, and serving.

There are six conditions for bacterial growth in foods. These conditions are:

1. The nutrient level of the food

2. The acidity of the food

3. The temperatures at which food is maintained during processing, storage, preparation, and serving

4. The time that food is held at temperatures favorable for pathogenic bacterial growth

5. The oxygen demand of the specific pathogenic bacteria

6. The amount of moisture available in food to support pathogenic bacteria growth

---

[1]Technically, a toxin-mediated infection is a disease due to a preformed toxin (toxin formed outside the body) for example, *S. aureus* and botulism (*Clostridium botulinum*) and a disease caused by toxin formation during infection such as *Clostridium perfringens*.

In the food service industry the six conditions for favorable growth of pathogenic bacteria are known as **FAT-TOM**. This acronym stands for Food, Acidity, Time, Temperature, Oxygen, and Moisture.

Food   Bacteria require nutrients to grow. Therefore, foods that are high in protein and carbohydrates such as meat, poultry, dairy products, seafood, rice, and beans can support growth of food-borne bacteria. Foods that are very low in or lack proteins and carbohydrates cannot usually support the growth of food-borne bacteria.

Acidity   The acidity and alkalinity of a food will determine whether the food is desirable for the growth of food-borne bacteria. The acidity and alkalinity of a food is measured on a pH scale. The pH scale has a range from 0 to 14.0 with 7.0 representing a neutral value. Most pathogenic bacteria experience a higher growth rate in a neutral pH environment. However, most bacteria can grow well in a pH that ranges between 4.0 and 9.0.

Time   The amount of time that food is kept in a favorable temperature range for growth is a significant factor in causing food-borne illness. Given a favorable environment in food and sufficient time, pathogenic bacteria can grow in the numbers from the lag phase or slow growth phase to the log phase where rapid growth occurs. It is during the log phase that a pathogenic food-borne bacteria can double in numbers every 15 to 20 minutes and quickly reach the quantity of the bacteria required for an infectious dose when the food is consumed.

Temperature   Temperature is probably the most important condition that must be monitored and controlled if food-borne illness is to be prevented. Pathogenic food-borne bacteria will grow well when held at temperatures between 41°F and 140°F. This temperature range is known as the "temperature danger zone." Below a temperature of 41°F there will be slow growth or no growth for most pathogenic food-borne bacteria. Studies have shown that *Listeria monocytogenes* will continue to grow slowly at temperatures below 41°F. Above a temperature of 140°F most pathogenic bacteria are destroyed.

Oxygen   Food-borne bacteria are classified by their oxygen demand. Bacteria are classified as either aerobic, anaerobic, or facultative anaerobes. Aerobic bacteria require oxygen to survive and grow. Anaerobic bacteria cannot grow in an environment with free oxygen but will thrive in an environment that is depleted of free oxygen. Facultative anaerobes can grow in either an aerobic or anaerobic environment.

Moisture   Bacteria cannot grow without available moisture. In foods, a water activity level (A_w) above 0.85 is required for pathogenic food-borne bacteria to grow. Water activity levels range between 0.0 and 1.0 and is a measure of the available water for bacterial growth. In fact, one of the oldest methods of food preservation is to dry food.

The concept of FAT-TOM is important in the food service industry because it allows the food service manager to easily understand the control techniques necessary to prevent an outbreak of food-borne illness in the food facility.

■ TABLE 11.1 ■

SOME COMMON POTENTIALLY HAZARDOUS FOODS (PHF)

Meats, Poultry, and Fish (Raw or Heat Treated) balloon
Dairy Products–Milk and Milk Products
Shellfish
Eggs and Shelled Eggs
Cooked Rice
Tofu and Soy Protein Foods
Sprouts and Raw Seeds
Sliced Melons
Baked and Boiled Potatoes
Garlic and Oil Mixtures

Potentially Hazardous Foods (PHF)

Foods that have the ability to support rapid growth of pathogenic food-borne bacteria are called **potentially hazardous foods (PHF)**. These foods usually are nutrient rich in proteins and carbohydrates *and* have a pH above 4.6 *and* a water activity level above 0.85. Some of the more commonly known and not so commonly known potentially hazardous foods are listed in Table 11.1.

In recent years quite a few foods that were previously considered as nonhazardous have been implicated in outbreaks of food-borne illness. In fact, the number of potentially hazardous foods has grown to such a degree that the National Sanitation Foundation (NSF) has developed a standard for nonpotentially hazardous foods.

Description of Food-Borne Diseases by Classification and Species

The following descriptions of various food-borne diseases are based directly on information from the Centers of Disease Control and Prevention, National Center for Infectious Diseases and the Food & Drug Administration, Center for Food Safety & Applied Nutrition, Bad Bug Book.

PATHOGENIC BACTERIA

Salmonella spp.

Etiologic agent: *S. typhi, S. enteritidis*—Enterobacteriaceae of the genus *Salmonella*, a gram-negative rod-shaped bacilli. Approximately 2,000 serotypes cause human disease.

Occurrence: Widespread occurrence in animals, especially in poultry and swine. Environmental sources of the organism include water, soil, insects, factory surfaces, kitchen surfaces, animal feces, raw meats, raw poultry, and raw seafood, among others.

Symptoms: Fever, abdominal cramps, and diarrhea (sometimes bloody). Occasionally can progress to sepsis.

Onset time (incubation): 6–48 hours

Infective dose: As few as 15–20 cells; depends upon age and health of host, and strain differences among the members of the genus.

Duration of symptoms: Acute symptoms may last for 1 to 2 days or may be prolonged, again depending on host factors, ingested dose, and strain characteristics.

Incidence of disease: 2 to 4 million cases of Salmonellosis occur in the United States annually.

Risk groups: Affects all age groups. Groups at greatest risk for severe or complicated disease include infants, the elderly, and persons with compromised immune systems.

Associated foods: Raw meats, poultry, eggs, milk and dairy products, fish, shrimp, frog legs, yeast, coconut, sauces and salad dressing, cake mixes, cream-filled desserts and toppings, dried gelatin, peanut butter, cocoa, and chocolate. *S. enteritidis* is also found inside the egg, in the yolk.

Clostridium botulinum

Etiologic agent: A potent neurotoxin produced from *Clostridium botulinum*, an anaerobic, spore-forming bacterium. Food-borne botulism is a severe type of food poisoning caused by the ingestion of foods containing the potent neurotoxin formed during growth of the organism. The toxin is heat labile and can be destroyed if heated at 80°C for 10 minutes or longer.

Occurrence: Approximately 10 to 30 outbreaks are reported annually in the United States. Inadequately processed, home-canned foods, but occasionally commercially produced foods have been involved in outbreaks.

Symptoms: Early signs of intoxication consist of marked lassitude, weakness, and vertigo, usually followed by double vision and progressive difficulty in speaking and swallowing. Difficulty in breathing, weakness of other muscles, abdominal distention, and constipation may also be common symptoms.

Onset time (incubation): Onset of symptoms in food-borne botulism is usually 18 to 36 hours after ingestion of the food containing the toxin, although cases have varied from 4 hours to 8 days.

Infective dose: A few nanograms of toxin can cause illness.

Duration of symptoms: Depending on the severity of the illness, it may take an extended period of time to recover. Survival also depends on the early administration of botulinal antitoxin (available from CDC) and intensive supportive care (including mechanical breathing assistance).

Incidence of disease: The incidence of the disease is low, but the disease is of considerable concern because of its high mortality rate if not treated immediately and properly.

Risk groups: All persons.

Associated foods: Almost any type of food that is not very acidic (pH above 4.6) can support growth and toxin production by *C. botulinum*. Botulinal toxin has been demonstrated in a considerable variety of foods, such as canned corn, peppers, green beans, soups, beets, asparagus, mushrooms, ripe olives, spinach, tuna fish, chicken and chicken livers, liver pate, luncheon meats, ham, sausage, stuffed eggplant, lobster, and smoked and salted fish. Sausages, meat products, canned vegetables, and seafood products have been the most frequent vehicles for human botulism.

Staphylococcus aureus

Etiologic agent: *S. aureus* is a spherical bacterium (coccus). Some strains are capable of producing a highly heat-stable protein toxin that causes illness in humans.

Occurrence: Staphylococci exist in air, dust, sewage, water, milk, and food or on food equipment, environmental surfaces, humans, and animals. Humans and animals are the primary reservoirs. Staphylococci are present in the nasal passages and throats and on the hair and skin of 50% or more of healthy individuals. Food handlers are usually the main source of food contamination in food poisoning outbreaks. Equipment and environmental surfaces can also be sources of contamination with *S. aureus*.

Symptoms: The most common symptoms are nausea, vomiting, retching, abdominal cramping, and prostration. Some individuals may not always demonstrate all the symptoms associated with the illness. In more severe cases, headache, muscle cramping, and transient changes in blood pressure and pulse rate may occur.

Onset time (incubation): 1 to 6 hours after ingestion of food containing the toxin.

Infective dose: A toxin dose of less than 1.0 microgram in contaminated food will produce symptoms of staphylococcal intoxication. This toxin level is reached when *S. aureus* populations exceed 100,000 per gram.

Duration of symptoms: Recovery generally takes two days, However, it is not unusual for complete recovery to take three days and sometimes longer in severe cases.

Incidence of disease: The true incidence of staphylococcal food poisoning is unknown.

Risk groups: All people.

Associated foods: Foods that are frequently incriminated in staphylococcal food poisoning include meat and meat products; poultry and egg products; salads such as egg, tuna, chicken, potato, and macaroni; bakery products such as cream-filled pastries, cream pies, and chocolate eclairs; sandwich fillings; and milk and dairy products. Foods that require considerable handling during preparation and that are kept at slightly elevated temperatures after preparation are frequently involved in staphylococcal food poisoning.

Campylobacter jejuni

Etiologic agent: *Campylobacter jejuni* is a gram-negative slender, curved, and motile rod. It is a microaerophilic organism, which means it has a requirement for reduced levels of oxygen. It is relatively fragile and sensitive to environmental stresses (e.g., 21% oxygen, drying, heating, disinfectants, acidic conditions). Because of its microaerophilic characteristics, the organism requires 3% to 5% oxygen and 2% to 10% carbon dioxide for optimal growth conditions.

Occurrence: Surveys show that 20% to 100% of retail chickens are contaminated. Raw milk is also a source of infections. The bacteria are often carried by healthy cattle and by flies on farms. Nonchlorinated water may also be a source of infections.

Symptoms: *C. jejuni* infection causes diarrhea, which may be watery or sticky and can contain blood (usually occult) and fecal leukocytes (white cells). Other symptoms often present are fever, abdominal pain, nausea, headache, and muscle pain.

Onset time (incubation): Symptoms usually occur 2 to 5 days after ingestion of the contaminated food or water.

Infective dose: The infective dose of *C. jejuni* is considered to be small. Studies suggest that about 400–500 bacteria may cause illness in some individuals, while in others, greater numbers are required.

Duration of Symptoms: Illness generally lasts 7 to 10 days, but relapses are not uncommon (about 25% of cases).

Incidence of disease: *C. jejuni* is the leading cause of bacterial diarrhea in the United States. There are probably numbers of cases in excess of the estimated cases of salmonellosis (2,000,000 to 4,000,000 per year).

Risk groups: All people. Children under 5 years and young adults (15–29) are more frequently afflicted than other age groups.

Associated foods: *C. jejuni* frequently contaminates raw chicken.

Listeriosis

Etiologic agent: *Listeria monocytogenes*, a gram-positive rod-shaped bacterium.

L. monocytogenes is quite hardy and resists the deleterious effects of freezing, drying, and heat remarkably well for a bacterium that does not form spores. Most *L. monocytogenes* are pathogenic to some degree.

Occurrence: Some studies suggest that 1% to 10% of humans may be intestinal carriers of *L. monocytogenes*. It has been found in at least 37 mammalian species, both domestic and feral, as well as at least 17 species of birds and possibly some species of fish and shellfish. It can be isolated from soil, silage, and other environmental sources.

Symptoms: The manifestations of listeriosis include septicemia, meningitis (or meningoencephalitis), encephalitis, and intrauterine or cervical infections in pregnant women, which may result in spontaneous abortion (2nd/3rd trimester) or stillbirth. The onset of the aforementioned disorders is usually preceded by influenza-like symptoms including persistent fever. It was reported that gastrointestinal symptoms such as nausea, vomiting, and diarrhea may precede more serious forms of listeriosis or may be the only symptoms expressed.

Onset time (incubation): The onset time to serious forms of listeriosis is unknown but may range from a few days to three weeks. The onset time to gastrointestinal symptoms is unknown but is probably greater than 12 hours.

Infective dose: The infective dose of *L. monocytogenes* is unknown but is believed to vary with the strain and susceptibility of the victim. From cases contracted through raw or supposedly pasteurized milk, it is safe to assume that in susceptible persons, fewer than 1,000 total organisms may cause disease.

Duration of symptoms: Depends on the severity of the disease.

Incidence of disease: Approximately 2,500 cases annually in the United States.

Risk groups: For invasive disease: immuno-compromised individuals, pregnant women and their fetuses and neonates, and the elderly.

Associated foods: *L. monocytogenes* has been associated with such foods as raw milk, supposedly pasteurized fluid milk, cheeses (particularly soft-ripened varieties), ice cream, raw vegetables, fermented raw-meat sausages, raw and cooked poultry, raw meats (all types), and raw and smoked fish. Its ability to grow at temperatures as low as 3°C permits multiplication in refrigerated foods.

Epidemic Cholera (*Vibrio cholerae O1* and *Vibrio cholerae non-O1*)

Etiologic agent: *Vibrio cholerae* O1 and *Vibrio cholerae* non-O1.

Occurrence: The cases between 1973 and 1991 were associated with the consumption of raw shellfish or of shellfish either improperly cooked or recontaminated after proper cooking. Environmental studies have demonstrated that strains of this organism may be found in the temperate estuarine and marine coastal areas surrounding the United States.

Symptoms: Symptoms of Asiatic cholera may vary from a mild, watery diarrhea to an acute diarrhea, with characteristic rice water stools. Abdominal cramps, nausea, vomiting, dehydration, and shock; after severe fluid and electrolyte loss, death may occur.

Onset time (incubation): Onset of the illness is generally sudden, with incubation periods varying from 6 hours to 5 days.

Infective dose: Human volunteer feeding studies utilizing healthy individuals have demonstrated that approximately one million organisms must be ingested to cause illness. Antacid consumption markedly lowers the infective dose.

Duration of symptoms: Depends on the severity of the case.

Incidence of disease: Over 200 proven cases of cholera have been reported in the United States since 1973, with 90% occurring within the last 5 years.

Risk groups: All people.

Associated foods: Sporadic cases occur when shellfish harvested from fecally polluted coastal waters are consumed raw. Cholera may also be transmitted by shellfish harvested from nonpolluted waters since *V. cholerae* O1 is part of the autochthonous microbiota of these waters.

Vibrio parahaemolyticus

Etiologic agent: *Vibrio parahaemolyticus*, a halophilic (salt-requiring) gram-negative bacterium naturally and commonly found in warm marine and estuarine environments.

Occurrence: This bacterium is frequently isolated from the estuarine and marine environment of the United States. Both pathogenic and nonpathogenic forms of the organism can be isolated from marine and estuarine environments and from fish and shellfish dwelling in these environments.

Symptoms: Watery diarrhea, often with abdominal cramping, nausea, vomiting, and fever.

Onset time (incubation): The incubation period is 4–96 hours after the ingestion of the organism, with a mean of 15 hours.

Infective dose: A total dose of greater than one million organisms may cause disease.

Duration of symptoms: Most persons recover after 3 days and suffer no long-term consequences. The median duration of the illness is 2.5 days. Bloodstream infections and death are uncommon and usually occur in persons with underlying medical conditions.

Incidence of disease: An average of 30 culture-confirmed cases, 10–20 hospitalizations, and 1 to 3 deaths are reported each year from the Gulf Coast region (reporting states are Alabama, Florida, Louisiana, Mississippi, and Texas). Nationwide, it is estimated that there are as many as 3,000 cases (most not culture confirmed), 40 hospitalizations, and 7 deaths.

Risk groups: All persons. Persons with underlying medical conditions, such as alcoholism and liver disease, may be at increased risk of infection and serious complications.

Associated foods: Consumption of raw, improperly cooked, or cooked, recontaminated fish and shellfish. A correlation exists between the probability of infection and the warmer months of the year. Improper refrigeration of seafood contaminated with this organism will allow its proliferation, which increases the possibility of infection.

Vibrio vulnificus

Etiologic agent: *Vibrio vulnificus*, a halophilic (salt-requiring) gram-negative bacterium naturally and commonly found in marine and estuarine environments.

Occurrence: It is found in all of the coastal waters of the United States.

Symptoms: Wound or soft tissue infections. In persons with underlying medical conditions, especially liver disease, can cause bloodstream infections characterized by fever, chills, decreased blood pressure, blistering skin lesions, and often death. In otherwise healthy persons, causes diarrhea, vomiting, and abdominal pain.

Onset time (incubation): In healthy individuals, gastroenteritis usually occurs within 16 hours of ingesting the organism. Ingestion of the organism by individuals with some type of chronic underlying disease may cause the "primary septicemia" form of illness. The mortality rate for individuals with this form of the disease is over 50%.

Infective dose: The infective dose for gastrointestinal symptoms in healthy individuals is unknown but for predisposed persons, septicemia can presumably occur with doses of less than 100 total organisms.

Duration of symptoms: Varies depending on the severity of the disease. Bloodstream infections in persons with liver disease are fatal approximately 50% of the time. Persons who recover suffer no long-term consequences.

Incidence of disease: An average of 40 culture-confirmed cases, 35 hospitalizations, and 12 deaths are reported each year from the Gulf Coast region (reporting states are Alabama, Florida, Louisiana, Mississippi, and Texas). Nationwide, there are as many as 95 cases (half of which are culture confirmed), 85 hospitalizations, and 35 deaths.

Risk groups: All persons. Persons with underlying medical conditions, especially liver disease, may be at increased risk of infection and serious complications.

Associated foods: This organism has been isolated from oysters, clams, and crabs. Consumption of these products raw or recontaminated may result in illness.

Clostridium perfringens

Etiologic agent: *Clostridium perfringens* is an anaerobic, gram-positive, spore-forming rod (anaerobic means unable to grow in the presence of free oxygen).

Occurrence: It is widely distributed in the environment and frequently occurs in the intestines of humans and many domestic and feral animals. Spores of the organism persist in soil, sediments, and areas subject to human or animal fecal pollution.

Symptoms: The common form of perfringens poisoning is characterized by intense abdominal cramps and diarrhea.

Onset time (incubation): 8–22 hours after consumption of foods containing large numbers of those *C. perfringens* bacteria capable of producing the food poisoning toxin.

Infective dose: The symptoms are caused by ingestion of large numbers (greater than 10^8) vegetative cells.

Duration of symptoms: The illness is usually over within 24 hours but less severe symptoms may persist in some individuals for 1 or 2 weeks.

Incidence of disease: CDC estimates that about 10,000 actual cases occur annually in the United States.

Risk groups: All persons.

Associated foods: The symptoms are caused by ingestion of large numbers (greater than 10^8) vegetative cells.

Bacillus cereus

Etiologic agent: *Bacillus cereus* is a gram-positive, facultatively aerobic spore-former whose cells are large rods. *B. cereus* food poisoning is the general description, although two recognized types of illness are caused by two distinct metabolites. The diarrheal type of illness is caused by a large molecular weight protein, while the vomiting (emetic) type of illness is believed to be caused by a low molecular weight, heat-stable peptide.

Symptoms: Watery diarrhea, abdominal cramps, and pain. Nausea may accompany diarrhea, but vomiting (emesis) rarely occurs.

Onset time (incubation): 6–15 hours after consumption of contaminated food.

Duration of symptoms: Symptoms persist for 24 hours in most instances.

Risk groups: All persons.

Associated foods: A wide variety of foods including meats, milk, vegetables, and fish have been associated with the diarrheal type food poisoning. The vomiting-type outbreaks have generally been associated with rice products; however, other starchy foods such as potato, pasta and cheese products have also been implicated. Food mixtures such as sauces, puddings, soups, casseroles, pastries, and salads have frequently been incriminated in food poisoning outbreaks.

Shigella spp.
Shigella: *boydii, dysenteriae, flexneri*, and *sonnei*.

Etiologic agent: *Shigella* are gram-negative, nonmotile, nonspore-forming rod-shaped bacteria.

Occurrence: *Shigella* rarely occurs in animals; principally a disease of humans except other primates such as monkeys and chimpanzees. The organism is frequently found in water polluted with human feces.

Symptoms: Abdominal pain; cramps; diarrhea; fever; vomiting; blood, pus, or mucus in stools; tenesmus.

Onset time (incubation): 12 to 50 hours.

Infective dose: A small inoculum (10 to 200 organisms) is sufficient to cause infection.

Duration of symptoms: Varies depending on the severity of disease

Incidence of disease: Approximately 14,000 laboratory confirmed cases of shigellosis and an estimated 448,240 total cases (mostly due to *S. sonnei*) occur in the United States each year. In the developing world, *S.flexneri* predominates. Epidemics of *S. dysenteriae* type 1 have occurred in Africa and Central America with case fatality rates of 5% to15%.

Risk groups: In the United States, groups at increased risk of shigellosis include children in child-care centers and persons in custodial institutions, where personal hygiene is difficult to maintain; Native Americans; orthodox Jews; international travelers; men who have sex with men; and those in homes with inadequate water for hand washing.

Associated foods: Salads (potato, tuna, shrimp, macaroni, and chicken), raw vegetables, milk and dairy products, and poultry. Contamination of these foods is usually through the fecal-oral route. Fecally contaminated water and unsanitary handling by food handlers are the most common causes of contamination.

Enterovirulent *Escherichia Coli* Group (EEC group)

Escherichia coli -enterotoxigenic (ETEC)

Escherichia coli -enteropathogenic (EPEC)

Escherichia coli -enteroinvasive (EIEC)

(Escherichia coli 0157:H7 will be discussed separately.)

Etiologic agent: There are four recognized classes of enterovirulent *E. coli* that cause gastroenteritis in humans.

Occurrence: Associated with contaminated food and water worldwide.

Symptoms: Watery diarrhea, abdominal cramps, low-grade fever, nausea, and malaise.

Onset time (incubation): Usually between 12 and 72 hours.

Infective dose: Volunteer feeding studies indicate that a relatively large dose (100 million to 10 billion bacteria) of enterotoxigenic *E. coli* is probably necessary to establish colonization of the small intestine, where these organisms proliferate and produce toxins that induce fluid secretion. With a high infective dose, diarrhea can be induced within 24 hours. Infants may require fewer organisms for infection to be established.

Duration of symptoms: Varies depending on severity of disease.

Incidence of disease: Very limited in the United States.

Risk groups: Infants and travelers to underdeveloped countries are most at-risk of infection.

Associated foods: ETEC is not considered a serious food-borne disease hazard in countries having high sanitary standards and practices. Contamination of water with human sewage may lead to contamination of foods. Infected food handlers may also contaminate foods. These organisms are infrequently isolated from dairy products such as semi-soft cheeses. Common foods implicated in EPEC outbreaks are raw beef and chicken, although any food exposed to fecal contamination is strongly suspect.

Escherichia coli 0157:H7 enterohemorrhagic (EHEC)

Etiologic agent: A minority of *E. coli* strains are capable of causing human illness by several different mechanisms. *E. coli* serotype 0157:H7 is a rare variety of *E. coli* that produces large quantities of one or more related, potent toxins that cause severe damage to the lining of the intestine. These toxins [verotoxin (VT), shiga-like toxin] are closely related or identical to the toxin produced by *Shigella dysenteriae*.

Occurrence: Usually 12 to 72 hours.

Symptoms: The illness is characterized by severe cramping (abdominal pain) and diarrhea that is initially watery but becomes grossly bloody. Occasionally vomiting occurs. Fever is either low-grade or absent. Some individuals exhibit watery diarrhea only. Hemolytic uremic syndrome (HUS): Persons with this illness have kidney failure and often require dialysis and transfusions. Some develop chronic kidney failure or neurologic impairment (e.g., seizures or stroke). Some have surgery to remove part of the bowel. Estimated 61 fatal cases annually; 3% to 5% with HUS die.

Onset time (incubation): Not given.

Infective dose: Unknown, but from a compilation of outbreak data, including the organism's ability to be passed person-to-person in the day-care setting and nursing homes, the dose may be similar to that of *Shigella spp.* (as few as 10 organisms).

Duration of symptoms: The illness is usually self-limited and lasts for an average of 8 days.

Incidence of disease: An estimated 73,000 cases occur annually in the United States. Uncommonly reported in patients in less-industrialized countries. Hemorrhagic colitis infections are not too common.

Risk groups: All persons. Children <5 years old and the elderly are more likely to develop serious complications.

Associated foods: Undercooked or raw hamburger (ground beef) has been implicated in many of the documented outbreaks, however *E. coli* 0157:H7 outbreaks have implicated alfalfa sprouts, unpasteurized fruit juices, dry-cured salami, lettuce, game meat, cheese curds, and raw milk.

VIRUSES

Hepatitis A virus

Etiologic agent: Hepatitis A virus (HAV) is classified with the enterovirus group of the Picornaviridae family.

Occurrence: Hepatitis A has a worldwide distribution occurring in both epidemic and sporadic fashions. Hepatitis A is endemic throughout much of the world.

Symptoms: Hepatitis A is usually a mild illness characterized by sudden onset of fever, malaise, nausea, anorexia, and abdominal discomfort, followed in several days by jaundice.

Onset time (incubation): The incubation period for hepatitis A, which varies from 10 to 50 days (mean 30 days), is dependent upon the number of infectious particles consumed.

Infective dose: The infectious dose is unknown but presumably is 10 to 100 virus particles.

Duration of symptoms: When disease does occur, it is usually mild and recovery is complete in 1 to 2 weeks. Occasionally, the symptoms are severe and convalescence can take several months.

Incidence of disease: About 22,700 cases of hepatitis A representing 38% of all hepatitis cases (5-year average from all routes of transmission) are reported annually in the United States. In developing countries, the incidence of disease in adults is relatively low because of exposure to the virus in childhood.

Risk groups: All people who ingest the virus and are immunologically unprotected are susceptible to infection. Disease, however, is more common in adults than in children.

Associated foods: Cold cuts and sandwiches, fruits and fruit juices, milk and milk products, vegetables, salads, shellfish, and iced drinks are commonly implicated in outbreaks. Water, shellfish, and salads are the most frequent sources. Contamination of foods by infected workers in food processing plants and restaurants is common. HAV is primarily transmitted by person-to-person contact through fecal contamination, but common-source epidemics from contaminated food and water also occur. Contamination occurs when HAV is excreted in feces of infected persons via sewage or food to susceptible individuals.

Norwalk virus group

Etiologic agent: Norwalk virus is the prototype of a family of unclassified small round structured viruses (SRSVs), which may be related to the caliciviruses.

Occurrence: The disease occurs worldwide.

Symptoms: The disease is self-limiting, mild, and characterized by nausea, vomiting, diarrhea, and abdominal pain. Headache and low-grade fever may occur.

Onset time (incubation): A mild and brief illness usually develops 24 to 48 hours after contaminated food or water is consumed.

Infective dose: The infectious dose is unknown but presumed to be low.

Duration of symptoms: The disease lasts for 24 to 60 hours.

Incidence of disease: Only the common cold is reported more frequently than viral gastroenteritis as a cause of illness in the United States. Although viral gastroenteritis is caused by a number of viruses, it is estimated that Norwalk viruses are responsible for about 1/3 of the cases not involving the 6 to 24-month age group.

Risk groups: All individuals who ingest the virus and who have not (within 24 months) had an infection with the same or related strain, are susceptible to infection and can develop the symptoms of gastroenteritis. Disease is more frequent in adults and older children than in the very young.

Associated foods: Norwalk gastroenteritis is transmitted by the fecal-oral route via contaminated water and foods. Secondary person-to-person transmission has been documented. Water is the most common source of outbreaks and may include water from municipal supplies, wells, recreational lakes, swimming pools, and water stored aboard cruise ships. Shellfish and salad ingredients are the foods most often implicated in Norwalk outbreaks. Ingestion of raw or insufficiently steamed clams and oysters poses a high risk for infection with Norwalk virus. Foods other than shellfish are contaminated by ill food handlers.

PARASITIC PROTOZOA AND WORMS

Giardia lamblia

Etiologic agent: *Giardia lamblia* (*intestinalis*) is a protozoan.

Occurrence: Giardiasis is the most frequent cause of nonbacterial diarrhea in North America.

Symptoms: Symptoms include diarrhea, loose or watery stool, stomach cramps, and upset stomach. These symptoms may lead to weight loss and dehydration. Some people have no symptoms.

Onset time (incubation): 1 to 2 weeks after being infected.

Infective dose: Ingestion of one or more cysts may cause disease.

Duration of symptoms: Normally illness lasts for 1 to 2 weeks, but there are cases of chronic infections lasting months to years.

Incidence of disease: The overall incidence of infection in the United States is estimated at 2% of the population.

Risk groups: Giardiasis occurs throughout the population, although the prevalence is higher in children than adults.

Associated foods: Giardiasis is most frequently associated with the consumption of contaminated water. Food contaminated by infected or infested food handlers, and the possibility exists of infections from contaminated vegetables that are eaten raw.

Entamoeba histolytica

Etiologic agent: *Entamoeba histolytica* is a single-celled parasitic protozoan. Amebiasis (or amoebiasis) is the name of the infection caused by *E. histolytica*.

Occurrence: Worldwide cysts survive outside the host in water and soils and on foods, especially under moist conditions on the latter.

Symptoms: (1) no symptoms, (2) vague gastrointestinal distress, (3) dysentery (with blood and mucus). Most infections occur in the digestive tract, but other tissues may be invaded.

Onset time (incubation): Usually 1 to 4 weeks.

Infective dose: The ingestion of one viable cyst can cause an infection.

Duration of symptoms: Infections may sometimes last for years.

Incidence of disease: Infrequent in the United States; more common among homosexual men.

Risk groups: All people are believed to be susceptible to infection.

Associated foods: Fecal contamination of drinking water and foods.

Cryptosporidium parvum

Etiologic agent: *Cryptosporidium parvum*, a protozoan. The sporocysts are resistant to most chemical disinfectants, but are susceptible to drying and the ultraviolet portion of sunlight.

Occurrence: *Cryptosporidium* sp. infects many herd animals (cows, goats, sheep among domesticated animals, and deer and elk among wild animals).

Symptoms: Intestinal cryptosporidiosis is characterized by severe watery diarrhea but may, alternatively, be asymptomatic. Pulmonary and tracheal cryptosporidiosis in humans is associated with coughing and frequently a low-grade fever; these symptoms are often accompanied by severe intestinal distress.

Onset time (incubation): 2 to 10 days.

Infective dose: Less than 10 organisms and, presumably, one organism can initiate an infection.

Duration of symptoms: Intestinal cryptosporidiosis is self-limiting in most healthy individuals, with watery diarrhea lasting 2 to 4 days. In some outbreaks at day-care centers, diarrhea has lasted 1 to 4 weeks.

Incidence of disease: Direct human surveys indicate a prevalence of about 2% of the population in North America. Serological surveys indicate that 80% of the population has had cryptosporidiosis. Incidence is higher in child day care centers that serve food.

Risk groups: Although all persons are at risk, children are more susceptible. Immunodeficient individuals, especially AIDS patients, may have the disease for life, with the severe watery diarrhea contributing to death.

Associated foods: *Cryptosporidium sp.* could occur, theoretically, on any food touched by a contaminated food handler. Fertilizing salad vegetables with manure is another possible source of human infection.

Cyclospora cayetanensis

Etiologic agent: *Cyclospora cayetanensis* is a unicellular coccidian parasite.

Occurrence: Usually found in people who lived or traveled in developing countries.

Symptoms: Watery diarrhea, with frequent, sometimes explosive, bowel movements. Other symptoms can include loss of appetite, substantial loss of weight, bloating, increased gas, stomach cramps, nausea, vomiting, muscle aches, low-grade fever, and fatigue. Some infected person do not show symptoms.

Onset time (incubation): Approximately 1 week.

Infective dose: Unconfirmed.

Duration of symptoms: A few days to several months

Incidence of disease: Since 1990, at least 11 food-borne outbreaks of cyclosporiasis, affecting approximately 3,600 persons, have been documented in the United States and Canada.

Risk groups: People of all ages are at risk for infection.

Associated foods: Fresh produce and water.

Anisakis sp. and related worms

Etiologic agent: *Anisakis simplex* (herring worm), *Pseudoterranova (Phocanema, Terranova) decipiens* (cod or seal worm), *Contracaecum spp.*, and *Hysterothylacium (Thynnascaris) spp.* are anisakid nematodes (roundworms).

Occurrence: These parasites are known to occur frequently in the flesh of cod, haddock, fluke, pacific salmon, herring, flounder, and monkfish.

Symptoms: Affected individual feels a tingling or tickling sensation in the throat and coughs up or manually extracts a nematode. In more severe cases, there is acute abdominal pain.

Onset time (incubation): Symptoms occur from as little as an hour to about 2 weeks after consumption of raw or undercooked seafood.

Infective dose: One nematode is the usual number recovered from a patient.

Duration of symptoms: Anisakids rarely reach full maturity in humans and usually are eliminated spontaneously from the digestive tract lumen within 3 weeks of infection.

Incidence of disease: Fewer than 10 cases are diagnosed in the United States annually. However, it is suspected that many other cases go undetected.

Risk groups: Consumers of raw or under-processed seafood.

Associated foods: The principal source of human infections with these larval worms is through the consumption of raw or undercooked seafood or improperly frozen and stored fish and shellfish.

Ascaris lumbricoides and *Trichuris trichiura*

Etiologic agent: Humans worldwide are infected with *Ascaris lumbricoides* and *Trichuris trichiura*; the eggs of these roundworms (nematodes) are "sticky" and may be carried to the mouth by hands, other body parts, fomites (inanimate objects), or foods.

Occurrence: These infections are cosmopolitan.

Symptoms: Vague digestive tract discomfort sometimes accompanies the intestinal infection, but in small children with more than a few worms there may be intestinal blockage because of the worms' large size. The larvae of ascarid species that mature in hosts other than humans may hatch in the human intestine and are especially prone to wander; they may penetrate into tissues and locate in various organ systems of the human body, perhaps eliciting a fever and diverse complications. *Trichuris sp.* larvae do not migrate after hatching but molt and mature in the intestine. Adults are not as large as *A. lumbricoides*. Symptoms range from inapparent through vague digestive tract distress to emaciation with dry skin and diarrhea (usually mucoid). Toxic or allergic symptoms may also occur.

Onset time (incubation): Varies depending on infective dose.

Infective dose: Infection with one or a few *Ascaris sp.* may be inapparent unless noticed when passed in the feces, or, on occasion, crawling up into the throat and trying to exit through the mouth or nose. Infection with numerous worms may result in a pneumonitis during the migratory phase when larvae that have hatched from the ingested eggs in the lumen of the small intestine penetrate into the tissues and by way of the lymph and blood systems reach the lungs.

Duration of symptoms: Both infections may self-cure after the larvae have matured into adults. In severe cases, surgical removal may be necessary. Allergic symptoms (especially but not exclusively of the asthmatic sort) are common in long-lasting infections or upon reinfection in ascariasis.

Incidence of disease: Ascariasis is more common in North America and trichuriasis in Europe. Relative infection rates on other continents are not available. Although no major outbreaks have occurred in the United States, there are many individual cases. The occurrence of large numbers of eggs in domestic municipal sewage implies that the infection rate, especially with *A. lumbricoides*, is high in the United States.

Risk groups: Usually consumers of uncooked vegetables and fruits grown in or near soil fertilized with sewage.

Associated foods: The eggs of these worms are found in insufficiently treated sewage-fertilizer and in soils where they embryonate (i.e., larvae develop in fertilized eggs). The eggs may contaminate crops grown in soil or fertilized with sewage that has received nonlethal treatment; humans are infected when such produce is consumed raw. Infected food handlers may contaminate a wide variety of foods.

NATURAL TOXINS

Ciguatera poisoning

Etiologic agent: The toxins are known to originate from several dinoflagellate (algae) species that are common to ciguatera endemic regions in the lower latitudes.

Occurrence: Ciguatera is a form of human poisoning caused by the consumption of subtropical and tropical marine finfish that have accumulated naturally occurring toxins through their diet.

Symptoms: Perioral numbness and tingling (paresthesia), which may spread to the extremities, nausea, vomiting, and diarrhea. Neurological signs include intensified paresthesia, arthralgia, myalgia, headache, temperature sensory reversal and acute sensitivity to temperature extremes, vertigo, and muscular weakness to the point of prostration. Cardiovascular signs include arrhythmia, bradycardia or tachycardia, and reduced blood pressure.

Onset time (incubation): Initial signs of poisoning occur within 6 hours after consumption of toxic fish.

Infective dose: Unknown.

Duration of symptoms: Ciguatera poisoning is usually self-limiting, and signs of poisoning often subside within several days from onset. However, in severe cases the neurological symptoms are known to persist from weeks to months. In a few isolated cases neurological symptoms have persisted for several years, and in other cases recovered patients have experienced recurrence of neurological symptoms months to years after recovery. Such relapses are most often associated with changes in dietary habits or with consumption of alcohol. There is a low incidence of death resulting from respiratory and cardiovascular failure.

Incidence of disease: The relative frequency of ciguatera fish poisoning in the United States is not known.

Risk groups: All humans are believed to be susceptible to ciguatera toxins.

Associated foods: Marine finfish most commonly implicated in ciguatera fish poisoning include the groupers, barracudas, snappers, jacks, mackerel, and triggerfish. Many other species of warm-water fish harbor ciguatera toxins. The occurrence of toxic fish is sporadic, and not all fish of a given species or from a given locality will be toxic.

Shellfish toxins (PSP, DSP, NSP, ASP)

Etiologic agent: Shellfish poisoning is caused by a group of toxins elaborated by planktonic algae (dinoflagellates, in most cases) upon which the shellfish feed. The toxins are accumulated and sometimes metabolized by the shellfish. The 20 toxins responsible for paralytic shellfish poisonings (PSP) are all derivatives of saxitoxin. Diarrheic shellfish poisoning (DSP) is presumably caused by a group of high molecular weight polyethers, including okadaic acid, the dinophysis toxins, the pectenotoxins, and yessotoxin. Neurotoxic shellfish poisoning (NSP) is the result of exposure to a group of polyethers called brevetoxins. Amnesic shellfish poisoning (ASP) is caused by the unusual amino acid, domoic acid, as the contaminant of shellfish.

Occurrence: Generally regarded as sporadic, continuous, and widespread.

Symptoms: In the case of PSP, the effects are predominantly neurological and include tingling, burning, numbness, drowsiness, incoherent speech, and respiratory paralysis. Less well characterized are the symptoms associated with DSP, NSP, and ASP. DSP is primarily observed as a generally mild gastrointestinal disorder, that is, nausea, vomiting, diarrhea, and abdominal pain accompanied by chills, headache, and fever. Both gastrointestinal and neurological symptoms characterize NSP, including tingling and numbness of lips, tongue, and throat, muscular aches, dizziness, reversal of the sensations of hot and cold, diarrhea, and vomiting. ASP is characterized by gastrointestinal disorders (vomiting, diarrhea, abdominal pain) and neurological problems (confusion, memory loss, disorientation, seizure, coma).

Onset time (incubation): PSP—(Symptoms of the disease develop fairly rapidly, within 0.5 to 2 hours after ingestion of the shellfish, depending on the amount of toxin consumed. NSP—(Onset of this disease occurs within a few minutes to a few hours. DSP—(Onset of the disease, depending on the dose of toxin ingested, may be as little as 30 minutes to 2 to 3 hours. ASP—(The toxicosis is characterized by the onset of gastrointestinal symptoms within 24 hours; neurological symptoms occur within 48 hours.

Infective dose: Ingestion of contaminated shellfish results in a wide variety of symptoms, depending upon the toxins(s) present, their concentrations in the shellfish and the amount of contaminated shellfish consumed.

Duration of symptoms: NSP—(few hours to several days; DSP—(2 to 3 days.

Incidence of disease: Unavailable.

Risk groups: All humans are susceptible to shellfish poisoning. Elderly people are apparently predisposed to the severe neurological effects of the ASP toxin.

Associated foods: All shellfish (filter-feeding molluscs) are potentially toxic. However, PSP is generally associated with mussels, clams, cockles, and scallops; NSP with shellfish harvested along the Florida coast and the Gulf of Mexico; DSP with mussels, oysters, and scallops, and ASP with mussels.

Scombroid Poisoning

Etiologic agent: Scombrotoxin (histamine poisoning).

Occurrence: Worldwide.

Symptoms: Initial symptoms include a tingling or burning sensation in the mouth, a rash on the upper body and a drop in blood pressure. Frequently, headaches and itching of the skin are encountered. The symptoms may progress to nausea, vomiting, and diarrhea and may require hospitalization.

Onset time (incubation): Acute onset ranging from immediate to 30 minutes.

Duration of symptoms: Usually 3 hours, but some cases may last as long as 3 days.

Incidence of disease: One of the most common forms of fish poisoning in the United States.

Risk groups: All humans are susceptible to scombroid poisoning.

Associated foods: Fish of the Scombroid family, including tuna, mahi mahi, bluefish, sardines, and mackerel.

OTHER PATHOGENIC AGENTS

Prions

Etiologic agent: Proteinaceous infectious agent; Prions are associated with a group of diseases called transmissible spongiform encephalopathies (TSEs). In humans, the illness suspected of being food-borne is variant Creutzfeldt-Jakob disease (vCJD). The human disease vCJD and the cattle disease, bovine spongiform encephalopathy (BSE), also known as "mad cow" disease, appear to be caused by the same agent.

Occurrence: The specific prions of interest in disease and their normally configured proteins are those found in mammals.

Symptoms: Cases of vCJD usually present with psychiatric problems, such as depression. As the disease progresses, neurologic signs appear—unpleasant sensations in the limbs and/or face. There are problems with walking and muscle coordination. Sometimes, late in the course of the disease, victims become forgetful and then experience severe problems with processing information and speaking. Uncontrolled muscle twitching and death follow.

Incidence of disease: There are no reported human cases of vCJD or bovine cases of BSE in the United States. In the United Kingdom, there have been 94 human cases of suspected or confirmed vCJD from 1993, when the illness was first recognized, through February 2001. Since 1986, more than 180,000 cases of BSE have occurred there in cattle, particularly dairy herds.

Risk groups: All cases of vCJD to date have occurred in individuals of a single human genotype that is methionine homozygous at codon 139. About 40% of the total human population belongs to this methionine-methionine homozygous state. The susceptibility of other genotypes is not yet known.

Associated foods: Contamination of meat products by central nervous system tissue (brain and spinal cord) during routine slaughter.

Protecting Food and Controlling Food-Borne Illness

The overall objective of any food protection program is to not only prevent the transmission of food-borne pathogens but to ensure that food is safe and will not cause harm to anyone resulting from its consumption. Therefore, effective food protection and safety programs are focused on preventing food-borne illness and ensuring that all food intended for human consumption is free of adulteration and contamination.

Within a conceptual framework for food safety, the most important factors that must be controlled at all times are the six conditions for bacterial growth in foods. These conditions are discussed above and are simply the nutrient level of the food; the acidity of the food; the temperatures that food is maintained during processing, storage, preparation, and serving; the time that food is held at temperatures favorable for pathogenic bacterial growth; the amount of moisture available in food to support pathogenic bacteria growth; and, the oxygen demand of the specific pathogenic bacteria. The principles of food safety are based on controlling these bacterial growth factors in food.

Principles of Food Safety

The principles of food safety are based on controlling the growth and transmission of food-borne pathogens that may be found in or on food intended for human consumption. They are presented here in a logical sequence.

Cleanliness Perhaps the most important principle in food protection safety is cleanliness. The concept of cleanliness goes to the heart of public health and is a way of life. Cleanliness means that food is stored, transported, processed, prepared, and served in an environment and facilities that are kept in a clean and sanitary manner. All areas of a facility that may come in contact with food in any manner must be kept clean at all times. A food facility is considered to be clean when there is no visible soil found on the surface of food equipment, utensils, and other food contact surfaces.

A food facility must be clean of litter, trash, and other debris inside and outside of the facility.

Litter, trash, and debris attract rodents and other vermin that may cause increased risk of food-borne illness associated with a facility.

Besides being clean, many areas within a food facility must be maintained in a sanitary condition. A sanitary condition exists when food contact surfaces and equipment are cleaned with a chemical sanitizing solution of chlorine, quaternary ammonia, or iodine that lowers the amount of bacteria present to levels that reduce the risk of disease transmission to acceptable levels.

Temperature Control Probably the most important aspect of preventing food-borne illness within a food facility is maintaining proper temperature control for all potentially hazardous food (PHF) at all times.

Potentially hazardous foods must be held at temperatures of either *41°F or lower* or *140°F or above*. Maintaining PHF at these temperatures will either kill any existing pathogen in the food or inhibit its further growth. However, food is usually not prepared or handled at these temperatures and most causes of food-borne illness are attributed to the reheating of stored food for serving or the cooling of hot cooked foods for storage or holding.

When prepared hot foods are cooled or when stored cold foods are being reheated, the food product's temperature passes thorough a temperature zone known as the "danger zone." The danger zone is the range of temperatures between 41°F and 140°F and constitutes the temperature range that food-borne pathogens can survive and multiply or grow. Although all PHFs exist for various periods of time in the danger zone during their processing, storage, preparation, and serving, it is important to minimize the period of time that a food product is in the danger zone.

The intent of temperature management of food is to prevent or minimize any food-borne pathogens that may exist on the food from entering the bacterial growth phase called the "log phase" in which rapid bacterial growth occurs. It is when bacterial pathogens in food enter the log phase of growth that the numbers of bacteria present can quickly multiply and reach a large enough number that is necessary for an infectious dose. Obviously, temperature control of PHF throughout the entire period that food is handled and prepared is critical in the control of food-borne illness.

Cross-Contamination occurs when bacteria or other harmful substances that exists in one food product is transferred to another food product, causing that product to become contaminated. The direct or indirect contamination of a food product can occur from contact with contaminated food contact surfaces, including equipment, utensils, and employee's outer garments or hands. Cross-contamination can be prevented by the following procedures:

- Clean and sanitize all equipment, utensils, and food contact surfaces between uses.

- Prepare raw foods in areas that are separate from cooked foods or produce.

- Use specific equipment for preparing different types of foods.

- Only use designated wiping cloths or towels for cleaning food spills.

- Use good food-handling techniques at all times when preparing or serving food.

Personal Hygiene Food service employees are probably the most important link in the scheme to ensure food safety. They are responsible for handling food and maintaining the food facility in a clean and sanitary condition. They are trained to follow specific procedures that are intended to ensure that food is handled properly and within the guidelines specified by law.

The food service employee is also the source, even if not always the cause, of food-borne illness. Employees who fail to wash their hands after using the restroom or between the handling of PHF often contaminate the food product resulting in food-borne illness. Employees are often the source of food-borne illness whose mode of transmission is the "fecal-oral" route. Food-borne

pathogens commonly attributed to employees are *Staphylococcus aureus* and *Shigella spp*.

Employers should check their employees daily for any apparent illnesses and adequate personal hygiene.

Food Safety Management Although not considered to be a true principle of food safety, the management of the food facility is actually the most important factor in food safety. The food facility owner or manager is responsible for ensuring that the facility is operating in full compliance of all food safety laws and regulations; that all food workers and managers are appropriately trained; that the food suppliers are delivering food products under the proper conditions; and that the flow of food in the food facility is properly managed and routinely checked and any corrections are immediately made by the food workers.

Maintaining any food service facility in a clean and sanitary manner at all times while ensuring that food workers are doing their part to prevent cross-contamination and properly managing food temperatures for all foods being handled and prepared is both an important responsibility and a necessity for adequately protecting the public's health.

Hazard Analysis Critical Control Point (HACCP)

Managing a food facility to assure that food-borne illness is prevented is very difficult without a system that helps food managers to identify potential problems before they occur and control or eliminate the problem. The system that has been developed and already implemented in most commercial food processing plants and a significant number of retail food facilities is the **Hazard Analysis and Critical Control Point (HACCP)** system.

The HACCP system consists of seven steps or principles as follows:

1. Hazard analysis consists of identifying potential food hazards including all potentially

hazardous foods, other biological hazards, chemical hazards, and physical hazards that must be identified and controlled.

2. Determine critical control points (CCP) in the food preparation process. A critical control point is usually the last point in the preparation of a food item where the foodborne pathogen can be destroyed or eliminated before the food is served. CCPs are established for each food item on the menu.

3. Establish critical limits for each critical control point. A critical limit is the standard that must be met to eliminate the hazard or reduce it to an acceptable level. Thoroughly cooking a food product to an internal cooking temperature that will destroy the specific pathogen associated with a particular food is the most common critical limit established for a CCP. For example, the CCP for chicken is to cook it until it meets the critical limit of an internal temperature of 165°F for at least 15 seconds.

4. Establish a monitoring system for each critical control point. Each CCP is monitored by making appropriate measurements or observations and documenting the findings.

5. Establish corrective actions. When monitoring detects that a critical limit was unmet, specific corrective action must immediately take place. Usually corrective actions are predetermined for each CCP.

6. Establish verification procedures. The HACCP plan must be verified at regular intervals to ensure that it is still functioning as designed and to make corrections or additions to the plan as conditions in the food facility change.

7. Establish documentation and recordkeeping. Recordkeeping is important in the HACCP system because it documents that the plan is being monitored and managed effectively. Examples of HACCP records are time-temperature logs, product specifications, logs of corrective action, and monitoring schedules.

When HACCP is properly implemented, supported by management and supervision, and followed by a well-trained food service staff, it has proven to be very effective in preventing foodborne illness and enhancing food safety.

The Regulatory Scheme for Food Safety

Various federal agencies have responsibilities for food safety. The principal federal agencies are the U.S. Department of Agriculture and the U.S. Food and Drug Administration.

The U.S. Department of Agriculture, Food Safety and Inspection Service (FSIS) is responsible for all inspection of meat, poultry, and egg products that will be marketed interstate. The Food and Drug Administration (FDA) is charged with protecting American consumers by enforcing the Federal Food, Drug, and Cosmetic Act and several related public health laws. The FDA is a public health agency within the Public Health Service, which in turn is a part of the Department of Health and Human Services.

The FDA has several important programs in food safety. They enforce requirements for registration, manufacturing, and process filing of low-acid canned foods (LACF) and acidified foods (AF) in hermetically sealed containers. The purpose of this program is to ensure safety from harmful bacteria or their toxins, especially the deadly *Clostridium botulinum* that may be present in these products.

The FDA's seafood HACCP program is designed to ensure the safety of seafood through HACCP. It's a mandatory program for all seafood processors under FDA regulatory control.

Another significant FDA program is the Model Food Code, which is a reference document designed for the more than 2,500 state and local regulatory agencies that enforce food safety in retail food facilities. Since the federal government lacks jurisdiction for food safety over states and local governments, the Food Code was developed to assist states with a model food law, which has the support of the federal government and the food service industry. State governments are encouraged to adopt it as state law.

The significance of the Food Code is that as it is adopted by the states, this country will eventually have a uniform food safety code. This will make it easier for the industry to comply with all food safety laws which is a problem for many of the national and multinational corporations involved in food service. The Food Code is updated every two years to reflect the changing needs of the food industry and to incorporate the most recent scientific information. This is important if this country is to meet its goal of having a "science-based food safety system."

FOOD SAFETY SURVEILLANCE

The inspection of food facilities and processors is important to ensure that the food supply is safe. However, it is critical to have a food safety surveillance system capable of detecting and identifying problems before they reach critical levels when controlling the problem becomes very costly.

The CDC, FDA, and USDA have developed several food safety surveillance systems that are intended to monitor specific problems. One of these monitoring systems is the National Antimicrobial Resistance Monitoring System.

The National Antimicrobial Resistance Monitoring System Enteric Bacteria (NARMSEB) is intended to detect emerging drug resistance among food-borne pathogens. In cooperation with the FDA, CDC, and USDA, a nationwide monitoring system has been created which will alert CDC and FDA of any change in bacterial response to antibiotics used in people. This information allows public health officials, animal producers, drug manufacturers, and veterinarians to use this information to control and prevent further harm to public health from the use of antimicrobials in food animals.

Another food safety surveillance program is PulseNet, which is also a collaborative project between CDC, FDA, USDA, and state health departments. PulseNet uses dedicated, high-speed Internet connections for the rapid comparison of DNA fingerprints of food-borne bacteria with those in CDC's database. This allows for the quick detection and response to emerging pathogens in the food supply. Many public health officials believe that PulseNet will prove to be essential to preventing widespread food-borne illness.

OTHER FOOD SAFETY REGULATIONS

In addition to the Food Code and state and local laws and regulations that are intended to protect the public from food-borne hazards, several other regulations also play an important role in protecting the country's food supply. One important area of regulation is imported food products. All imported products are required to meet the same food safety standards as domestic goods. As specified in law all imported foods must be pure, wholesome, safe to eat, and produced under sanitary conditions in accordance with the Food, Drug and Cosmetic Act. This law also requires that all imported products must contain "informative and truthful labeling in English." Under the Food, Drug and Cosmetic Act, the FDA has the right to refuse entry to this country of any food product that appears to be in violation of the act. The FDA's inspection and enforcement procedures for food imports are coordinated with the U.S. Customs Service.

Another area of concern that poses a threat to food safety are pesticides, which are used by most farmers. All pesticides are evaluated and registered for use by the U.S. Environmental Protection Agency (U.S. EPA). Before a pesticide can be approved for use, the manufacturer must show that the pesticide will not pose an unreasonable risk to farm workers, consumers, or the environment. While most foods have very little or no detectable pesticide residue when it reaches the consumer, the position of those who have studied the health risk assessments of residual pesticides find that the benefits of consuming fresh fruits and vegetables clearly outweigh any associated risk from exposure to trace levels of pesticide residues.

Are pesticides a real threat to food safety? According to the state of California's Department of Pesticide Regulation (Cal-DPR), about 1% of samples they have tested have illegal residues. No residues were detected in about 65% of samples tested by Cal-DPR. The remaining samples were found to have mostly trace levels that were well below the legally allowable limits.

ENFORCEMENT OF FOOD SAFETY REGULATIONS

How are public health laws such as pesticide regulations enforced by the regulating governmental agency? For pesticides, agricultural inspectors take samples of produce from the fields before harvest, from wholesale and retail markets, packing sheds, processing plants, and even ports of entry. Food samples are then analyzed with a screening test that can detect the presence of different pesticides. When a food product, usually produce, is tested positive for illegal pesticide residues it is immediately tracked back to the grower. If the crop is still in the field, the harvest is stopped and the regulator may order the crop destroyed. Should it be found that the illegal crop has been harvested and shipped to market, the illegal crop may be quarantined and destroyed if necessary. Growers who violate the law may lose their crop and be subject to civil and criminal prosecution, which may result in fines, jail, and other penalties.

Enforcement of food safety regulations in other areas usually proceed in the same manner as the example given above with pesticide regulations. It should be noted that if a violation of a food safety regulation occurs, it is common practice under administrative law to issue a compliance order to the owner or manager of the business. Should the party cited immediately correct the violation then all further enforcement activities will cease. It is the threat of enforcement and the resulting consequences that motivate many food service operators to comply with the law. Without a strong and effective public health enforcement program many food safety laws would go unheeded by food service operators.

Public health law is usually classified as administrative law as opposed to criminal law. When administered properly, it is very effective in eliminating public health nuisances. In fact, most public health laws are considered to be nuisance laws because just the presence of a public health nuisance can bring harm and even the death of someone. Unfortunately, this is a condition we observe all too frequently today, especially in the area of food.

SUMMARY

The same food that is a necessity of life can lead to deterioration of life through disease-causing agents. Thus, food quality management is an important component of public and environmental health programs, and preventing the entrance of food-borne pathogens is of major concern. It involves monitoring food from its agriculture origin, through harvest, processing, storage, and transportation, to food preparation and consumption.

Food-borne diseases are of two main types: food-borne infections and chemical food poisoning. Preventive measures include sanitary handling, the application of heat, and refrigeration. Food preservation methods include temperature control (**pasteurization**, cooking, **canning**, refrigeration, or freezing), **drying**, chemical treatment (**osmotic balance disturbance** and pH reactions such as **pickling**) and **fermentation**, the process used in making cheese, vinegar, and sauerkraut.

Food additives are placed in foods intentionally to improve appearance, flavor, texture, or storage properties. These include vinegar, sugar, salt, nitrites and nitrates, sulfites, and coloring agents, among many others. The entities largely responsible for monitoring foods are the U.S. Department of Agriculture (particularly milk) and Public Health and Environmental Health agencies (restaurant inspection).

KEY TERMS

Adulteration, p. 173

Bovine spongiform
  encephalopathy
  (BSE), p. 174

Canning, p. 197

Contamination,
  p. 173

Creutzfeldt-Jakob
  disease, p. 174

Drying, p. 197

REFERENCES

FDA/CFSAN. *Bad Bug Book: Introduction to Food-borne Pathogenic Microorganisms and Natural Toxins*. Centers for Disease Control and Prevention/National Center for Infectious Diseases, *http://www.cdc.gov/ncidod/diesases/cjd/*

FDA/CFSAN. *Food Safety Initiative Constituent Update: Diagnosis and Management of Food-Borne Illness: A Primer for Physicians*; Federal Food Safety Strategic Plan. MMWR, November 5, 1982, 31(43); 580, 585.

FDA/CFSAN. *Managing Food Safety: A HACCP Principles Guide for Operators of Food Establishments at the Retail Level*. MMWR, March 17, 2000, 49(10): 201–5 Preliminary FoodNet Data on the Incidence of Food-borne Illnesses—Selected Sites, United States, 1999.

FDA/CFSAN. Progress and Perspective—Food Safety Initiative FY 1999 Annual Report.

Food and Drug Administration. *What Consumers Should Know About Food Additives*. (Leaflet No. 10). Washington, DC.

Longree, Karla. 1996. *Quantity Food Sanitation*, 5th ed. John Wiley and Sons, New York.

Longree, Karla, and Gertrude G. Blaker. 1971. *Sanitary Techniques in Food Service*. John Wiley and Sons, New York.

NASD: Consumer Fact Sheet, "Pesticides and Food Safety."

Potter, Norman N. 1986. *Food Science*, 4th ed. AVI Publishing, Westport, CT.

Public Health Service. 1995. *Food Service Code*. U.S. Government Printing Office, Washington, DC.

———. 1965. *Grade A Pasteurized Milk Ordinance*. U.S. Government Printing Office, Washington, DC.

Tartakow, Jackson, and John H. Vorperian, 1981. *Food-borne & Water-borne Diseases*. AVI Publishing, Westport, CT.

Taylor, R. J. 1980. *Food Additives*. John Wiley and Sons, New York.

12

SHELTER ENVIRONMENTS

Joe Beck

Eastern Kentucky University

....

INTRODUCTION

The way housing is used at the start of the new millennia has evolved significantly; no longer is housing viewed as primary shelter from the elements but increasingly as a place where one goes after work or where we may even work. We now often fulfill our socialization, recreation, and entertainment desires in our new age shelter.

In the past, a person worked all day, came home at night, ate dinner, read awhile, and went to sleep. Today, we have hot tubs, entertainment centers with hundreds of TV channels, high definition flat screen television, and we are capable of calling around the world on our telephones without being constrained by wires. Our homes are sometimes wired with high-speed cable and equipped with state-of-the-art computer systems. Seldom do our

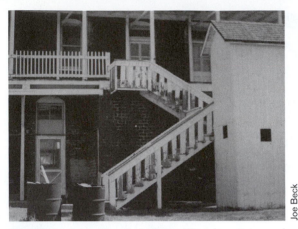

Substandard housing–"when recycling is not a good thing." Two-story pit privy serving four apartment units in central Illinois. Water used for drinking came from dug well 25′ deep 5′ to the left of the outhouse.

Joe Beck

neighborhoods have sidewalks, people no longer sit on their porches and greet their neighbors, and children no longer have the free run of the neighborhood. At the same time we are bewildered that more of our children exhibit antisocial behavior, gain excess weight, watch TV all the time, play with their violent computer games, or lock themselves in their rooms and talk on their cell phones to other children just down the block in their equally wired homes. As these quality-of-life issues impact health they also become a concern for the environmental health professional that is responsible for designing housing codes and other building standards that affect health.

. . . .

THE MODERN HOME

The modern home has a plethora of furnishings that requires both awareness of their hazards and considerable competence and education in their safe operation and maintenance. Examples of these may include home swimming pools, hot tubs, electronic air cleaners, ozone and ion emitting devices, ultraviolet water and air cleaners, microwave cooking devices, cell phones emitting microwave radiation, computers, home theater systems, powerful home

cleaning agents and deodorizers, pesticides, humidifiers, trampolines, power-washers, and highly complex home exercise equipment. The above list is not meant to imply that we all possess all of these items or that all have been named. Each of the above presents potential environmental health hazards if misused and some are not proven safe at this time. The following is a short description of some of the potential problems with their use.

Swimming Pools and Hot Tubs

Their proper operation requires considerable knowledge of water chemistry and the impact of pH on the effectiveness of disinfectants. The hot tubs require an understanding of the impacts of heated liquids on disinfectant and the potential of the warm water to grow bacteria like a warm organic soup. Many of the chemicals used in both pools and hot tubs are highly reactive and potentially explosive.

Electronic Air Filters and Ion Creation Devices

Some electronic air filters have only roughing filters and charcoal as filter media, and present no hazard of significance. Other units create ozone by fracturing the O_2 molecule into **ozone** (O_3). The creation of the ozone is facilitated by either ultraviolet light or a corona discharge process. If inhaled, the ozone can do serious lung damage from tissue exposure to the highly reactive ozone molecule.

Ultraviolet Water and Air Cleaners

Ultraviolet light (UV) is often used to disinfect air, water, and certain types of equipment. The disinfection is provided by the high energy of the ultra blue spectrum of light. This is the same type of radiation that results in most sunburns acquired beside the pool or at the beach. While these devices have a proven track record of reducing viral or bacterial bioload in water and air, they do require routine maintenance. The wavelength of the UV emissions does shift over time and becomes ineffective, and the bulbs attract dust and soil particles due to static charge. The dirty bulbs, if not cleaned, result in reduced effectiveness of the device. Looking at the bulbs can result in serious eye damage.

Microwave Ovens and Cell Phones

Microwave ovens use electromagnetic radiation for the purpose of vibrating the water molecules in food. The vibration of these water molecules results in heat generation that cooks the food. The ovens must be maintained without damage to the seals on the unit to ensure that microwaves do not leak from the unit. While unproven to some scientists, some researchers are concerned that cell phones that use microwaves may prove to impact the brain cells as a result of prolonged exposure.

Microwave radiation impacts tissue by causing the water molecule to move at high speed. The water molecule is dipolar, meaning that one side of the molecule is charged opposite of the other. When this dipolar molecule is placed in a magnetic field that is modulating or shifting, it will cause the water molecule to spin, creating friction with other surfaces. It is this friction that results in the generation of heat and it is that heat that cooks the food or damages tissue.

Computers

The electrical components of computers create extensive electromagnetic fields that can impart static charges to users (transfer of electrons). This charge can result in skin rashes and eye irritation due to allergens in the air being attracted to the exposed charged surfaces of the body.

Ergonomics

Ergonomics is the study of human interactions with equipment or workstations. The relationship of workstations and human health must not be underestimated. The home workstation is often one in which we skimp expenses and as a result may incur tremendous long-term cost. The nature of the computer user is that they often spend many hours in front of a bright screen and use an inadequate desk and chairs that are often improperly adjusted. This can result in major damage to the skeletal structure and considerable eyestrain.

Home Theater Systems

The use of earphones and high technology speaker systems allow even the mature or conservative user to cause permanent damage to their hearing. This happens due to the fatigue of the cochlea cilia and results in temporary threshold hearing loss. This temporary loss results in the user increasing the volume. This increase in volume eventually results in an increased pace of permanent hearing damage. We are now seeing evidence of this damage and expecting to see an entire generation of hearing problems as a result of the lack of understanding of this new technology.

Cleaning Agents, Deodorizers, and Pesticides

Most of the cleaning agents, deodorizers, and pesticides are required by law to be used in accordance with the product labels. Misuse of these products can result in fines or imprisonment and more importantly, damage to both the environment and the humans who come in contact with the materials.

Humidifiers

Humidifiers are used to increase the moisture level of the air of a building. The ideal **humidity** level for homes is 40% to 60%. If the humidity level is below this level, irritation to the skin and nasal membranes can result. Another consequence of low humidity is the buildup of static electricity that can cause damage to electronic devices. Excessive humidity provides an excellent source of moisture for molds and bacteria. The humidifier has been proven to be a powerful breeding and dispersal system for dangerous bacteria and fungi. This discovery requires tremendous care in the routine disinfection of the unit and its use.

Power-Washers

Power-washers present in many homes are used to clean decks, homes, and cars by taking water from the utility and putting it under high pressure by the use of a compressor. These devices can create a major risk by sucking water from the utility and exceeding the flow rate of the utility fixture. This creates a vacuum in the water line with the potential of pulling contamination into the water lines from commonly used items such as pesticide sprayers, chemical tanks, septic tanks, and anything to which a water hose might be connected.

Trampolines and Home Exercise Equipment

Even though we all agree that routine exercise is essential for good health the devices we use can also result in serious risk to both health and life. When trampolines and exercise equipment are used in a gym, supervision is almost always present. When in use at home the user may not be observed and is at serious risk if clothing becomes caught, if falls occur, or if a heart attack occurs.

Don't Eat the Paint

Lead is everywhere around us. Although some lead comes from natural sources, most is caused by human activities. Lead has been used in making batteries, pottery, solder, pesticides, cooking utensils, plumbing, and—what has received so much recent attention—household paint. Another source of lead in the environment has been leaded gasoline.

The amount of lead, even in remote areas such as Greenland, has been increasing since about 800 B.C., when people began mining and using lead. The amount of lead in the environment increased sharply during the Industrial Revolution and even more with the coming of the internal combustion engine. The latter increase occurred because manufacturers began putting lead in gasoline as an antiknock additive.

Lead is one of the oldest known toxic materials. Some historians believed it hastened the fall of the Roman Empire. During the Romans' reign, many people in the ruling class suffered from stillbirths, sterility, and brain damage—attributable, it is believed, to lead poisoning from lead cooking pots, wine vessels, and drinking water that came from waterlines that contained lead. The high concentration of lead found in the bones of some an-

cient Romans support this theory. Probably many house painters, as well as artists such as the Spanish painter Goya, died of lead poisoning. Some painters put the brushes in their mouths to shape them—thus ingesting lead.

Before 1940, lead was used in house paint in the United States. Later, and largely as a result of children ingesting paint, lead poisoning became a national concern. In 1971 the Lead Poisoning Prevention Act was passed, setting permissible levels of lead for paint.

Children are particularly vulnerable to lead poisoning because they are more likely to swallow things that contain lead. Examples are ingesting paint chips and lead-laden dirt, inhaling or eating street dust, color magazines, newspaper, wallpaper, wrapping paper, and snow and icicles containing lead. Also, children may lick their hands after playing in the streets where auto exhaust has deposited lead. Approximately 15,000 children are treated for lead poisoning each year.

Lead is a cumulative poison. Except when exposed to high levels, such as in lead smelters and battery plants, lead usually is excreted from the body in the urine. Small amounts, however, are deposited in bones, replacing calcium. Cortisone therapy can cause a release of lead into the blood at toxic levels. The United States has had the highest levels of lead in the world except Japan—because of automobiles releasing lead into the air. Unleaded gas is alleviating that problem.

Wooden Decks and Playground Equipment

An emerging issue currently deals with the types of preservatives used in wood on outdoor decks, landscaping materials, and playground equipment. Some of these preservatives are powerful toxins such as lead arsenate, creosote, and other pesticides. They may leach from the preserved product and absorb into the ground and/or the skin of an individual coming into contact with the product or ground. This is an area that the consumer should follow as new research emerges that more fully defines the degree of hazard presented by the preservatives.

Electrical Safety

As the availability of consumer appliances has increased over the years, so has the potential risk of accidental electrocution and fire from those appliances increased. Electrical current flows from higher potential to lower potential just as water flows down hill. The trick is to ensure that it does not flow through the human body in the process. Table 12.1 describes the exposure levels of electricity, which may vary dynamically under varied environmental conditions.

We now have televisions and telephones in bathrooms, computers in bedrooms, and electric gadgets of every description and purpose in every room of the house. Even though new homes traditionally have electrical plug-ins every 10 feet, some find that this amount is not enough. Some people will foolishly run extension cords under carpets and throw rugs. This practice is a major risk due to two issues: (1) the cord under the carpet may become damaged and the damage not visible, and (2) the heat from the current flowing through the extension cord may result in decomposition of the cord and result in fire or electrocution.

Electrical wiring in the United States is sized based on the **American Wiring Gauge (AWG)**. The larger the wiring size (AWG) numbers, the smaller the gauge of the wire. AWG 14 wire is only designed to carry 15 amperes safely, AWG 12 is only designed to carry 20 amperes safely, and AWG 10 will safely carry up to 30 amps. It is not difficult to calculate the amperage draw from an appliance, all you must do is use the formula: volts × amperes = watts. Most appliances list the number of watts that they use on their specification plate; the typical line voltage for most small household appliances is 110 volts. Therefore, the manipulation of the formula to watts divided by volts will equal the amperes drawn by the appliance. Because many appliances require more energy to charge their systems a shortcut would be to use the ratio that 100 watts = 1 ampere in a 110-volt system. The volt is typically considered a unit of electrical pressure, the ampere an indication of electrical intensity, and the watt as a unit of power required.

Modern appliances are generally equipped with a cord that has three prongs on the electrical plug. Two of the prongs carry current that moves from higher potential to lower potential. The third prong, typically the round one that is located at the bottom of the plug, is known as the **appliance ground** connection. This appliance ground is intended to ground the conductive sections of the appliance to the house or building ground. This grounding provides a much more efficient way for the electricity to reach ground than through the body in the event that an electrical short circuit occurs in the appliance. While not foolproof, this appliance ground has saved many lives without the benefactor even being aware that they were at risk.

A recent innovation to the improvement of electrical safety, both in and outside of the home, is the **ground fault interrupter**, also known as a **GFI** (Figure 12.1). These devices contain electronic sensing elements that detect very small amounts of leakage of electricity between the two prime conductors. When the difference of electrical flow between the two becomes great enough, an internal switch is thrown in the GFI resulting in the termination of the flow of electricity. These GFIs are now required by most electrical codes to be installed in kitchens, bathrooms, and on outside appliances. These units will sometimes activate from excess moisture in the air but this is a small price to pay for the safety provided by the units. Many people mistakenly believe that the breaker or the fuse box for the home provides protection against life-threatening shock. This is not the case; these are designed to protect the electrical system from overheating that would damage the conductors or result in fire.

■ TABLE 12.1 ■

EXPOSURE LEVELS OF ELECTRICITY

Exposure level	Impact
Less than 1mA	Barely perceptible
1 to 8mA	Strong surprise
8 to 15mA	Unpleasant, victim able to detach
Greater than 15mA	Muscular freeze, victim cannot let go
Greater than 75mA	Usually fatal

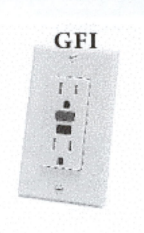

FIGURE 12.1 GFI.

. . . .

HOUSING HISTORY

I hope by now it is obvious that being an effective homeowner increasingly requires considerable education. It is also important to view today's homes in view of their evolution. The following history of housing in the United States has been excerpted from the manual "Basic Housing Inspection" developed in 1976 by the Office of Housing and Urban Renewal and the Centers for Disease Control. The following is a modified part of that history narrative.

Wooden Chimneys

Fire control resulted in some of the first public policies on housing in this country, established during the colonial period. Many of the early houses were constructed with wooden chimneys and thatched roofs. Plymouth Colony, in 1626, passed a law stipulating that new houses should not be thatched but roofed with either board or a similar fire-resistant material. In 1648, in New Amsterdam, chimneys on existing houses were required to be inspected regularly. Charlestown's general assembly in 1740 passed an act that declared that all buildings should be built of brick or stone, that all "tall" wooden houses must be pulled down by 1745, and that the use of wood was to be confined to window frames, shutters, and to exterior work. This law was obviously unenforceable because, as we learn from other publications during that period, more Charlestown houses were made of timber than of brick.

Living in Caves

Social control over housing was exerted in other ways. Early settlers in Pennsylvania frequently dug caves out of the banks of the Delaware River and used these as primitive-type dwellings. Some of these shelters were still in use as late as 1687 when the Provincial Council ordered inhabitants to provide for themselves other habitations, in order to have the said caves or houses destroyed. In some New England communities, around the turn of the 18th century, standards were raised considerably higher by local ordinances. In East Greenwich, it had been the custom to build houses 14 feet square with posts 9 feet high; in 1727 the town voted that houses shall be built 18 feet square with posts 15 feet high with chimneys of stone or brick as before.

Water-Carried Sewage

During the early days of this country, basic sanitation was very poor, primarily because outdoor privies served as the general means of sewage disposal. The principal problems created by the use of these privies involved their nearness to the streets and their easy accessibility to hogs and goats. In 1652, Boston prohibited the building of privies within 12 feet of the street. The Dutch of New Amsterdam in 1657 prohibited the throwing of rubbish and filth into the streets or canal and required the householders to keep the streets clean and orderly.

First Housing Authority

During the early part of the 19th century, the only housing control authority was vested in the fire wardens, whose objective was to prevent fires, and the health wardens, who were charged with the enforcement of general sanitation. In 1867, with the passing of the Tenement Housing Act, New York City began to face the problem of substandard housing. This law represented the first comprehensive legislation of its kind in this country. The principal features of the act are summarized as follows: for every room occupied for sleeping in a tenement or lodging house, if it does not connect directly with the external air, a ventilating or transom window to the neighboring room or hall; a proper fire escape on every tenement or lodging house; the roof to be kept in repair and the stairs to have banisters; water closets or privies—at least one to every twenty occupants for all such houses; after July 1, 1867, permits for occupancy of every cellar not previously occupied as a dwelling; cleansing of every lodging house to the satisfaction of the Board of Health, which is to have access at any time; reporting of all cases of infectious disease to the Board of Health by the owner or his agent; inspection and, if necessary, disinfection of such houses; and vacating buildings found to be out of repair. There were also regulations governing distances between buildings, heights of rooms, and dimensions of windows. The terms "tenement house," "lodging house," and "cellar" were defined.

Although this act had some beneficial influences on overcrowding, sewage disposal, lighting, and ventilation, it did not correct the evils of crowding on lots and did not provide for adequate ventilation for inner rooms. In 1879, a second tenement act, amending the first, was passed adding restrictions on the amount of lot coverage and providing for a window opening of a least 12 square feet in every room. Several attempts in 1882, 1884, and 1895 were made to amend this original act and provide for occupancy standards, but they were relatively unenforceable. While these numerous acts remedied only slightly the serious problems of the tenements, they did show the city's acknowledgment of the problems.

This public acknowledgment, however, was seldom shared by the owners of the tenements, or, in some cases, by the courts. The most famous case, in 1892, involved Trinity Church, at that time one of the largest owners of tenements in New York City. In the case, the city of New York accused Trinity Church of violating provisions of the Act of 1882 by failing to provide running water on every floor of its buildings.

A district court levied a fine of $200 against the church, which in turn appealed to the Court of Common Pleas to have the law set aside as unconstitutional. Incredibly, the court agreed unanimously to uphold the landlord's position, stating "there is no evidence nor can the court judicially know that the presence and distribution of water on the several floors will conduce to the health of the occupants . . . there is no necessity for legislative compulsion on a landlord to distribute water through the stories of his building; since if tenants require it, self-interest and the rivalry of competition are sufficient to secure it . . . now, if it be competent for the legislature to impose an expense upon a landlord in order that tenants be furnished with water in their rooms instead of in the yard or basement, at what point must this police power pause? . . . A conclusion contrary to the present decision would involve the essential principle of that species of socialism under the regime of which the individual disappears and is absorbed by a collective being called the 'state', a principle utterly repugnant to the spirit of our political system and necessarily fatal to our form of liberty." Fortunately, three years later, the city health department was granted an appeal from the court order, and eventually the constitutionality of the law was upheld.

The Battle for Improving Living Conditions

Jacob A. Riis, Lawrence Veiller, and others did much during this period to champion the cause of better living conditions. Their efforts resulted in the Tenement House Act of 1901, a milestone in housing and an extremely comprehensive document for its time. It began with concise definitions of certain terms that were to become important in court actions. It contained provisions for protection from fire, requiring that every tenement erected thereafter, and exceeding 60 feet in height, should be fireproof. In addition, there were specific provisions regarding fire escapes on both new and existing houses. More light and ventilation were required; coverage was restricted to not more than 70% on interior lots and 90% on corner lots. There were special provisions governing rear yards, inner courts, and buildings on the same lot with the tenement house. At least one window of specified dimensions was required for every room, including the bathroom. The minimum size of rooms was specified, as were certain characteristics for public halls. Significantly included were provisions concerning planning for the individual apartments in order to assure privacy. One of the most important provisions of the Tenement Act was the requirement for running water and water closets in each apartment in new tenement houses. Special attention was given to basements and cellars, the law requiring not only that they be damp-proof but also that permits be obtained before they were occupied. One novel section of this act prohibited the use of any part of the building as a house of prostitution.

The basic principles and methodology established in the Tenement Act of 1901 still underlie much of the housing efforts in New York City today. Philadelphia, a city that can be compared with New York from the standpoint of age, was fortunate to have farsighted leaders in its early stage of development. Since 1909, with the establishment of the Philadelphia Housing Association, the city has had almost continual inspection and improvement.

Although Chicago is almost two centuries younger than New York, it enacted housing legislation as early as 1889 and health legislation as early as 1881. Regulations on ventilation, light, drainage, and plumbing of dwellings were put into effect in 1896. Many of the structures, however, were built of wood, were dilapidated, and constituted serious fire hazards.

Before 1892, all government involvement in housing was at a local level. In 1892, however, the federal government passed a resolution authorizing investigation of slum conditions in cities containing 200,000 or more inhabitants. At that time, these included the cities of Baltimore, Boston, Brooklyn, Buffalo, Chicago, Cincinnati, Cleveland, Detroit, Milwaukee, New Orleans, New York, Philadelphia, Pittsburgh, St. Louis, San Francisco, and Washington. Much controversy surrounded the involvement of the federal government in housing. The Commissioner of Labor was forced to write an extensive legal opinion concerning the constitutionality of expenditures by the federal government in this area. The result was that Congress appropriated only $20,000 to cover the expenses of this project. The

lack of funds limited actual investigations to Baltimore, Chicago, New York, and Philadelphia and did not cover housing conditions within these cities. Facts obtained from the investigation were very broad, covering items such as the number of arrests, distributions of males and females, proportion of foreign-born inhabitants, degree of illiteracy, kinds of occupations of the residents, conditions of their health, their earnings, and the number of voters.

The Feds Get Involved in Housing

The 20th century started off rather poorly in the area of housing. No significant housing legislation was passed until 1929 when the New York state legislature passed its Multiple Dwelling Law. This law continued the Tenement Act of New York City but replaced many provisions of the 1901 law with less strict requirements. Other cities and states followed New York State's example and permitted less strict requirements in their codes. This decreased what little emphasis there was in enforcement of building laws so that during the 1920s the cities had worked themselves into a very poor state of housing. Conditions in America declined to such a state by the 1930s that President Franklin D. Roosevelt's shocking report to the people was "that one-third of the nation is ill-fed, ill-housed, and ill-clothed." With this the federal government launched itself extensively into the field of housing. The first federal-housing law was passed in 1934. One of the purposes of this act was to create a sounder mortgage system through the provision of a permanent system of government insurance for residential mortgages. The Federal Housing Administration was created to carry out the objectives of this act.

Many other federal laws followed: the Veterans Administration became involved in guaranteeing of loans, the Home Loan Bank Board, Federal National Mortgage Association, Communities Facilities Administration, Public Housing Administration, and the Public Works Administration. With the U.S. Housing Act of 1937, the federal government entered the area of slum clearance and urban renewal, requiring one slum dwelling to be eliminated for every new unit built under the Federal

Housing Administration program. It was not until the passage of the Housing Act of 1949 that the federal government entered into slum clearance on a comprehensive basis.

The many responsibilities in housing administered by various agencies within the federal government proved to be unwieldy. Hence, in 1966, the Department of Housing and Urban Development was created to have prime responsibilities for the federal government's involvement in the field of housing.

Role of Health Agencies in Housing

Up until the end of World War II, the health departments carried on most local housing hygiene programs. After WW II, health agencies began to drift away from the field of housing hygiene. This gap was filled by a variety of other city agencies including building departments, police departments, fire departments, and more recently created departments of licenses and inspections. Regardless of which department administers the housing code, the health department, if it is to live up to its responsibilities of protecting the public health, must have an involvement in housing. A general statement of public health policy is that the basic responsibility of health agencies, with regard to housing is to see to it that local and state governments take action to ensure that all occupied housing meets minimum public health standards. This basic responsibility falls upon federal, state, and local health agencies alike.

How Government Controls Housing Standards

Several kinds of governmental action are required. These include: (1) adoption of minimum standards in housing, (2) conduct of a program to achieve and maintain these standards, (3) periodic evaluation of the standards to ensure their current adequacy, and (4) monitoring of the standards enforcement effort to guarantee that public health values are provided. Health agencies, in order to meet their responsibilities, must accept the role of either stimulating or carrying out these four required kinds of governmental action.

In communities that have neither standards nor programs, the health agency has the responsibility of initiating both by stimulating the required governmental action. Stimulation may be direct, through elected or appointed officials, or indirect, by generating public support that will trigger official action.

The principal function of a house is to provide protection from the elements. In its current stage, however, our civilization requires that a home not only provide shelter but also privacy, safety, and reasonable protection of our physical and mental health. A living facility that fails to offer these essentials through adequately designed and properly maintained interiors and exteriors cannot be termed "healthful housing."

One of the major global public health concerns of the 20th century is pollution. In simple terms, pollution can be defined as contamination of the environmental air with substances/items that have adverse effects on human health. Shelter and protection against unfavorable elements in the environment are a basic need of humans. Extremes in temperature, ionizing radiation, animals, insects, noise, sunrays, and wind are examples of unfavorable elements in the environment against which humans must be protected. Shelters include private homes, hotels, hospitals, nursing homes, jails, prisons, motels, mobile homes, ships, mental institutions, schools, universities, military bases, camps, and housing for migrant workers and senior citizens. Housing or shelters should minimize the risk of accidents and the spread of disease while keeping humans safe, happy, and productive. The four fundamental needs that housing (shelters) should provide are: (1) fundamental **physiological needs**, (2) fundamental psychological needs, (3) protection from causative agents of disease, and (4) protection against accidents (discussed in Chapter 2).

. . . .

BUILDING STANDARDS

Three primary sets of standards govern housing in the United States. These are building codes, housing codes, and zoning regulations. The building codes regulate the building methods and materials used in construction. The housing codes regulate the way we live in homes and maintain those homes, and the zoning regulations are enforced to ensure that the comprehensive land use plan for the community is followed.

Structural Standards for Housing

These standards are essential to ensure that housing meets minimum standards for safety, protection, and privacy. The person responsible for building code enforcement must be well qualified in build-

ing techniques and familiar with the positive and negative traits of the various types of building materials. Figure 12.2 is an example of those structural elements not visible through the brick or siding of a modern home. Each number represents a structural component of the home. The failure to consider any defect in relationship to the whole structure can result in catastrophic failure of the building. The house must be built on a strong, secure footing that

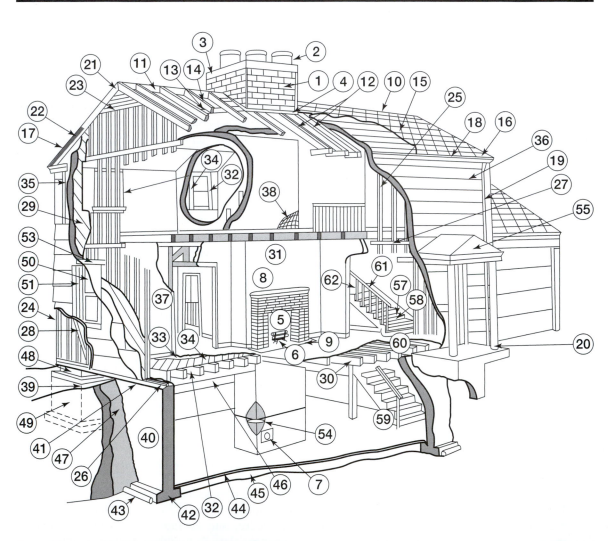

Source: Basic Housing Inspection Manual, CDC 1975.

FIGURE 12.2 Housing structure. The modern home is a complex structure with many interrelated structural elements.

is capable of both bearing the weight of the structure and will not slip or move. Such movements will eventually ruin the building and result in damage that will take from the value or structural safety of the building. These footers must also have drains called **footing drains** to drain away accumulated moisture from the structure. The failure to do so can result in sinking of the foundation, or provide moisture for the development of hazardous life-forms such as molds, fungus and bacteria that could impact the health of the residents. The foundation wall should be equipped with a **termite shield** to provide a first line of defense against these highly destructive pests. The termite shield is nothing more than a piece of copper or similar metal that prevents the termite from burrowing into the wood of the structure from the tunnels they build up the side of the foundation.

How many people who have chimneys realize that the chimney must extend a full 3 feet above the highest point of the house or any structure within 20 feet of the building (Figure 12.3)? This is essential to prevent drafts of air from flowing backwards down the chimney. The back draft can occur due to shifting winds and as a result blow ash, live coals, or toxic gas back into the house with disastrous results to the occupants.

If the chimney is not of sufficient height, the lower edge of the gust of wind will slow due to friction with the surface of the roof or nearby structure and as a result will drag the direction of the wind downward resulting in a downdraft.

Have you ever walked into a home that has been uninhabited for a while and notice the very strong odor of rotten eggs or a sulfurous smell? If so, you have just been taught one of your first plumbing lessons. The smell is probably originating in the sewer of the home and then entering the home through dried out **P traps.** The P traps are the piping below sinks (sometimes called U traps) and lavatories that look like a P lying on its side (see Figure 12.4). The P trap is designed to provide a water seal between the inside of the home and the sewer. There are many reasons to provide this barrier between the sewer and the home but two reasons are critical to the protection of health and prevention of home explosions. Gases are formed in sewers that represent major hazards to

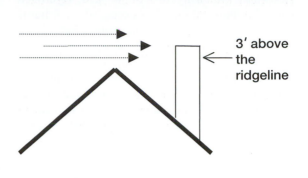

FIGURE 12.3 Desired chimney height above roof of building.

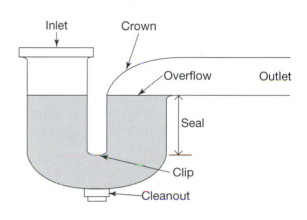

FIGURE 12.4 Diagram of a P trap. The P trap is used in conjunction with proper venting of the waste system to keep harmful material from entering into the home through the use of a water seal. This trap is also called a U trap.

home occupants; sewer gas is made up of explosive methane and hydrogen sulfide gas. Hydrogen sulfide gas is a colorless, extremely poisonous gas that has a very disagreeable odor, much like that of rotten eggs. It is slightly soluble in water and is soluble in carbon disulfide. Dissolved in water, it forms a very weak dibasic acid that is sometimes called hydro sulfuric acid. Hydrogen sulfide is flammable; in an excess of air it burns to form sulfur dioxide and water, but if not enough oxygen is present, it forms elemental sulfur and water. It is formed in the sewer as a result of biological waste decomposition. While the smell is very noticeable at low concentrations, at concentrations high enough to present immediate danger it paralyzes the olfactory epithelium cells (sense of smell) and as a result the human can no longer detect the hazard.

Water-Heating Devices

One of the true conveniences of modern living is the flow of both hot and cold running water to our lavatories, showers, and bathtubs. Like all technology, even this that we take for granted has hidden hazards. Domestic water heaters, when they are appropriately installed, are very safe and reliable and will typically provide about 10 years of trouble-free operation. When it is time to replace them, they tend to be replaced due to major leaks developing in the water-holding tanks. These leaks often develop because we forget that they also need to be serviced and maintained. Murphy's law dictates that these critical elements of our home's infrastructure will fail at the worst possible time, which in my family's case would be a weekend with a large contingent of stay-over guests in the house. It is at these times that our thinking often becomes fuzzy and we become driven by expediency rather than intellect or wisdom. New water heaters are generally sold without a critical safety device called the temperature pressure relief valve (also called the TPR valve or sometimes the T&P). This safety valve is essential for preventing the water heater from turning into an explosive device, which can occur if the sensor for the heating unit fails and results in the heating unit failing to shut off. Such an explosion is certainly life threatening and has been known to level homes to their foundation.

Figure 12.5 shows a typical electric water heater and where the TPR valve is located therein. The TPR valve is a safety device that releases water if the pressure or temperature in the tank reaches

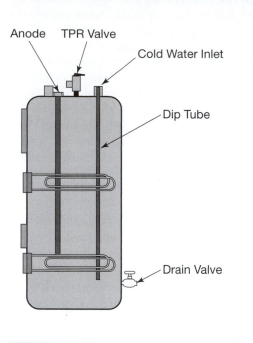

FIGURE 12.5 Home water heater—a potential explosion hazard.

unsafe levels. Located on the TPR valve is a manual release lever. The valve should be tested by periodically lifting the manual release. Failure of the valve may be indicated if water fails to discharge or if the valve continues to leak after the release, indicating a need for replacement. Due to the scalding potential of the discharge from the TPR valve, the outlet from the valve should be piped to a safe area. Figure 12.5 also shows that often the discharge pipe for the TPR valve is forgotten (see drain valve in the lower right). Typically they are piped down to within 6 inches of the floor or even outside of the dwelling at near ground level. Check with your local building department for local building code requirements. Of additional concern is the potential burn hazard from the superheated water produced by water heaters. Scalds can occur much faster than most people recognize and at some surprising water temperatures (Table 12.2).

LENGTH OF TIME FOR HOT WATER TO CAUSE SCALDING

125°F	1½ to 2 minutes
130°F	About 30 seconds
135°F	About 10 seconds
140°F	Less than 5 seconds
145°F	Less than 3 seconds
150°F	About 1 ½ seconds

· · · · · · · · · · · · · · ·

PHYSIOLOGICAL NEEDS

By altering the environment, putting on and taking off clothing, people can live in very cold and very hot environments. The first modern endeavors to alter the environment included opening windows, designing draft systems, and burning wood in fireplaces. Now sophisticated air-conditioning systems have been developed to cool the indoor environment when it is too hot, creating an environment that permits adequate heat loss. In many places the fireplace has been replaced by elaborate, convenient, heating systems that protect the body from undue heat loss. Many people are not aware of the fact that the leading cause of weather-related deaths in the United States is not hurricanes, tornados, or lightning but as a result of heat.

Temperature and Humidity

These systems usually control humidity as well as temperature. Humidity control is important in maintaining a comfortable environment. For example, one might be comfortable in a room that is 78°F (25.5°C) with 50% humidity, whereas with 90% humidity the same room at 78°F (25.5°C) would be uncomfortable. Hence, the American Public Health Association's Committee on the Hygiene of Housing has recommended temperatures and humidity levels. A temperature of 65°F (18.3°C) is recommended for working and sleeping areas. Temperature readings should be made 18 inches (45.7 cm) above floor level. If young chil-dren are playing on the floor, that temperature should be 70°F (21.1°C) at 18 inches (45.7 cm) above the floor. Hot and humid environments cause one to feel sluggish. Dry, cooler environments stimulate people. Low humidity (less than about 20%), however, can cause nosebleeds and chills because the body's mucous linings dry out as a result of loss of moisture to the dry air, which predisposes one to communicable disease. That is why between 40% and 60% humidity is desirable.

VENTILATION

An unventilated room, when occupied by people, will undergo changes. The temperature will increase because the body is exothermic and radiates the excess heat to the environment, thus warming the air. The body loses excess heat by conduction, convection, radiation, and evaporation. If one sits on a block of ice, the body will lose heat as the ice absorbs it. Heat flows from hot to cold. When hot and perspiring, we like to stand in the breeze and lose heat by convection. This is what happens when we create a draft by a fan. The body loses some heat by radiation. When the body cannot lose the excess heat in the above-mentioned ways, we perspire (sweat). If the body does not lose the excess heat, the body temperature will become elevated, with associated problems, and even brain damage in extreme cases. Thus, to exchange air and prevent drafts, air movement is recommended to be less than 500 feet per minute at the dust exit.

Second, an unventilated room will increase in humidity. The body loses moisture by perspiration and by breathing. When air is pulled into the lungs, it picks up moisture. This phenomenon, plus radiated body heat, accounts for a room that was at first comfortable, eventually becoming too warm and humid. It is recommended that a room's air be exchanged every hour.

Third, an unventilated room will retain odors. In food establishments, the main reason for ventilation is to remove food odor. Other changes taking place in an unventilated room may be a decrease in the amount of oxygen and an increase in the amount of carbon dioxide and possibly carbon monoxide, as humans breathe in O_2 and exhale CO_2.

The failure to control both temperature and humidity in a home can result in considerable health risk. Often people fail to replace their water heaters when the warranty expires and they wake up some night or come home from a long trip to discover a flooded home. The damage done to these homes can be at times irresolvable, due to the growth of molds between the walls and other inaccessible areas of the home. The New York City Department of Health, Office of Environmental and Occupational Epidemiology provided the following information concerning **house molds** in a brochure entitled "Facts About Mold," which addresses some of the most common questions and concerns regarding mold.

What is black mold and where is it found?

Mold (fungi) is present everywhere—indoors and outdoors. There are more than 100,000 species of mold. At least 1,000 species of mold are common in the United States. Some of the most commonly found are species of *Cladosporium*, *Penicillium*, and *Aspergillus*. Mold is most likely to grow where there is water or dampness—such as in bathrooms and basements.

How can mold affect your health?

Most types of mold that are routinely encountered are not hazardous to healthy individuals. However, too much exposure to mold may cause or worsen conditions such as asthma, hay fever, or other allergies. The most common symptoms of overexposure are cough, congestion, runny nose, eye irritation, and aggravation of asthma. Depending on the amount of exposure and a person's individual vulnerability, more serious health effects—such as fevers and breathing problems—can occur but are unusual.

How can you be exposed to mold?

When moldy material becomes damaged or disturbed, spores (reproductive bodies similar to seeds) can be released into the air. Exposure can occur if people inhale the spores, directly handle moldy materials, or accidentally ingest it. Also, mold can sometimes produce chemicals called mycotoxins. Mycotoxins may cause illness in people who are sensitive to them or who are exposed to large amounts of them in the air. Large exposures are typically associated with certain occupations (for example, agricultural work).

How does mold grow?

All molds need water to grow. Mold can grow almost anywhere there is water damage, high humidity, or dampness. Most often molds are confined to areas near the source of water. Removing the source of moisture—such as through repairs or dehumidification—is critical to preventing mold growth.

What is *Stachybotrys chartarum*?

Stachybotrys chartarum (also known as *Stachybotrys atra*) is a type of mold that has been associated with health effects in people. It is a greenish-black mold that can grow on materials with a high cellulose content—such as drywall sheetrock, dropped ceiling tiles, and wood—that become chronically moist or water-damaged, due to excessive humidity, water leaks, condensation, or flooding.

How can you tell if *Stachybotrys chartarum* is present in your home?

Many molds are black in appearance but are not *Stachybotrys*. For example, the black mold commonly found between bathroom tiles is not *Stachybotrys*; *Stachybotrys* can be positively identified only by specially trained professionals (for example, mycologists) through a microscopic exam.

How can *Stachybotrys chartarum* affect your health?

Typically, indoor air levels of *Stachybotrys* are low; however, as with other types of mold, at higher levels health effects can occur. These include allergic rhinitis (cold-like symptoms), dermatitis (rashes), sinusitis, conjunctivitis, and aggravation of asthma. Some related symptoms are more general—such as inability to concentrate and fatigue. Usually, symptoms disappear after the contamination is removed.

There has been some evidence linking *Stachybotrys* with pulmonary hemosiderosis in infants who are generally less than six months old. Pulmonary hemosiderosis is an uncommon condition that results from bleeding in the lungs. In studied cases of pulmonary hemosiderosis, the exposure to *Stachybotrys* came from highly contaminated dwellings, where the infants were continually exposed over a long period of time.

What should you do if mold is present in your home or apartment?

Although any visible mold can be sampled by an environmental consultant and/or analyzed by a laboratory specializing in microbiology, these tests can be very expensive—from hundreds to thousands of dollars. There is no simple and cheap way to sample the air in your home to find out what types of mold are present and whether they are airborne. Even if you have your home tested, it is difficult to say at what levels health effects would occur. Therefore, it is more important to get rid of the mold rather than find out more about it. The most effective way to treat mold is to correct underlying water damage and clean the affected area.

How should mold be cleaned?

Mold should be cleaned as soon as it appears. Persons cleaning mold should be free of symptoms and allergies. Small areas of mold should be cleaned using a detergent/soapy solution or an appropriate household cleaner. Gloves should be worn during cleaning. The cleaned area should then be thoroughly dried. Dispose of any sponges or rags used to clean mold.

If the mold returns quickly or spreads, it may indicate an underlying problem such as a leak. Any underlying water problems must be fixed to successfully eliminate mold problems. If mold contamination is extensive, a professional abatement company may need to be consulted.

Will your health or your child's health be affected, and should you see a physician?

If you believe that you or your children have symptoms that you suspect are caused by exposure to mold, you should see a physician. Keep in mind that many symptoms associated with mold exposure may also be caused by many other illnesses. You should tell your physician about the symptoms and about when, how, and for how long you think you or your children were exposed.

FAVORABLE ENVIRONMENT

Protection against unfavorable elements, so as to maintain or enhance health, is necessary in all types of shelters, where creating an environment favorable for habitation is paramount. By favorable environment, we mean adequate space, a safe water supply, approved means of sewage and solid waste disposal, the absence of pests (such as insects and rodents), the absence of excessive noise and ionizing radiation, a favorable thermal environment, a means of protecting the food supply, the absence of indoor and outdoor air pollution, a structural design that will reduce the likelihood of injuries, and the absence of toxic materials.

Proper lighting is a need of humans. If light is insufficient, eyestrain and fatigue may result. Proper lighting can be accomplished by using either natural or artificial lighting. Those who recognize the need for energy conservation advocate the use of natural light and natural ventilation as much as possible.

Protection against excessive noise is another human need. Housing in noisy environments requires soundproofing materials to reduce the noise. Hearing the neighbor's television while you are studying or doing work that requires concentration is annoying. Housing regulations should require soundproofing in all multi-unit dwellings. (Noise is discussed further in Chapter 15.)

Regardless of the type of shelter, whether it is a house or a penal institution, adequate space is a basic physiological need. Opportunities for physical exercise and recreation, for adults and children alike, are essential for physical, mental, and social well-being. In planning shelter environments, the provision of recreational space often is omitted because of cost, shortage of space—and many times a lack of understanding as to the role of exercise and recreation in maintaining health. Housing projects, prisons, nursing homes, schools, day-care centers, and so forth should provide adequate space activity. At least 22 square feet should be provided for each student in a classroom. For physiological and psychological needs, houses should provide at least 10 square feet per person, with one room having at least 150 square feet. To reduce the spread of com-

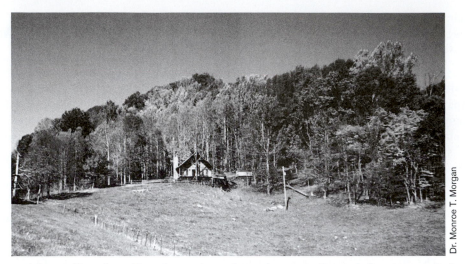

A cabin in the mountains provides a favorable environment away from noise, congestion, and other stress-producing agents.

municable disease, approximately 400 cubic feet of space is needed.

....

FUNDAMENTAL PSYCHOLOGICAL NEEDS

To many people, the word "home" signifies the place where they can isolate themselves from the world. Privacy is a basic need, and adequate housing should provide a means of fulfilling that psychological need. In rural areas this need is not as great, because people can find privacy. In cities, however, the home is a refuge from the noise, tension, crime, and other stress-producing agents of a crowded environment. For psychological and sociological health, housing authorities recommend that a house have a living room where youth can meet and socialize with different age groups and sexes.

Psychiatric opinion holds that children over age 2 years should sleep in a room separate from their parents. The need for privacy in bathrooms and bedrooms is also a psychological and social requirement of housing. It is recommended that only children of the same sex sleep in a bedroom after they reach 8 years of age. Also, most standards are based on no more than two people per bedroom.

Because of the psychological and social values that result from participating in normal community life, family housing should be in a community that permits easy access to basic institutions of culture, commerce, and employment. Community facilities that should be convenient to the home areas include schools, churches, shopping centers, entertainment facilities, libraries, medical care facilities, and recreation facilities. Unfortunately, "normal community life" is not possible in some large, crowded areas that are plagued with problems associated with overcrowding. Drugs and crime force some people to live behind locked doors. Society tries to correct this problem by putting those causing the problem behind the locked doors of prisons.

A psychological as well as physical need for humans is the provision of facilities that will maintain cleanliness of the dwelling and the person. Baths, showers, and lavatories are needed for keeping the body clean. Some shelters have mop sinks, vacuum systems, and other facilities to promote cleaning. These systems require running water and electricity. Some homes, however, do not have electricity and running water; brooms, mops, and standpipes (a water spigot in the yard) are used and water is heated on the stove. In some countries a standpipe serves several homes and a central community shower (bathhouse) fulfills the need for personal cleanliness.

PROTECTION AGAINST CAUSATIVE AGENTS OF DISEASE

Communicable Diseases

Chapter 2 discusses the causative agents of disease. Chapter 3 groups the communicable diseases by their mode of transmission. A potable water supply, as discussed in Chapter 4, should be provided to prevent the spread of water-borne infectious diseases. Plumbing should be constructed to prevent cross-connections where the water supply can be contaminated by sewage, chemicals, or other contaminants. Adequate toilet facilities should be provided to prevent the spread of communicable disease. In areas where, for geological or financial reasons, flush toilets are not available, pit privies may be used. Toilets and privies should be constructed, as discussed in Chapter 6, to prevent the spread of disease by flies, roaches, water, or direct contact.

Another basic need for housing is to exclude vermin from the shelter. Rats and other vermin spread disease, in addition to destroying property, as discussed in Chapter 8. Hence, "building them out" is desirable. This can be accomplished (as described in Chapter 8) by screening doors and windows and using hardware cloth over openings.

Adequate space for each person housed in a facility is necessary to prevent the spread of respiratory diseases. An example would be the sleeping and living space allocated in barracks and dormitories. This translates to more than 6 feet (1.82 m) between the center of adjoining cots or a space of more than 50 square feet (4.64 m) per bed. Approximately 400 cubic feet (1–1.3 m) per occupant in sleeping areas is desirable. If ventilation is inadequate, more space should be provided.

Asbestos

The presence of asbestos is undesirable in shelter environments. **Asbestos** is a mineral mined in much the same way as other minerals. However, asbestos crystals are fiber-shaped rather than crystal-shaped like those of table salt. Three common varieties of asbestos are chrysotile, amosite, and crocidolite. All three varieties are resistant to chemicals, making them popular for a variety of industrial and commercial uses. Asbestos has been used in more than 3,000 products and was first recognized has a major heath hazard in 1840.

The three major health problems associated with asbestos are asbestosis, lung cancer, and mesothelioma. Asbestosis was first recognized in the 1920s, but no maximum allowable concentration for safety was determined. In 1986, the Occupational Safety and Health Administration (OSHA) set the occupational exposure limit at 0.2 fibers per cubic centimeter. Asbestosis-related lung cancer was detected during the 1930s and 1940s, and mesothelioma (a crocidolite and amosite asbestos-related lung disease) was reported in the 1960s.

Exposure to airborne asbestos continues to be a major area of occupational health concern. Material containing asbestos has been used widely for thermal insulation, fireproofing, sound absorbents, and aesthetic purposes. **Friable** materials such as insulation, fireproofing, and decorative materials containing asbestos can endanger employees if they are damaged, exposed, or disturbed in some way. A material is considered friable if it can be crumbled, pulverized, or reduced to a powder by hand. Generating any amount of airborne asbestos is significant because of the serious potential health hazard posed to any person exposed to it. The hazard is long range or chronic and may not manifest itself for as long as 25 to 40 years after exposure.

Generally, the amount of asbestos that may be present in materials used for fireproofing or insulating ranges from 10% to 80% of total dry weight. Friable asbestos insulation can be found in any structure regardless of the year of construction or type of insulation. If asbestos is present, special procedures and precautions must be followed to protect employee health and comply with OSHA and EPA regulations. Regardless of the amount of asbestos-containing materials removed, EPA notification is required. If insulation or other material containing asbestos is damaged, handled, demolished, or removed, appropriate procedures must be followed to ensure adequate employee protection and compliance with government regulations.

Asbestos minerals are classified as one of two groups: serpentine and amphiboles.

1. The *serpentine* group has only one member, chrysotile, which constitutes about 90% of the asbestos used in the United States. Chrysotile comes primarily from Quebec, Canada, but deposits in British Columbia also are a source. Arizona has a deposit that is superior for electrical uses, and chrysotile also has been mined in Vermont and California.

2. The *amphiboles* group has three members of commercial importance: crocidolite, amosite, and anthophyllite. Tremolite and actinolite also are members of the amphiboles group, but these occur primarily as contaminants in other minerals. Although their chemical and physical properties differ, all amphiboles are crystalline, fibrous, and noncombustible. Amosite and crocidolite come primarily from South Africa, although materials from Bolivian sources have been used in the United States. Anthophyllite derives from several deposits in Georgia. Tremolite occurs as an impurity in commercial talc and other minerals.

An important property of asbestos, especially chrysotile, is fiber length. All asbestos is graded by fiber length, depending on the amount passing three screens—half-inch, 4-mesh, and 10-mesh. Chrysotile has the finest fibers and is more flexible so that it can be most easily spun and woven into cloth. The amphiboles minerals differ from one another, but unlike chrysotile, they are all acid-resistant. Although all types of asbestos can cause the lung disease asbestosis, they differ in their ability to cause cancer, particularly mesothelioma. All asbestos varieties are heat-resistant, with a melting point of 1200°F to 1500°F.

Asbestos can be made into weavings, yarn, cloth, tape, and braided tubes. Because of its excellent thermal and electrical resistant properties, asbestos textiles have been used for a diversity of fire- and heat-resistant applications: clothing, welding blankets, high-temperature insulation coverings, and many others.

The largest use of asbestos in tonnage has been in asbestos cement. Because of its superior strength, asbestos cement has been used for roofing, wallboard, drainage pipe, pressure pipe, laboratory hoods, ventilation ducts, and many other products. Although amounts vary, most final products using asbestos cement are only 10% to 25% asbestos. The second most common use of asbestos, after cement, has been in friction products—disk brakes, drum brakes, jaw and band brakes, and dry and oil clutches.

The fibrous mineral nature of asbestos makes it appropriate for sealants and gaskets, and, like other fibrous materials, it can be made into paper. As an electrical resistor, asbestos has been used as roving or braid around electrical wires, as a board in electrical apparatus, and as the strengthening agent in high-pressure laminates. Asbestos used as filler is found in roofing compounds, gasket cement, floor tiles, and plastic products.

In the past, asbestos was mixed with a variety of rubbers to make gasket materials. It has been used as paper, cloth, and raw fiber to form the gaskets and sealants that can be made to resist any material for high-pressure or high-temperature use. For thermal insulation, asbestos has been used as a spray, magnesia block, calcium silicate block, and Marinite. Sprayed asbestos is characterized by its homogeneity, seamless surface adherence to any surface, ability to be formed, and capacity to improve acoustic properties of walls and ceilings.

A special use of crocidolite, anthophyllite, or amosite asbestos was in the acid-resistant construction material Haveg, used for pipes, tanks, valves, reaction vessels, acid towers, and pump housing. It consisted of asbestos with a penthol of furane resin and hardening agent. Virtually all uses of asbestos, of course, are being phased out in the United States.

Carbon Monoxide

Carbon monoxide is a colorless, odorless, tasteless gas produced from the incomplete burning of fuels containing carbon. Exhaust from the internal combustion engine is the principal contemporary anthropogenic source of carbon monoxide. Motor vehicle exhaust falls into this category.

Other man-made sources of carbon monoxide include industrial processes, agricultural burning, fuel combustion in stationary sources, solid waste disposal, and cigarette smoking. Natural sources include volcanic activity, natural occurrence in the ground, and photochemical degradation of certain organic compounds. Rising carbon monoxide levels are undesirable because they affect human health adversely. To explain how carbon monoxide harms health, some basic physiological processes follow.

■ The human respiratory and cardiovascular systems, working together, normally transport oxygen from the atmosphere to the various tissues of the body at a rate sufficient to maintain tissue **metabolism**. Oxygen in ambient air is inhaled into the lungs, where the bloodstream absorbs it. The oxygen becomes bound to the hemoglobin in red blood cells and may be transported from the lungs to the extra-pulmonary tissues.

■ Carbon monoxide harms health by competing with oxygen for binding sites on the hemoglobin molecule. Because the affinity of hemoglobin for carbon monoxide is more than 200 times that for oxygen, carbon monoxide, even at low partial pressures, can impair the transport of oxygen from the blood into body tissues. When the gas combines with hemoglobin, it forms a compound called carboxyhemoglobin, which prevents oxygen from being transported to and utilized by the body's cells.

■ Adverse physiological effects begin at carboxyhemoglobin levels of approximately 2.5%. Exposure to air with 50 ppm of carbon monoxide for 90 minutes, or 15 ppm for 10 hours, is enough to reach this level. Carbon monoxide exposure producing carboxyhemoglobin levels as low as 3% was found to result in adverse effects on complex mental functions such as concentration and memory. Epidemiological evidence also has linked the incidence of myocardial infarction to the concentration of carbon monoxide in the air. The current EPA standard for carbon monoxide is justified mainly on the basis of preventing adverse effects in persons with cardiac and peripheral vascular disease.

■ Manifestations of carbon monoxide poisoning include brain functioning impairment, irregular heart functioning, dizziness, blurred vision, headache, seizures, vomiting, and coma. Skin color of the affected person varies from normal (in more than half of the cases) to flushed, cyanotic (bluish) or cherry-pink. Blisters and bulbous lesions also may occur. After apparent recovery, persistent neurological complications are common. At very high concentrations (such as 1500 ppm for 1 hour), death may occur. Fetuses and the very young are especially susceptible to the toxic effects of carbon monoxide and the resulting lower oxygen saturation.

In treating carbon monoxide exposure, high concentrations of oxygen are administered. This hastens elimination of the carbon monoxide gas from the body. Although outdoor carbon monoxide concentrations are a cause for concern, indoor concentrations may be even more important. Not only does the average person spend most of his or her time indoors, but also high carbon monoxide levels indoors generally are not diffused readily into the atmosphere. Most buildings today have been weatherproofed, or sealed tightly. These buildings do not allow adequate air exchange between the indoor and outdoor environments. In attempting to make homes and other buildings energy-efficient, we may be exposing ourselves to dangerous levels of carbon monoxide, as well as other pollutants.

Some possible sources of indoor carbon monoxide production are cooking appliances such as gas stoves, space heaters, furnaces, fireplaces, wood-burning stoves, and cigarette smoking. An inadequate supply of air for combustion—that which occurs in "airtight" wood-burning stoves and improperly maintained gas stoves and gas and oil furnaces—greatly increases the rate of carbon monoxide emission. If set wrong, flues and dampers restrict the flow of carbon monoxide and other combustion products to the outside, causing a potentially harmful buildup indoors.

Two types of indoor environments that are more likely to have higher than normal carbon monoxide concentrations are (a) indoor garages and buildings with attached indoor parking areas, and (b) residences with improperly ventilated space-heating equipment. These settings often maintain carbon monoxide concentrations as high as 100 ppm. Cigarette smoking also can produce high concentrations of carbon monoxide. Mainstream cigarette smoke contains up to 40% carbon monoxide.

Because of the potential for serious health problems resulting from carbon monoxide exposure, measures should be taken to decrease indoor levels. One method to stabilize indoor carbon monoxide levels is to remove the source of contamination. Preferably, the garage is separated from the house. Combustion appliances can be replaced with cleaner devices that perform the same function. For example, electric appliances or solar heating systems can be used in place of combustion appliances such as gas stoves. A source may be altered by a change in design. An example of this is using an electric ignition rather than a gas pilot light in gas stoves. Spatial confinement also may be utilized to decrease carbon monoxide exposure in a home. This can be accomplished by placing combustion appliances in isolated rooms. Oil and gas combustion heating units may be placed outside of the house. Timing the production of contaminants to periods of non-occupancy also reduces carbon monoxide exposure.

One simple and effective method of decreasing carbon monoxide exposure is to avoid cigarette smoke—not to smoke and to stay away from those who are smoking. People are justified in not allowing smoking in their home and insisting on the separation of smokers and nonsmokers in their place of employment. Most businesses and public agencies now have smoking policies.

Ventilation or general air exchange between inside and outside air is another uncomplicated method of reducing indoor carbon monoxide levels. A local ventilation device such as a simple exhaust fan can be used for combustion appliances. The general public is largely unaware of the dangers of carbon monoxide exposure, especially indoor concentrations. People need to be educated as to what produces carbon monoxide within their own homes and how to prevent dangerous levels from forming. Regulation of combustion appliances, such as gas stoves and kerosene heaters, is helpful, but they must be properly installed and maintained to prevent them from becoming health hazards. CO detectors might be used in sleeping areas of shelter environments.

The two main factors that could help us all breathe a little easier are increased public education and enforcement of regulations (such as building codes and consumer-product requirements).

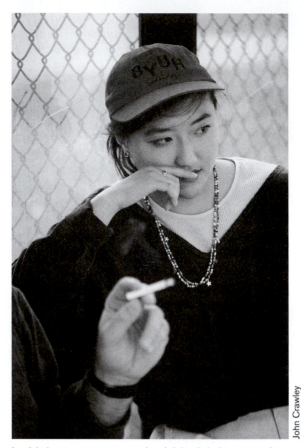

John Crawley

Legislation to protect nonsmokers' rights is being stepped up.

•••••••••••••••

SICK BUILDING SYNDROME

Of the air most individuals breathe, 80% to 90% is indoor air. The air, sometimes clean, sometimes polluted, is modified in composition because of confinement. With the onset of the energy crisis in the 1970s, buildings (commercial, nonresidential, and residential) in advanced countries were constructed to be energy-efficient with less air exchange between them and their surroundings. Among the problems that arose in these buildings as a result of this energy-efficient mindset were:

- Retention of higher temperatures
- Higher humidity levels
- Decreased ventilation
- Increased odor retention

The advent of higher temperatures and increased humidity levels in buildings gave birth to the proliferation of microorganisms in indoor environments. In addition, certain synthetic materials used to construct the buildings, as well as some furnishings, were found to produce volatile organic compounds, all of which have adverse effects on human health. These factors have created indoor air pollution, a term used interchangeably with the term adverse indoor air quality.

The EPA estimates that indoor air pollutants cause 6,000 cancer deaths each year. This estimate may be a reason for indoor pollution-control ballooning into a billion-dollar-a-year business. The average holding time for airborne substances is of the utmost importance in indoor pollution. The air in a room must be exchanged with an open atmosphere via open doors, windows, a variety of leaks, and by ventilating fans and ducts. Exchange is measured by the time required for full replacement of air. Half an hour to 5 hours is the average turnover time for residential buildings. Houses built by conventional standards show values of 50 to 100 minutes, excluding conditions created by unusual winds or extreme contrasts in temperature. Larger buildings have required forced ventilation by design.

An ancient source of particulate additions to indoor air was *combustion*. Today, most combustion products are vented directly outdoors by way of a chimney or hood. Cigarettes produce high levels of indoor air pollutants and emit in excess of 300 toxic gases.

A study done in India of the typical kitchen with a housewife or cook demonstrated particulate concentrations more than two dozen times the U.S. open-air standard for 24-hour exposure. Even the most inefficient natural-gas stove is less noxious than that. Direct analysis of even a small sample of houses displays wide sources of contamination. Vapors and degradation products result from pesticides used to preserve wood structure, organic sprays, and solvents. The concentrations of these organic air contaminants are low but appear to be higher in summer than in winter. This finding is contrary to the belief that open windows and doors (in the summer season) are effec-

tive in decreasing the concentrations because of more circulation and outside air transfer. The higher vapor pressures and higher reaction rates of warm weather more than offset the better summer ventilation.

Fatal lung cancer incidents are rising in direct relation to smoking. The factor is a 10% to 12% increase among pack-a-day smokers. The effect of smoke on nonsmokers has yet to be established. One research study showed that a couple of smokers in a modest room could raise particulate counts close to or beyond the legal standards for outside air. Another study showed that Boston children and adult French women who lived in a household among smokers had a poorer measured lung function than those who did not. Other studies of nonsmoking women married to heavy smokers, showed a doubling of the rate of lung cancer in these populations.

Air pollution, biological hazards, and toxic chemicals, if not ventilated properly, contribute to many maladies suffered by workers in new and old office buildings. The World Health Organization has estimated that as many as 30% of new and old renovated office buildings emit various toxic substances.

Volatile organic compounds (VOCs) can be found in the air of new buildings in concentrations as much as 100 times higher than those found outdoors, and they can remain elevated for 6 months after construction. Pollutants classified as VOCs

---

SYMPTOMS COMMONLY ASSOCIATED WITH SICK-BUILDING SYNDROME INCLUDE:

- Headaches
- Fatigue
- Nausea
- Nosebleeds
- Nasal congestion
- Difficulty breathing
- Dry skin
- Irritability
- Flu-like symptoms

Source: Medical Laboratory Observer, 1996

are found in cleaning solvents, glue, and paint. (Outdoor sources of VOCs include automobile exhaust and vapors from engine refueling.) In a study conducted by the EPA, the most common VOCs were benzene, toluene, chloroform, acetone, styrene, and ethylene oxide. The 1982 study was prompted by increasing reports and complaints of **sick building syndrome** (Table 12.3).

Fifty building materials were studied for emission of one or more target chemicals. The highest emitters were molding and carpet adhesives, latex caulks and paints, and vinyl rubber moldings. Proper ventilation systems can control the emission of these particulates. Heating, ventilation, and air-conditioning (HVAC) systems often are linked to respiratory ailments and complaints when they do not function consistently. The systems, sometimes invaded by mold, mildew, and bacteria, must be serviced and cleaned to maintain function. Other particulates include airborne fibers from common fabrics such as cotton, wool, nylon, and rayon.

Sick building syndrome is not created solely by the structure itself but, for the most part, from the activities of its occupants. Sources of sick building syndrome include tobacco smoke, use of appliances, power equipment, equipment chemicals, bacteria and other organisms in the air, wear and tear of structural materials, radon, chemicals in building material, and intrusion of outside chemicals. These sources, many of which are inevitable, magnify a problem when there is improper ventilation. National Institute of Occupational Safety and Health research studies indicate that about 50% of all sick building syndrome problems are the result of inadequate ventilation. Consequently, the first step in rectifying the phenomenon is to check the ventilation system and proceed accordingly.

Most indoor pollutants are invisible and odorless. They tend to be emitted at low levels, which make them hard to track down. Once the culprit is identified, however, the remedy is usually straightforward. Remedies include cleaning ventilation systems, replacing carpets, and replacing and segregating office machines in a single, well-ventilated room. If the problem comes from the outside, outdoor air-intake ducts may be moved away.

INFECTIOUS DISEASES TRANSMITTED VIA INDOOR AIR

Opportunistic Obligate Pathogens

Bacterial
Anthrax
Brucellosis
Legionella sp.
Legionnaire's disease
Pontiac fever
Pseudomonas sp.
Streptococcal pneumonia
Tuberculosis

Viral
Common cold
Chicken pox (Varicella)
Influenza
Herpes
Shingles (Zoster)
Measles
Rubella
Hantavirus
Aspergillosis
Cryptococcosis

Fungal
Blastomycosis
Candida sp.
Coccidioidomycosis
Histoplasmosis
Mucormycosis
Phycomycosis

Protozoal
Cryptosporidiosis
Pneumocystis
Pneumonia

Source: Medical Laboratory Observer, 1996

Formaldehyde

Formaldehyde is a gas with a pungent smell that is water-soluble and colorless at room temperature. Frequently it is marketed in the form of an aqueous solution labeled "formalin." Formaldehyde has a wide variety of industrial uses. It often is used in the manufacture of plastics and resins, photographic chemicals, paints and glue, rubber, synthetic textiles,

■ TABLE 12.3 ■

EXAMPLES OF BUILDING-RELATED ILLNESSES

Disease	Cause
Pontiac Fever An acute, self-limited, febrile, nonpneumonic illness with an incubation period of 36 hours. Attack rate: 90%–100%	*Legionella sp.* (bacteria)
Legionnaire's Disease Life-threatening bronchopneumonia with an incubation period of 2 to 10 days. Attack rate: 5%–10%	*Legionella pneumophila* (bacteria)
Hypersensitivity Pneumonitis Acute extrinsic alveolitis. Chronic form may have characteristics of an interstitial fibrotic pneumonitis. Genetics may influence attack rate.	Fungi, bacteria, organic dust, organic chemicals, aerosolized protein, etc.
Humidifier Fever A type of hypersensitivity pneumonitis characterized by an acute febrile attack accompanied by malaise, cough, and dyspnea. Chronic form is called humidifier lung. Genetics may influence attack rate.	Fungi, bacteria, protozoa, microbial endotoxins, mycotoxins, arthropods.

Source: Medical Laboratory Observer, 1996

explosives, and various types of building materials and insulation. Formaldehyde is a component of cigarette smoke, automobile exhaust, diesel exhaust, photochemical smog, and out-gases from some urea foam insulation, particleboard, and other building materials. The average person may come into contact with these quite frequently.

The extensive use and presence of formaldehyde in everyday occupational, recreational, and domestic activity has received quite a bit of attention recently because of its irritant effect on the respiratory tract, eyes, and exposed skin surfaces. Much concern has been raised over the potential carcinogenic effects of formaldehyde, as well as its effects on actual lung function and neurological changes. The most common complaints of people frequently exposed to formaldehyde or formalin are:

■ Irritation of the upper airway

■ Burning of eyes and nasal passages

■ Skin irritation and rashes

■ Chronic bronchitis

■ Shortness of breath

In addition, depression, headache, chest tightness, nausea, irritability, memory dysfunction, and anorexia have been linked to prolonged exposure to formaldehyde. In many instances where lung function tests have been performed in direct association with formaldehyde exposure, a slight decrease in lung function has been found with short-term, acute exposure, which usually is transient in nature. A much more significant decrease is found with prolonged, repeated exposure. This, too, usually can be reversed with absence of exposure for several weeks. Carcinogenic effects, particularly nasal cancer, are being studied.

Various occupations with high exposure rates to formaldehyde or formalin include hair stylists, wood workers, workers in plants producing acid-curing paints, workers in an industry producing phenol-formaldehyde-plastic components of fiberglass, histology technicians, and funeral service workers. People living in homes insulated with urea formaldehyde foam also are at high risk.

A 1980 study examined the effect of formaldehyde on workers in a wood product manufacturing plant that produced kitchen cabinets coated with veneer that was glued on with a urea resin. The hardening process and subsequent processes released formaldehyde, to which employees were directly exposed. Researchers measured exposure, studied lung functions, conducted spirometric tests, and interviewed workers. (The researchers used a control group of nonexposed workers in whom factors such as smoking and age were taken into account.) The study established a dose-response relationship. Slight impairment of lung function, as well as upper airway and mucous membrane irritation, occurred after only one 8-hour shift, but the effects were transient. A 5-year follow-up study of these same exposed workers revealed a significant decrease in lung function that would reverse itself after 4 weeks of nonexposure.

Complaints of histology technicians at hospitals in Los Angeles and a request for inquiry into the effect of solvents and fixatives used in their laboratories led to a study involving 76 women who were histology technicians in hospitals and laboratories in that city. Researchers used a control group of the same number of clerical workers and secretaries in the same hospitals. The researchers studied the effect of formaldehyde and xylene exposures on respiratory and neurobehavioral symptoms. They found that disturbances of memory, mood, equilibrium, and sleep occurred simultaneously with headache and indigestion. The women working in histology who were exposed daily to xylene, toluene, and other agents incurred irritation of eyes, upper airway, and trachea much more often.

Studies done to determine the effect of residing in homes insulated with urea formaldehyde showed results similar to those done in industrial settings. The most significant symptoms by the homeowners were eye irritation, upper airway irritation, headaches, depression, and skin rashes. Lower airway and lung function impairment showed a correlation. A dose-response relationship was demonstrated. The support for a causal relationship between impaired health and living in urea-formaldehyde foam-insulated residence

was established to be moderately strong. The demonstrated adverse effects, however, were considered to be generally minor in nature.

In 1987, EPA classified formaldehyde as a "probable human carcinogen" under conditions of unusually high or prolonged exposure. The International Agency for Research on Cancer also concluded that formaldehyde is a probable human carcinogen. The OSHA and EPA concluded that new rules governing exposure limits were necessary. In November 1987, OSHA proposed that the occupational standard for formaldehyde exposure be reduced from 3 parts per million (ppm) to 1 ppm, averaged over an 8-hour workday; this proposal became law the following month. In May 1992, the law was amended, and the formaldehyde exposure limit was reduced to 0.75 ppm.

The EPA was created many years ago to serve the United States as a controller of outdoor air pollution. Today, the concern of greater import is indoor air pollution, which studies have shown can be many times the acceptable level of its outdoor counterpart.

The average white-collar worker may be exposed to benzene from cleaning solutions, toluene from rubber-cement solvent, ozone from copying machines, hydrocarbons from typewriter correction fluids and copy papers, bacteria and fungi from ventilation systems, and insecticides. Most office workers have no reaction to these substances, but as many as 10% could be chemically sensitive. The symptoms can be mild and flu like or debilitating, respiratory attacks.

Radon

Radon is a colorless, odorless, tasteless, naturally occurring radioactive gas that is a product of uranium decay. Uranium tends to concentrate in rock formations and deposits such as granites and shale. When these rocks are heated in the presence of a liquid, the uranium flows with the liquid until it cools. This accounts for the widespread distribution of uranium soils and rocks across the United States. When uranium begins to decay, it gives off a lower atomic weight radioactive element—radon gas. Because radon is a gas, it tends to enter the atmosphere. It rises from the soil beneath buildings and enters these structures through their foundations. The gas is still radioactive when it enters the building. Radon remains radioactive until it decays in a sequence that includes a number of radionuclides, finally reaching a stable isotope of lead. Before becoming stable, radon decays to radioactive particulate substances that attach themselves to particulate matter in the air. These combined particles, if inhaled, concentrate in the lungs, where they become inactive isotopes of lead, which can lead to lung cancer.

Radon emits alpha particles, which are more damaging biologically than beta particles or gamma radiation. Therefore, the risk of cancer increases in the presence of radon. Radon tops the list of indoor hazards, along with accidents from falls and fires. Because radon occurs naturally, it also is considered more dangerous than asbestos, pesticides, and other pollutants. The EPA has estimated that 20,000 deaths have been caused by radon. Radon tends to be more lethal to men than to women, and also more lethal to smokers than to nonsmokers. Many scientists believe that smoke-damaged respiratory tracts cannot clear the alpha particles effectively, permitting longer time for the cells to be exposed to the carcinogen. According to Jacob Fabrikant of the University of California at Berkeley, a person who spends 12 hours a day in the presence of excess radon levels increases his or her risk of lung cancer by 50%.

Radon is more dangerous indoors than outdoors because diffusion within the air dilutes outdoor radon. Outdoor radon measures approximately 0.2 picocuries per liter of air. Outdoor levels vary widely depending on geographical location (and thus geology), permeability of the soil, energy-efficiency of the building, presence of a water well, and the use of stone building materials. The EPA has set a guideline for indoor radon levels at 4 picocuries per liter. An estimated 8 million homes in the United States have radon levels high enough above the guideline to cause lung cancer.

The radon rising from the earth tends to be pulled into the house because of less pressure inside the home. This vacuum action is stronger when the house is more energy-efficient and lacks ventilation. The most effective way to reduce this vacuum is to reverse the airflow. Drilling through the basement floor and installing a system to diffuse the air away from the house can achieve this. This system costs up to $2,500 plus electricity to operate the system. Cheaper methods include sealing walls and floors, which should be tried first.

Radon concentrations usually are highest in the basement, attic, and closed-in places with little ventilation. Radon also rises with groundwater tables. Therefore, if the water supply originates from a well, the gas may enter through the plumbing, causing a high concentration in closed-in shower stalls.

TESTING

Radon concentration in the home is about 60% higher, on the average, in the winter when windows and doors are likely to be closed. Therefore, when testing for radon, the test kit should be set up in one of these potentially high-concentration areas, and testing should be done in winter.

The EPA recommends that all homes be tested. If radon levels exceed 20 picocuries per liter, the test should be repeated. One of the most common tests is the alpha track detector. Alpha radiation is given off as radon breaks down. These alpha particles etch tracks across the film in the test kit. The radon level is determined by counting the marks left on the film, which is done professionally. Another common test involves use of a charcoal canister. In this test, the alpha particles are absorbed by the activated charcoal and then analyzed by professionals to determine radon levels. Reliable tests usually require 2 to 3 days. The EPA warns consumers to beware of test kit vendors who promise quick results.

PREVENTIVE MEASURES

If the test results show a high level of radon, preventive measures should be taken. These include sealing cracks in the foundation and walls, increasing ventilation by opening a window or installing vents, installing a fan to create cross-ventilation, and putting in gas drains. If these measures do not decrease the radon levels to within desired limits, a more sophisticated system may be installed to diffuse the gas away from the house.

INSTITUTIONAL ENVIRONMENTS

Environmental health plays an increasingly prominent role in the institutional environment. These environments include, but are not limited to health care, day care, nursing homes, research, educational, jail, and correctional facilities. The person responsible for environmental health in institutions must plan, provide oversight, and develop solutions for conditions that may result in biological, chemical, or physical threats to the well being of workers, patients, and guests of the facilities. Infections occurring in such facilities are referred to as **nosocomial** in nature. This means that they have been contracted in-house. The institutional environmental health officer must be able to integrate knowledge to recommend improvements, maintain, or improve the following:

- Potable water supplies, including in-house treatment systems for hardness and purification
- Lead poisoning control, monitoring, and prevention
- Food management, transportation, storage, preparation, personal hygiene
- Solid, hazardous, infective, and radioactive waste management and disposal
- Biohazard safety, blood-borne pathogen control, and infection control techniques
- Engineered systems such as water treatment, anesthesia gases, storage, ventilation, fire control, and plumbing
- Structural issues that threaten health and safety
- Laundry
- Central supply
- Equipment and supply storage, decontamination, and reuse
- Universal body fluid protection standards
- Occupational health and industrial hygiene
- Hazardous chemical and material management
- Quality assurance and TQM systems
- Radiological material management
- Noise and sound stress management

What Institutions Have in Common

The unique and difficult nature of institutional environmental health is in part due to the lack of specific standards for the various types of institutions and the extreme latitude of discretion of interpretation of any standards that do exist. It is logical that infections occur with greater frequency in health care institutions than those that do not deal with individuals with compromised health conditions and weakened biological immunity. The four factors that must guide the decision-making processes of the institutional environmental health professional are as follows:

- Current best practice and legal compliance.
- The susceptibility to disease of the population served by the institution.
- The numerous potential routes of disease transmission and the degree of biological invasiveness of those routes.
- The quality of potential exposure of the institutional dependent and the workers of the institution to disease, chemical, or injury-causing elements.

Clean vs. Sanitary

When talking to health care workers the words clean, sanitary, and sterile have very specific meanings. **Clean** is a term that refers to the visual state of a surface; it has no apparent material adhering to its visible surfaces. The term **sanitary** is used to define a relative state of contamination generally considered to be safe. The term **sterile** is used to define the total absence of life forms or active virus particles. It is very difficult to achieve a sterile surface and is typically achieved by the use of a combination of heat, pressure, and steam and for surfaces that cannot be heated, ethylene oxide (ETO) gas is used. **Ethylene oxide** is a powerful carcinogen, mutagen, and a teratogen; therefore, it must be used with extreme caution in the health care environment.

Antisepsis is a term used to describe the use of a chemical agent applied to tissue for the purpose of reducing infective agents to a level not capable of causing infection. Pasteurization is a term that describes the use of heat for the purpose of disinfecting food and other such materials taken by mouth. It is generally used on things such as milk, fruit juices, and other such food products rather than inanimate objects.

Microbiostasis is a term that describes the act of preventing microbial growth. This is often attempted though the use of chemical agents or toxic metals. The term fomites applies to inanimate objects such as soap, tissue, and other such objects that have the potential of being a carrier of infectious agents.

The **general principles of** (chemical) **disinfection** can be summarized as follows:

1. Concentration of disinfectant
2. Type and number of microbial agents present
3. Cleanliness of the surface
4. Time allowed for contact of the disinfectant with the surface
5. Temperature of the surface and agent
6. pH of the surface and other chemical influences on the disinfectant

Before a surface can be disinfected or sterilized a surface must be first cleaned. If not cleaned first the contaminating materials may provide a protective surface for the life forms we are seeking to kill. In achieving this state a sterile surface is extremely difficult and seldom maintained for long.

Common classes of disinfectants include but are not limited to the following materials:

Alcohol	Best used at concentrations between 70%–90% and also used as an antiseptic.
Chlorine	Best used for a disinfectant at concentrations between 4% and 5%.
Iodine	Used as both a disinfectant and as an antiseptic, does stain surfaces.
Phenolics	Used as a disinfectant on smooth hard surfaces, can be toxic and corrosive.
Quaternary ammonium compounds	Currently one of the more popular classes of disinfectants, generally not corrosive or irritating to tissue. They also often have strong odor reduction properties.

Universal Precautions

In 1991, the Occupational Safety and Health Administration (OSHA) in collaboration with the Centers for Disease Control (CDC) issued regulations designed to protect health care workers from occupational exposure to and infection from blood-borne pathogens. These regulations require that employers have a Hepatitis B Virus (HBV) vaccination and post-exposure follow-up program for all employees who anticipate contact with blood or fluids requiring universal precautions. Specific HBV post-exposure guidelines are covered in a separate document (Hepatitis B Immunization Program, CDC Occupational Health Clinic). If the source fluid is known to be infected with HIV, or needs to be evaluated for that possibility, this document provides the protocol that should be followed. Because post-exposure use of zidovudine is a consideration that requires prompt action, employees who handle blood or any specimens requiring universal precautions should be familiar with this protocol. The post-exposure period is not the optimal time to first consider the use of zidovudine.

To expedite the appropriate procedures following an occupational exposure to HIV, supervisors and employees should be familiar with the actions outlined in this document for exposures during duty hours and nonduty hours. Ideally, the employee should immediately notify the supervisor (or someone who can act on behalf of the supervisor), who should accompany the employee to the clinic as quickly as possible. The employee should move expeditiously to the clinic, even if there is no one to accompany him/her.

BASIC PRINCIPLES OF A SOUND UNIVERSAL PRECAUTIONS PROGRAM

Universal precautions are intended to prevent infection by the following routes:

1. Parental (e.g., inoculation)
2. Mucous membrane (e.g., splash onto mouth)
3. Conjunctival (e.g., spray into eye)
4. Non-intact skin (e.g., contamination of cut on hand)

Precautions must be applied to all persons being treated to protect workers from known and unknown blood-borne pathogens in persons under their care. The main principles are:

1. Handwashing after any contamination of hands
2. Care of intact normal skin
3. Protection of damaged skin by covering with a waterproof dressing or by gloves
4. Proper handling and disposal of sharps
5. Good hygiene practices to prevent most infections

There must be containment of all blood and body fluids, that is, confining spills, splashes, and contamination of the environment and workers to the smallest amount possible.

Each workplace must ensure that appropriate and adequate equipment (such as gloves and aprons) is available at strategic points. Employee education and training in prevention measures should be carried out and standard operating procedures developed for all activities having the potential for exposure. Supervision has an important role in maintaining procedures and employees have a duty to follow the agreed procedures.

Research and Health-Care Facilities

These institutions, due to their specific nature of activity in controlling or researching the nature of disease causing organisms, present significant risk to the workers, patients and communities in which they are located. In order to mitigate these risks, the Centers for Disease Control has established levels and standards of operation for controlling what can be high-risk factors. The four levels are as follows:

BIOHAZARD LEVELS

1. Not known to cause disease in healthy adults.
2. Associated with human disease, hazard from auto-inoculation, ingestion, mucous membrane exposure.
3. Indigenous or exotic agents with potential for aerosol transmission, disease may have serious or lethal consequences.
4. Dangerous/exotic agents that pose a high risk of life-threatening disease, aerosol-transmitted lab infections, or related agents with unknown risk of transmission.

Detention and Correctional Institutions

The typical American correctional facility is often in a state of stress resulting from underfunding, overcrowding, or a confused mission. The mission confusion is due to the ambiguity about whether its prime purpose of the facility is to be detention, punishment, or rehabilitation, or for the accomplishment of all three. The person responsible for environmental health and safety needs to understand the differences between the various types of correctional facilities. They range from juvenile, work release, halfway houses, county jails, state farms, state prisons, to the many different types of federal prisons. There are many variations of facilities contained in even those limited categories. The facilities must be viewed from three separate and distinct perspectives—that of the prisoner, the public, and the correctional workers. The safety and health concerns of all three must be balanced. We must recognize the safety and health issues related to the prisoners' contact with other prisoners as well, for they are in an extremely hazardous, high-risk environment. Key issues range from industrial hygiene (hazards in the work environment) to sanitation. The conditions of the facilities vary due to the age and societal values under which they were constructed. Society often moves from states of compassion to anger in the way that they desire that prisoners should be managed. The environmental health officer and the correctional staff must be the buffer to such public temperament shifts based on the best long-range needs of society.

Critical Concerns When Doing Jail and Correctional Facility Inspections

- Written policies and procedures on prisoners with special health needs are identified and maintained.
- Written policies and procedures that ensure a prisoner's health is protected during periods of lockdown or for the protection of prisoners with specific behavior modification techniques.
- Written policies and procedures to protect the health care rights of prisoners in the detention facilities.
- Protocols for ensuring personal hygiene for prisoners.

- Arrangements for the issuance, maintenance, and disinfecting of bedding, linen, clothing, and pillows.

- Procedures for controlling pediculosis and other insect infestations.

- The cells must provide ample floor space (ACA requirements) per prisoner to reduce respiratory disease contagion.

- Cleaning and shop materials that can be made into explosives or propellants must be carefully controlled.

- Work areas must be monitored for radiation, air pollutants, and other safety hazards, and the inmates must be trained in safety techniques.

Other Public Facilities of Environmental Health Interest

The environmental health professional must design and conduct inspections and investigations of a variety of public institutions including: multi-purpose and community buildings, bingo, casinos, tanning salons, cosmetology salons, tattoo parlors, and massage clinics, to name just a few. Culture-based fads, such as skin piercing, tanning and tattooing, have increased in popularity in recent years. With the increased awareness of the health impacts of exposure to chemicals, the potential of transmission of bloodborne disease, and the cancer risk of ultraviolet light (UV radiation) exposure, strategies must be developed to protect the health of the public.

One major example of hidden risk is the case of formaldehyde. This chemical was discussed earlier in this chapter as an indoor air pollutant in housing. A little recognized source of the chemical formaldehyde is from cosmetics found in the many products used within barbershops and cosmetology salons. These products range from many shampoos, lotions, coloring agents, and disinfectants to the materials used to construct the facility. The presence of high levels of moisture and the use of non-moisture-retardant construction materials increase the natural release of these agents from the plywood, particleboard, and certain types of insulation. The level of formaldehyde sometimes approaches critical levels, capable of causing serious respiratory damage in both patrons and workers of barbershops and cosmetology salons.

Tattoo and Body Piercing Facilities

The skin of the human body is an intricately designed barrier designed to protect the organs of the body from deadly infections. It can be argued that any unnecessary penetrations of the body should be avoided due to the potential of compromising this elaborately designed defense system, but if history is any indication, such arguments will be lost to individual desire and the unnecessary risk will be taken. The regulation of such facilities should be undertaken with extreme care and viewed as any surgical procedure interims of infection control. At minimum, aseptic control techniques for tattooing or body piercing should be followed, and they include:

- Appropriate use of sterile gloves
- Proper handwashing techniques
- Processes for disinfection of equipment
- Acceptable environmental conditions for process
- Minimal training needed for process
- Appropriate use of Universal Body Fluid Precautions measure

SUMMARY

The advent of higher temperatures and increased humidity levels in buildings gave birth to the proliferation of microorganisms in indoor environments. Also, certain synthetic materials used in building construction and furniture were found to have organic compounds with adverse effects on health by creating indoor air pollution.

Houses should be designed to allow for fundamental physiological needs such as advantageous lighting, ventilation, soundproofing, and space, as well as psychologically enhancing features such as privacy and proximity to community facilities. The control of communicable diseases is a major goal of housing design and maintenance. Some chemical and physical agents of disease are in the earth or in the building material. Pollutants that have been addressed specifically through legislation and testing procedures include asbestos, carbon monoxide, and lead.

KEY TERMS

Antisepsis, p. 224

American Wiring Gauge (AWG), p. 203

Appliance ground, p. 203

Asbestos, p. 215

Biohazard levels, p. 226

Carbon monoxide, p. 216

Clean, p. 224

Ergonomics, p. 201

Ethylene oxide, p. 224

Friable, p. 215

Footing drain, p. 209

General Principles of Disinfection, p. 225

Ground fault interrupter (GFI), p. 203

House molds, p. 212

Humidity, p. 201

Lead, p. 202

Microbiostasis, p. 225

Metabolism, p. 217

Nosocomial, p. 224

Ozone, p. 200

Physiological needs, p. 207

P trap, p. 209

Sanitary, p. 224

Sterile, p. 225

Sick building syndrome, p. 220

Termite shield, p. 209

Ultraviolet light, p. 200

Volatile organic compounds (VOCs), p. 219

REFERENCES

Am. Ind. Hyg. Association Tech. Committee on Indoor Environmental Quality. 1993. *The Industrial Hygienist's Guide to Indoor Air Quality Investigations*, ed. P. J. Rafferty, Am. Ind. Hyg. Association, Fairfax, VA.

American Public Health Association. 1954. *Basic Principles of Healthful Housing*. New York.

American Society of Heating, Refrigerating and Air-Conditioning Engineers. 1989. "Ventilation for Acceptable Indoor Air Quality." ASHRAE Standard 62–1989, Atlanta.

Apter, A., A. Bracker, M. Hodgson, J. Sidman, and W. Y. Leung. 1994. "Overview: Epidemiology of the Sick Building Syndrome." *Journal of Allergy Clinics Immunology*, 94(2):277–88.

Batterman, S. A. and H. Burge. 1995. "HVAC Systems as Emissions Sources Affecting Indoor Air Quality: Critical Review." *HVAC & Refrig. Res.* 1, no. 1:61–80.

Beck, J. E., and Joseph Salvato. 1994. *Environmental Health and Engineering, New Tools for Engineers and Environmental Health Specialists*. Wiley and Sons.

Beck, J.E., et. al. 2000. "Environmental Health Specialist, REHS/RS Study Guide." National Environmental Health Association/National Assessment Institute, 2nd ed.

Blum, Steven. 2000. "Pesticides in Urban Housing." *Journal of Housing and Community Development*. 52, no. 5(Sept–Oct): 38.

Bond, R., G.Michaelsen, and R. DeRoos. *Environmental Health and Safety in Health-Care Facilities*, Macmillan Publishing Company, New York, 55–56.

Brief, R. S., and T. Bernath. 1988. "Indoor Pollution: Guidelines for Prevention and Control of Microbiological Respiratory Hazards Associated with Air-Conditioning and Ventilation Systems." *Appl. Indus. Hyg.* 3, no. 3:5–10.

Burge, H. A., and M. E. Hoyer. 1990. "Indoor Air Quality." *Appl. Occup. Env't. Hyg.* 5 no. 2:84–93.

Clayton, G., and F. Clayton. 1978. *Patty's Industrial Hygiene and Toxicology*. John Wiley and Sons, New York.

Godish, T. 1995. *Sick Buildings: Definition, Diagnosis and Mitigation*. Lewis Publishers, Boca Raton, FL.

Greene, Robert E., and Philip Williams. 1996, October. "Indoor Air Quality Investigation Protocols." *Journal of Environmental Health*. 59, no. 3.

Hansen, S. J. 1991. *Managing Indoor Air Quality*. Failmont Press, Lilburn, GA.

Hicks, J. B. 1984. "Tight Building Syndrome: When Work Makes You Sick." *Occupational Safety & Health*. 53, no. 1:51–56.

Jones, J. R. 1994. *Solving Indoor Air Quality Problems: The Work Environment*, Vol. 3, ed. D.J. Hansen. Lewis Publishers, Boca Raton, FL.

Kohuth, Barbara, and Boyd Mansh. 1974. *An Education Guide for Planning an Improved Human Environment*. Inner Circle Press, Hudson, OH.

Kreiss, K. 1989. "Epidemiology of Building-Related Complaints and Illness." *Occup. Med.* 4, no. 4:575–592.

Lane, C. A., J. E. Woods, and T. A. Bosman. 1989. "Indoor Air Quality Procedure for Sick and Healthy Buildings." *ASHRAEJ* 31, no. 7:48–52.

Light, E. N., and N. Presant. 1994. "Investigation of Indoor Air Quality Complaints." *Immunol. Aller. Clinics N. Am.* 14, no. 3:659–678.

Lippy, B. E., and R. W. Turner. 1991. "Complex Mixtures in Industrial Workspaces: Lessons for Indoor Air Quality Evaluations." *Environmental Health Perspective*. 95:81–93.

Mariso, L. 1994. "Cleaning the Air: IAQ Emerges as a Major Health Issue of the 90's." *The Synergist*. 5, no. 10:8–9.

Melius, J., K. Wallingford, R. Keenlyside, and J. Carpenter. 1984. "Indoor Air Quality: The NIOSH Experience." *Annals Am. Conf. Gov't. Ind. Hyg.* 10:3–7.

Mobile Home Manufacturers Association. 1960. *Mobile Home Park Sanitation*.

Morey, P. R., M. J. Hodgson, W. G. Sorenson, G. J. Kullman, W. W. Rhodes, and G. S. Visvesvara. 1984. "Environmental Studies in Moldy Office Buildings: Biological Agents, Sources and Preventive Measures." *Annals Am. Conf. Gov't. Indus. Hyg.* 10:21–35.

National Safety Council. 1983. *Fundamentals of Industrial Hygiene*, Chicago.

New York City Department of Health, Office of Environmental and Occupational Epidemiology. Brochure–Facts About Mold.

Passon, Theodore Jr., James W. Brown, and Seth Mante. 1996, July. "Sick-Building Syndrome and Building-Related Illness." *Medical Laboratory Observer* 28, no. 7.

Public Health Service. *Environmental Engineering for the School*. Government Printing Office, Washington, DC.

Quinlan, P., J. M. Macher, L. E. Alevantis, and J. E. Cone. 1989. "Protocol for the Comprehensive Evaluation of Building-Associated Illness." *Occup. Med: State of the Art Rev.* 4, no. 4:771–779.

Salvato, Joseph A. 1992. *Environmental Engineering and Sanitation*, 4th ed. John Wiley and Sons, New York. 1241–1247.

Tamblyn, B. T., and S. Khandekar. 1994. "IAQ: An Operation and Maintenance Perspective." *ASHRAEJ.* 36, no. 7:37–42.

U.S. Public Health Service, Centers for Disease Control. "Universal Blood and Body Fluid Precautions," *MMWR* 38:26–36.

U.S. Environmental Protection Agency. 1991. *Building Air Quality* (EPA/400/1–91/003). Washington, DC.

U.S. Public Health Service. 1976. *Basic Housing Inspection*. Government Printing Office, Washington, DC.

13

ENVIRONMENTAL SAFETY

Trenton G. Davis, Dr.P.H.

East Carolina University

OBJECTIVES

- Understand the magnitude of the accident problem.
- Recognize the historical basis for environmental safety programs.
- Identify the major accident hazards in homes, recreational activities, and transportation.
- Identify major federal laws that relate to environmental safety programs.
- Discuss what individuals can do to prevent accidents.

Injuries continue to constitute a significant public health problem in the United States. Compounding the problem, safety and accident prevention programs tend to be underfunded in relation to the magnitude of the impact of injuries on public health, and safety programs generally do not have the same level of public support as many other public and environmental health programs. The public seems complacent when ranking the importance of injuries, possibly because the risk of injury often is accepted as a voluntary one for which the hazards are known.

Another factor may have to do with the public's perception of accidents as being random events over which they have no control. Most people do not understand that injuries are preventable. Injuries are considered to be accidents, and the term "accidents" implies that these events are not pre-dictable or preventable. To the contrary, research has shown that injuries are just as predictable and preventable as illnesses such as mumps, heart attacks, and lung cancer.

One example of the predictability and preventability of injuries that has been studied in some detail centers on motor vehicle injuries. One of the most important determinants of motor vehicle injury is driving after drinking alcohol. Drivers who have been drinking are much more likely to be involved in crashes than drivers who have not been drinking. Because people who drink and drive are more likely to do this at night and on weekends, more motor vehicle injuries occur at night and on weekends. If people could be prevented from drinking and driving, the motor vehicle injury death rate might be cut in half. Therefore, motor vehicle injuries are preventable. By getting drunk drivers off the road, the roads could be made safer for all drivers.

This way of thinking about injuries is not very different from the way we think about preventing measles or polio by immunizing children. Although preventing drinking and driving may not be as easy as giving immunizations, it is no less important.

Injuries may be intentional or unintentional. Intentional injuries include homicide, assault, suicide, child abuse, rape, and other acts of violence. Unintentional injuries are those that frequently are referred to as accidental injuries because they do not involve someone attempting to inflict harm on another person. This chapter focuses on unintentional injuries that occur outside of workplace environments.

For years, the category of **unintentional injuries** has been the leading cause of death in the United States for individuals between the ages of 1 and 34 and the fourth leading cause of death overall. Cancer is the leading cause of death for individuals between the ages of 35 and 64, while heart disease is the leading killer for individuals 65 years of age and older.

More than 60 million Americans incur nonfatal injuries each year. Nonfatal injuries are those usually defined as being severe enough to cause a person to seek medical treatment or to be unable to perform usual activity for a day or longer.

Another way to consider the magnitude of injury mortality is to review data pertaining to **years of potential life lost (YPLL)** published by the Centers for Disease Control and Prevention, National Center for Health Statistics. YPLL before 65 is a measure of mortality that reflects deaths occurring before age 65. In 1988, unintentional injury was the leading cause of YPLL before age 65, accounting for 2,319,400 years of life lost, or 18.9% of the total years of potential life lost. This is followed by cancer at all sites (14.7%), diseases of the heart (11.9%), suicide and homicide (11.1%), and congenital anomalies (5.5%). YPLL before age 65 caused by AIDS has become a leading cause of years of potential life lost, especially in some age groups, and may impact the leading causes of YPLL in the near future.

Over the years, many investigators have contributed to greater understanding of injury causation and prevention. In 1961, J. J. Gibbons observed that all injury events involve the harmful effects of only five agents, which are all forms of physical energy:

1. Kinetic or mechanical energy
2. Chemical energy
3. Electricity
4. Radiation
5. Thermal energy

Injury thus is physical damage to the body that results when energy is transferred to the body in amounts greater than it can withstand, such as fires or poisons, or when the body is deprived of sufficient energy, such as oxygen or heat. Because the absence of needed energy also may lead to physical damage to the body, drowning is considered to be an injury, as is suffocation. Any number of events potentially can transfer energy to the body. All of the human and environmental components thought previously to be the agents of injuries now are recognized as either vehicles or vectors—enabling factors for the real agents.

John E. Gordon wrote, in 1948, that application of **epidemiology** techniques was an appropriate way to increase understanding of the causes of injury, and thus prevent or reduce accidents. He suggested that injuries involve much more than the agent; rather, they involve a combination of forces from at least three sources: the host, the agent, and the environment in which host and agent find themselves. Strategies to prevent injuries can be directed at any of the three factors.

Table 13.1 gives specific injury prevention strategies directed at the host, the agent of energy exchange, and the environment, for the three leading causes of unintentional childhood injury death in North Carolina.

In 1963, William Haddon, Jr. divided the injury event into three phases. During the pre-injury or pre-event phase, the energy source goes out of control. In the injury phase, the amount of energy released and the nature of its transfer to tissues de-

■ **TABLE 13.1** ■

PREVENTION STRATEGIES FOR MOTOR-VEHICLE INJURIES, FIRES, AND DROWNINGS

	Host	Agent	Environment
Motor-vehicle injuries	Persuade people to use seatbelts and child safety seats	Provides safety features such as airbags in automobiles	Modify roadways to include features such as guardrails, adequate lighting, and separate areas for cars, bicycles, and pedestrians
House fires	Teach families to develop and practice escape	Mandate fire-safe cigarettes (cigarettes that are less likely to ignite house fires)	Provide smoke detectors to alert household members of a fire
Drownings	Teach parents never to leave children unattended in the presence of water	Put child-resistant latches on toilet seats to prevent curious toddlers from falling in	Build fences around swimming pools, with self-closing and self-latching gates

Source: Saving Children's Lives: Preventing Childhood Injuries by J. D. Moore and L. W. Gardner, North Carolina Public Health Forum, 1994, Vol. 3, No. 1, p. 14.

■ **TABLE 13.2** ■

INJURY CONTROL STRATEGIES, BY RELATIONSHIP TO EVENT

Relationship to Event	Purpose of Strategies	Examples	
		Drowning	**Intentional Self-Poisoning**
Pre-event phase	To prevent events that may cause injuries	Four-sided fencing for pools	Diagnosing and treating depression
Event phase	To prevent injury when event occurs	Personal flotation devices	Limiting total amount of medication prescribed
Post-event phase	To prevent unnecessary severity or disability when an injury has occurred	Cardiopulmonary resuscitation	Removing toxic substance from the body by dialysis

Source: Saving Children: A Guide to Injury Prevention by M. H. Wilson, S. P. Baker, S. P. Teret, and J. Garbarino. Oxford University Press, 1991.

termine whether injury occurs and its severity. Finally, during the post-injury or post-event phase, personal homeostatic mechanisms and external factors, including the timing, quantity, and quality of emergency and rehabilitative care, contribute largely to the final outcome. Definition of the three phases made it evident that an injury event is not a simple occurrence in which a harmful outcome can be avoided by preventing the initial event. Strategies to prevent injuries can be directed toward preventing events that may cause injury (pre-event phase strategies); or toward protecting individuals against injury if a mishap occurs (event phase strategies); or toward minimizing the consequences following an injury through prompt and skilled emergency services and medical care. Table 13.2

In 1937, a drug manufacturer decided that the best way to capitalize on the popularity of the new sulfa drugs was to market them in a liquid, nonprescription form. He developed a product called Elixir Sulfanilamide, which combined a sulfa compound with diethylene glycol—a commercial solvent used in making antifreeze and brake fluid. Because the drug control laws of the time did not require safety testing, the manufacturer was free to put the product on the market, and he did so—with devastating results. Although only 2,000 pints of the elixir were produced and only 93 were consumed, 107 people died from effects of the solvent.

indicates how strategies from all three phases can be used to control selected injuries.

. . . .

CONSUMER PRODUCT SAFETY COMMISSION

In 1972, the U.S. Congress passed the Consumer Product Safety Act, which created the Consumer Product Safety Commission (CPSC) because "an unacceptable number of consumer products which present an unreasonable risk of injury are distributed in commerce." Before then, thousands of products intended for use by consumers were not regulated by any agency. These products were responsible for more than 20 million injuries in the United States each year in and around the home, more than 30,000 of which resulted in death.

The Consumer Product Safety Act authorizes the CPSC to ban hazardous consumer products, to initiate recalls for products that pose imminent or substantial hazards to the public, and to establish mandatory performance standards and warning and instruction requirements for consumer products. The act requires that a mandatory safety standard be "reasonably necessary to prevent or reduce an unreasonable risk of injury associated with such products." The CPSC also is responsible for administering and enforcing the Federal Hazardous Substances Act, the Poisoning Prevention Packaging Act, the Flammable Fabrics Act, the Refrigerator Safety Act, and the Child Protection and Toy Safety Act.

The CPSC was granted broad authority to issue and enforce standards over more than 10,000 consumer products—from toasters to cribs to lawn mowers. Exempted from the CPSC's authority are firearms, food, drugs, cosmetics, economic poisons, airplanes, motor vehicles, and boats, as they are covered by other regulatory agencies. The CPSC's overall contribution to a safer America has been positive. Consumer product standards have been established for a variety of products including children's sleepwear, bicycles, baby cribs, power mowers, matchbooks, swimming pool slides, and toys with small parts. Age restrictions have been applied to toys with sharp points. Warning labels and instructions have been required for items where misuse would be particularly harmful. And some extreme hazardous sources of injury, such as unstable refuse bins, flammable contact adhesives, and materials containing free-form asbestos, have been banned.

A study published in 1981 showed that in the 9 years after the CPSC came into existence, accidental household injuries fell more than 2.5 times faster than they did in the 9 years previous to the CPSC. Through the use of a **National Electronic Injury Surveillance System (NEISS)**, the CPSC has improved the state of knowledge of product-injury epidemiology and identified the most dangerous consumer products. The system monitors admissions to selected hospital emergency rooms daily for injuries involving consumer products. Then the CPSC supplements the emergency room data by conducting on-site investigations, after which a hazard index of product categories is published.

Bicycles had the dubious distinction of heading the first list as the consumer product that seemed to pose the greatest threat of injury to the American public. Today, bicycles rank low in the category of sports and recreational equipment because of widespread use of reflective devices to improve the visibility of bicycles at night, and the increased use of helmets by riders. Although accidents involving bicycles continue to occur, the severity has decreased.

In recent years, the effectiveness of the CPSC to function on behalf of the public has been questioned. The Commission's budget has been cut drastically, and the number of highly experienced technical specialists on staff has been reduced significantly. The number of reporting hospitals in the NEISS has been cut in half, thereby weakening the CPSC's major data-gathering activity. Finally, the CPSC has virtually ceased to promulgate regulations or to impose hazardous product bans. One can only wonder whether the public is now being adequately protected from consumer products that present an unreasonable risk of injury.

The CPSC is not the only agency that has responsibility for programs designed to reduce or prevent injuries. At the federal level, the U.S. Department of Transportation and the Division of Injury Control within the Centers for Disease Control and Prevention are involved in activities to develop a coordinated national injury agenda. At the level of state government, injury prevention activities are sponsored by a number of agencies including state health agencies. At the local level, many health departments have taken the lead in developing safety programs in their communities. Many nonprofit agencies and citizen groups, including the National Safety Council, are important contributors to efforts to prevent injuries.

. . . .

HOME SAFETY

Someone once wrote, "Your home may be your castle, but the enemy is not entirely outside the walls"—a thought-provoking statement, as more accidents occur in and around the home than in any other place.

To verify that the home is a hazardous place, one simply has to review annual statistics on home accidents. A home accident is defined as one that occurs on home premises to members of the family or invited guests. Excluded are individuals who are on home premises during the course of gainful employment, such as repair persons, postal workers, delivery persons, and the like.

A major portion of one's life is spent in and around the home setting. Young children spend nearly 90% of their time in home settings. As children enter school, they spend less and less time in the home environment. During the working years, the amount of time spent at home stabilizes, and with ensuing age, most people spend more of their nonworking hours in the home. In retirement, most people have gone full circle and again spend 90% of

their time at home. This means that the youngest and oldest members of our population are at greater risk from home accidents, in part because of the greater number of hours of exposure in home environments.

Falls

Falls are the leading cause of accidental death in the home, outpacing burns and all other causes combined. Among the elderly and children, falls top the home unintentional injuries list. In 1996 alone, over 14,000 deaths were attributed to falls. Approximately 42% of falls that result in death are attributed to stairs and steps. Falling out of bed accounts for 10% of falls, while ladders account for 9%. Only 4% of falls involve playing sports.

CHILDREN

In children, falls occur under a wide variety of circumstances, but the risk of death or permanent impairment is related strongly to the height of the fall and the nature of the material struck. Falls from windows—an especially serious problem during the summer among children younger than 5—increase in severity as the height of the window and the hardness of the surface increase. Falls from second-story windows usually are not fatal unless the child lands on concrete or other hard surface.

Many falls from children's furniture occur. Each year some 9,000 injuries are related to cribs, 8,000 to highchairs, and 22,000 to bunk beds. For each of these products, the majority of injuries are caused by falls. Children also fall from bassinets and shopping carts. Most falls down stairs do not have serious consequences, partly because the fall is broken by each step the child lands on. In contrast, when an infant in a baby walker falls down stairs, the fall may be unbroken until the bottom, in which case death or permanent brain injury can result, especially if the floor is concrete.

Many of the serious childhood injuries occurring on stairs are related to walkers. In 1991, of the 27,000 injuries to children up to 15 months of age that were related to baby walkers, 92% were to the head or face. Some experts suggest that because walkers are of no known developmental benefit, their use should be discouraged.

In the case of falls on the same level, sharp corners on furniture, glass coffee tables, and broken glass in play areas are some of the sources of injury.

Caregivers must be vigilant in their supervision of young children and anticipate that the young are interested in exploring their world and are highly active. Efforts must be made to remove hazards in their environment that may increase the risk of injury from falls.

OLDER ADULTS

Unlike fall victims who are children, older fall victims are much more likely to die from falls. Falls are the leading cause of injury or death for individuals over 65 years of age. The difference is that older individuals are unable to absorb as much physical trauma as the young. Children are more resilient and more readily able to recover from injury.

The death rate from falls among the elderly aged 75 and older is nearly 12 times greater than the rate for all other ages combined. The risk of hospitalization is nearly seven times as great.

Visual acuity and depth perception may be seriously diminished with aging. Physical responses become slower, and balance and coordination are impacted adversely to the extent that older adults may not be able to react quickly enough when they commence to fall or slip. The widespread use of drugs and medications by older adults has been associated with increased incidents of dizziness, loss of coordination, and falls.

PREVENTING FALLS

Stairways are the site of more than 750,000 fall injuries each year. Factors involved in these accidents include obscured vision, poor lighting conditions, obstacles on stairs, and slippery tread surface. To reduce accidental falls involving stairways, stairs should be well lighted, handrails should be provided, the height of steps should be no greater than 8.25 inches, tread width should be at least 10 inches, stairways should not be used as storage areas, and stair coverings should be composed of slip-resistant materials.

Falls also occur on floors and walkways and in bathtubs and showers. Efforts must be made to prevent conditions that may lead to slippery floors and walkways. Older adults must be especially cautious in bathrooms—one of the most hazardous areas in the home.

Although not as numerous as stairway accidents or falls on level surfaces, falls from ladders account for more than 100,000 injuries yearly. Falls from ladders can be reduced by selecting the proper ladder for the intended use and then using the ladder properly.

Fire and Burn Injuries

Despite continuing efforts to prevent injuries and deaths from fires and burns, fire still kills about 4,000 people in the United States annually—an average of 11 per day. This is one of the highest fatality rates in the industrialized world.

Fire kills disproportionately. People who are black, poor, old, or very young are two to three times more likely to die in fires than the national average. Most residential fires occur during December through March, a period of colder weather and longer darkness. Residential fires constitute the third leading cause of injury deaths (after motor vehicle–related injuries) of children aged 1 to 14 years and the sixth leading cause of such deaths in persons aged 65 years and older.

In 1991, 48% of fire deaths occurred during January, February, March, and December. The three leading causes of deaths of children younger than 5 years, were:

1. Children playing with fire-ignition sources, such as matches (37%)
2. Faulty or misused heating devices (19%)
3. Faulty or misused electrical distribution sources (11%)

For persons older than 70 years, the three leading causes were:

1. Careless smoking (33%)
2. Faulty or misused heating devices (19%)
3. Faulty or misused electrical distribution sources (12%).

Despite the 37% decline in rates of residential fire-related deaths from 1970 through 1991, the overall rate in 1991 (1.5 per 100,000 persons) exceeded the rate targeted by a national health objective for the year 2000 (reducing the rate of residential fire-related deaths to no more than 1.2 deaths per 100,000 persons). In particular, the rates for children younger than age 5 (3.7 per 100,000 children) and for persons age 65 and older (3.5 per 100,000)—the highest-risk groups—exceeded the age-group specific target goal of 3.3 per 100,000 for each group.

The increased occurrence of fire-related deaths during winter months reflects the seasonal use of portable heaters, fireplaces, chimneys, and Christmas trees. Fires associated with electrical portable heaters usually result from electrical shortages or device failures rather than from ignition of nearby materials such as draperies. Electrical cords for portable electric space heaters should be plugged directly into the wall and not linked through an extension cord, kept at least 3 feet from any combustible material, and unplugged when not in use. Fires attributed to the use of kerosene portable heaters usually result from using the wrong fuel, faulty switches and valves, and fuel leaks and spills that subsequently ignite. Kerosene heaters should be used only with K-1 kerosene, rather than gasoline or camp-stove fuel, and should be refueled outdoors after the heater has cooled. Chimney fires usually result from the buildup of creosote, a highly flammable by-product of wood fires. Chimneys should be cleaned or inspected annually to detect and prevent creosote buildup. A fire screen should be used in front of the fireplace. Wood stoves and fireplaces should burn only seasoned wood, not green wood, trash, or wrapping paper.

Fires related to Christmas trees usually result from electrical problems, such as overloaded electrical circuits caused by using several extension cords in one outlet, or frayed wire and cords. In 1991, of the four leading causes of residential fires, Christmas trees accounted for the lowest number of fires but a substantially higher proportion of deaths than the other types of residential fires. People in households with electric holiday decorations should examine the electric lights periodically and should not place trees near heating sources or fireplaces. In addition, live cut trees should be watered sufficiently to reduce drying.

To reduce the risk of death or injury resulting from fires, a smoke detector should be installed outside each sleeping area on every habitable level of a home, and the battery should be changed at least annually. Occupants should develop escape plans that include identifying two exits from every living area and should practice exit drills and meeting at a designated safe location sufficiently distant from the home. In addition, every home should have a multipurpose fire extinguisher conveniently available for use in extinguishing small fires. If a fire cannot be extinguished within 1 minute, the residence should be evacuated because of the rapid rate of accumulation of heat and toxic gases.

Children playing with fire-ignition sources were the leading cause of fires resulting in the deaths of children younger than 5 years. Therefore, children should be taught not to play with matches or lighters and these items should be stored out of the reach of young children.

Scalding rarely is a cause of death, but it is important because of its high incidence in young children and elderly adults. Hot tap water, coffee, and tea are the most common agents, and boiling water is the most damaging. Scalds occurring when children upset containers of hot liquid often affect the face and hands.

Tap water scalds can be reduced by setting thermostats on water heaters at a temperature no higher than 120°F in all residences and institutional dwellings. Water heated to 140°F can cause third-degree burns in only 2 seconds. Unfortunately, many water heaters are set at this temperature. When the water temperature is turned down to 120°, the same burn takes 5 minutes to occur.

Poisoning

In 1961, poisoning claimed the lives of 450 children under the age of 5. By 1989, that number had dropped to 42. This reduction in the age group at greatest risk is attributable to several factors including child-resistant packaging, better emergency care, more poison-control centers, reformation of some poisonous substances such as lead paint, reduced use of other substances such as kerosene, and parental education.

Despite the progress in reducing the number of deaths from poisoning, nonfatal poisonings still occur in a substantial number of children. Estimates indicate that for every death from poisoning in children younger than age 5, some 80,000 to 90,000 children will go to an emergency room for treatment, and approximately 20,000 will have to be hospitalized.

The substances that children ingest most commonly are aspirin, solvents and petroleum products, tranquilizers, and iron compounds. The highest rates are seen in children about 1 to 2 years of age; boys are at slightly higher risk than girls. Other substances ingested frequently include personal care products such as shaving cream, deodorants, bath oils, nail polish, and pediatric cough syrup.

A study by the CPSC revealed that 23% of oral prescription drugs ingested by children under age 5 belonged to someone who did not live with the children. Overall, 17% of the drugs ingested belonged to a grandparent or great-grandparent. Education of parents, grandparents, babysitters, day-care providers, and teachers is imperative if the accidental poisoning rates are to decrease significantly.

Parents and other caregivers must carefully assess the poisoning hazards in homes where young children live and take action to childproof those environments. The American Academy of Pediatrics offers the following recommendations:

- First and foremost, store household products and medicines out of reach of children, and use safety latches on all drawers and cupboards that contain potentially harmful substances.

- Keep products in their original containers. Never put products that can be poisonous in old food or beverage containers.

- Never call medicine "candy."

- Have syrup of ipecac available at home, and use it to induce vomiting if a child ingests a poisonous substance.

- Keep poison control and other emergency phone numbers near the telephone, and call immediately in an emergency.

- Leave original labels on all products.

- Clean out medicine cabinets periodically and discard unneeded and dated medications in a safe manner.

A number of poisonous plants found in and around the home are capable of causing severe itching, burning, and swelling of skin tissues on contact, or nausea and vomiting if ingested. These plants include poison ivy, mushrooms, azalea, oleander, dieffenbachia, rhododendron, and poinsettia. Parents and other caregivers should be knowledgeable about these and other poisonous plants and take the necessary precautions to protect children from accidental exposure.

Firearm Injuries

From 1968 through 1999, firearm-related deaths increased by 60% (from 23,875 to 38,317). Based on these trends, by the year 2003, the number of firearm-related deaths will surpass the number of motor vehicle–related deaths and firearms will become the leading cause of injury-related death. Firearm injuries usually have been divided into homicides, suicides, and unintentional shootings. This separation has masked the severity of the firearm problem as a major killer of children and young adults. In 1988, gunshot wounds were the eighth leading cause of unintentional injury deaths in all age groups in the United States and the third leading cause among children and teenagers aged 10 to 19 years. For males aged 10 to 19 years, the unintentional firearm-related death rate is seven to ten times that for females. Males aged 15 to 19 years are at higher risk than are males in any other age group. Children and teenagers living in the southern region of the country are at highest risk for dying from an unintentional gunshot wound; those living in the Northeast are at lowest risk. Within regions, white males aged 15 to 19 years are at greatest risk in the South; in all other regions, deaths are highest for black male teenagers. Overall, children and teens living in nonmetropolitan regions are more than twice as likely to die from an unintentional gunshot wound as those living in metropolitan areas.

The apparent intent of the shooter in firearm deaths varies with the age of the victim. At ages 0 to 4 the majority of firearm fatalities are homicides. At ages 5 to 9, most of firearm deaths are unintentional. At ages 10 to 14, deaths from guns are almost evenly divided among suicides, homicides, and unintentional shootings. For persons aged 15 and above, suicides and homicides are most commonly the intent.

A multifaceted approach to reduce firearm-related injuries should include at least three elements.

1. Foster changes in behavior through campaigns to educate and inform persons about the risks and benefits of possessing firearms and the safe use and storage of firearms.

2. Direct legislative efforts toward preventing access to or acquiring firearms by specific groups that should not have firearms (e.g., felons and children) and toward regulating the storage, transport, and use of firearms.

3. Make technologic changes to modify firearms and ammunition so as to render them less lethal (e.g., a requirement for childproof safety devices such as trigger locks).

Reduction of morbidity and mortality from unintentional firearm-related injuries among children and teenagers must emphasize limiting access to loaded weapons.

Nonpowder firearms (those using gas, air, or a spring to propel ammunition, including BB guns) cause more than 14,000 injuries annually among children younger than age 15, with boys accounting for over 80% of the injuries. Although nonpowder-firearm injuries generally are less severe than those from powder guns, fatalities and permanent disabilities do occur. Nonpowder firearms should be used only under responsible adult supervision and should be treated in much the same way as other firearms.

Power Lawn Mower Injuries

Power lawn mowers (walk-behind and ride-on) continue to be responsible for hundreds of injuries each year, in spite of the CPSC's longtime effort to reduce injuries associated with these laborsaving machines. Commencing in the late 1970s, manufacturers adopted numerous voluntary safety standards designed to reduce the risks, including reducing blade speed on rotary motors, installing blade control systems to prevent the blade from operating un-

less the operator actuates the control, installing deflector covers over discharge chutes, and using devices that cause the blade to stop within 3 seconds after the control is released. From 1983 to 1989, lawn mower injuries decreased by 38%.

Operators must recognize that power lawn mowers are extremely hazardous and must be operated safely. Further reduction in injuries through changes in design may not be effective without greater attention to safe operation.

Approximately half of all injuries that happen while using power lawn mowers are to persons under 16 or over 55 years of age. Though rare, deaths do occur from power lawn mower accidents. More than 60% of the deaths are children under age 5 and adults over 65 years of age. This means that the lawn-mowing task must not be assigned to young, inexperienced operators or to older adults who may not have the strength or reflexes necessary to operate a power lawn mower safely.

. . . .

RECREATIONAL SAFETY

Millions of Americans participate in leisure activities each year. These activities range from those that constitute a low risk of injury to those that may constitute a high risk. Among the features that may determine the degree of risk are the activity itself, the participant's age, skill level, and health, and the condition of the environment. No doubt, individuals who are skilled in an activity, who understand the risks, and who adhere to safe practices are at lower risk of being involved in injury-causing accidents. This section will highlight a few of the leisure activities in which Americans participate.

Swimming

Swimming is one of the most popular recreational activities in the United States, and also one of the most dangerous. Drowning, the fourth leading cause of childhood fatal injuries, is most common in children 4 years of age and males aged 15 to 19 years. In the latter group, drownings occur in a wide variety of environments and alcohol use is associated with an estimated 40% to 50% of these

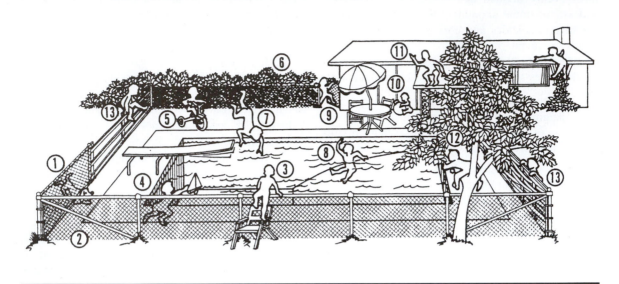

FIGURE 13.1 Each number represents an unsafe act or unsafe condition for a swimming pool area.

events. Drowning rates for black children are almost twice those for white children. In three states (Arizona, California, and Florida), drowning is the leading cause of fatal injuries for children 4 years of age. In all states, up to 90% of drownings among this age group occur in residential swimming pools. Alaska has the highest drowning rate in the country.

In a study of swimming pool drownings in Maricopa County, Arizona, 40% were attributed to a lapse in supervision, 35% to absence of a pool fence (a fence that completely encloses the pool and isolates it from the house and play area), 14% to an inadequate or unclosed gate or latch, 2% to an inadequate fence, and 9% to other causes.

Data from this study suggest that pool fencing, in combination with adequate gates and latches, could have prevented 51% of the drownings or near-drownings reported. Because so many incidents were attributed to a lapse in supervision (the supervisor's attention was diverted or a child was not observed momentarily while the adult performed a chore in the pool area), educating parents and caregivers about constant vigilance at a pool should complement an emphasis on passive barriers to the pool. Other measures may include instruction

on the maintenance of gates and latches, cardiopulmonary resuscitation classes, and improvement in the design and placement of pools. Figure 13.1 shows hazard areas in residential swimming pools.

Suction drains in spas, hot tubs, whirlpool baths, and swimming pools are extremely hazardous. They have proven fatal and caused injuries to children who have been sucked against the drain or had their hair drawn into the drain. Some states now require that all newly constructed pools be designed to reduce the risk of suction-drain injuries.

People who swim in natural bodies of water may be at greater risk than those who swim in residential-type swimming pools. Additional hazards include changing environmental conditions such as depth, currents, and weather; insufficient warning signs; murky or cloudy water, close proximity to water craft; and inaccessibility of emergency medical services.

In some states, laws have established basic safety requirements for natural swimming areas, including depth markings and warning signs, lifeguards, life-saving equipment, and first-aid supplies, telephones for emergency use, safety plans, and restrictions on the number of persons allowed in a specific swimming area.

In addition to drowning, many injuries are associated with water activities. The most serious are paralysis resulting from diving into shallow water in a pool, river, or other body of water. Propeller injuries to water skiers are too common and could be eliminated if propellers were shielded adequately. Hundreds of children are injured on swimming pool slides each year.

Recreational Boating

Recreational boating continues to grow in popularity each year, and with it comes a corresponding increase in risk. Recreational boats include canoes, rowboats, duckboats, sailboats, motorboats, yachts, jet skis, and kayaks.

A review of statistics on recreational boating fatalities in recent years indicates that fatalities are highest among the 20 to 28 age group, and that a high percentage of accidents occur on Saturday and Sunday. June and July are the months in which the greatest number of accidental boating deaths occur. In most cases, the watercraft were open outboard motorboats or boats less than 15 feet in length with no motor (excluding sailboats) and with only two persons aboard. The most frequent type of accident is capsizing while boating in nontidal, calm waters, with clear weather conditions and a light wind.

The greatest number of fatalities occur while the boat is cruising, which means that the vessel is proceeding normally and unrestricted, with no drastic rudder or engine changes at the time of the accident. The second largest number of fatalities occur while the boat is being used for fishing. Drifting, in which a vessel is carried along with the tide or wind, is the operational category accounting for the third largest number of fatalities. These three operations account for more than two-thirds of the fatalities each year.

One of the newest and fastest growing recreational boating activities involves personal watercraft or jet skis. These are small, agile boats powered by an inboard engine and a jet pump mechanism. Deaths and injuries involving personal watercraft have increased dramatically since the mid-1980s. In fact, the death rate per 100,000 registered boats is more than twice as high for personal watercraft as for all other types of boats.

Boaters should take the following precautions to reduce the risk of an accident:

- Be totally familiar with the boat's operation. This means that young, inexperienced operators should be supervised until they acquire skills necessary to be safe operators.

- Equip boats with approved personal flotation devices for each person, and with fire extinguishers and other safety equipment.

- Be familiar with all of the rules of safe boating.

- Avoid the use of alcoholic beverages. Studies conducted by the U.S. Coast Guard suggest that alcohol may be involved in as many as 60% of recreational boating fatalities.

. . . .

OTHER RECREATIONAL ACTIVITIES

Each year in the United States an estimated 30 million persons ride horses. The rate of serious injury per number of riding hours is estimated to be higher for horseback riders than for motorcyclists and automobile racers. Falls account for most horseback-riding injuries, and fewer than 20% of riders were wearing a helmet at the time of the fall. Even when riders wear headgear, it may be decorative or secured improperly, thereby providing limited or no protection. Horseback riders should wear properly secured hard-shell helmets lined with expanded polystyrene or similar material.

Horseback riders sometimes are injured when they collide with fixed objects, are dragged along the ground with a foot caught in a stirrup, are crushed between the horse and ground, or are trampled, kicked, or bitten. Equipment problems associated with injuries include improper boot stirrup fit, broken reins, bridles, or stirrup straps, and malfunctions of the stirrup-release mechanism. All equipment must be kept in good repair.

Recreational use of *snowmobiles* is extremely popular in many regions of the country. One study suggests that most fatal snowmobile incidents involve male operators in their twenties, use of alcohol, or excessive speed, and that half the persons killed sustained head injuries. It has been estimated that helmet use could reduce the risk for death among snowmobile users by approximately 42%

In 1962, Dr. William Hadden, Jr. developed a list of 10 strategies for injury prevention and control that still are applicable today. These are listed, with examples of current significance in parentheses.

1. Prevent the creation of the hazard. (Ban the production and sale of all-terrain vehicles.)
2. Reduce the amount of the hazard. (Package medicines in small amounts so the entire bottle, if ingested, is not a lethal dose.)
3. Prevent the release of a hazard that already exists. (Manufacture all cigarettes to be self-extinguishing when not inhaled.)
4. Modify the rate or spatial distribution of the hazard. (Require airbags in cars.)
5. Separate, in time or space, the hazard from that which is to be protected. (Use bicycle paths to separate bicycles from cars.)
6. Separate the hazard from that which is to be protected by a material barrier. (Build fences around swimming pools.)
7. Modify relevant basic qualities of the hazard. (Manufacture nonflammable upholstery.)
8. Make what is to be protected more resistant to damage from the hazard. (Prevent osteoporosis, which weakens hipbones and makes them susceptible to breaking.)
9. Begin to counter the damage already done by the hazard. (Provide emergency medical care.)
10. Stabilize, repair, and rehabilitate the object of the damage. (Provide acute care and rehabilitation services.)

Source: Injury in North Carolina

and could reduce the likelihood of head injury in a nonfatal incident by approximately 64%.

All-terrain vehicles (ATVs) are three- or four-wheeled vehicles designed mainly for recreational or agricultural off-road use. Licensing is not required in most states. Since ATVs became popular in the United States in 1982, more than 1,100 persons have died while operating them, and more than half of these deaths were among children under 16 years of age. In addition, nearly 420,000 nonfatal injuries have resulted nationwide from operation of these vehicles.

ATVs overturn easily, especially on rough terrain. Concern about instability and resulting injuries led to a ban on the sale of three-wheeled ATVs in December 1987.

Data support a strong recommendation prohibiting use of ATVs by children younger than 16 years. Certainly, children younger than 16 should not use adult-size ATVs. Helmets offer protection against head injury and should be required, but helmets cannot prevent spinal cord injury and other injuries associated with ATVs.

Firearm injuries associated with *hunting* appear to affect the young disproportionately. As many as 25% of hunting firearm injuries are fatal. One in seven shooters in hunting fatalities is a male younger than age 15. Hunting injuries could be reduced by encouraging hunters to participate in hunter safety instruction, requiring hunters to wear orange clothing while hunting, and prohibiting children under age 12 from hunting unless accompanied by an experienced adult.

· · · · · · · · · · · · · · · ·

TRANSPORTATION SAFETY INTRODUCTION

Over the past four decades, numerous interventions in motor vehicle and highway safety have contributed to reducing transportation injuries and deaths in the United States. These interventions have focused on a multifaceted, science-based approach to reduce mortality from motor vehicle crashes and have included public information programs, promotion of behavioral changes, changes in legislation and regulations, and advances in engineering and technology. These strategies have resulted in safer vehicles (e.g., the addition of laminated windshields and interior padding), safer driving practices (e.g., reduced occurrence of alcohol-impaired driving and increased use of safety belts), safer travel environments (e.g., construction of safer highways and roads), and improved emergency medical services.

Key elements of the science-based approach include the establishment of a national data-collection system to routinely monitor motor-vehicle-related deaths, identification of modifiable risk factors, design and implementation of preventive measures, and evaluation of the effectiveness of these measures. Since 1966, when the federal government identified transportation safety as a major goal and subsequently established the National Highway Traffic Safety Administration (NHTSA) to help reduce death and injury on the highway, the annual number of motor-vehicle-related deaths in the United States has decreased, even though the annual number of vehicle-miles traveled has increased more than 114%. From 1968 through 1991, motor-vehicle-related deaths decreased by 21%. Despite these considerable efforts and results, motor-vehicle injuries continue to be the leading cause of death (> 40,000 deaths annually) for people from 1 to 34 years of age and are the leading cause of work-related deaths. Of those who die, 15% are pedestrians. Motor-vehicle accidents also are the major cause of serious head and spinal cord injuries.

The impact of motor-vehicle injuries on certain groups is illustrated by the following:

- Motor-vehicle crash injuries claim the lives of more than 5,500 teenagers each year.
- More than over 2,200 children ages 0 to 12 die in motor-vehicle crashes annually.
- More than 40% of the deaths of 16- to 19-year-olds from all causes result from motor-vehicle accidents.
- Motor-vehicle accidents are the cause of about half of all child deaths from injury.
- Alcohol is involved in about half of all deaths from motor-vehicle crashes.
- Motor-vehicle crashes cause the deaths of more than 5,500 pedestrians each year.
- Motor-vehicle crashes cause 23% of all occupational injury deaths.
- Annually, motor-vehicle crashes are the cause of fatal injuries of more than 6,000 elderly people (65 years of age and older); 65% are passenger-car occupants and 20% are pedestrians.

Child Restraints

Although in recent years the increase in child safety seat use has saved lives of and prevented injuries to infants (children 1 year old and younger) and toddlers (children aged 1 to 4 years), the leading cause of death in children ages 1 to 4 years continues to be injuries to motor-vehicle occupants. These injuries account for the largest number of years of potential life lost before age 65 and the highest costs associated with pediatric injury.

In 1990, child safety seats were used with an estimated 83% of infants and 84% of toddlers, compared to 60% and 38%, respectively, in 1983. Despite this high level of use, 500 to 700 infants and toddlers died each year from 1983 through 1990 in traffic crashes. In 1990, NHTS reported that 624 children younger than 5 years of age were killed in motor-vehicle crashes, of whom 70% were not restrained. The evidence is clear that children who are not restrained may be at greater risk of involvement in a potentially fatal crash. Based on estimates from 1982 through 1990, the use of restraints (both child safety seats and adult safety belts) saved 1,546 lives of young children in passenger-vehicle crashes. Further reductions in child crash fatalities will require education and motivation of parents to use child safety seats and safety belts.

Pedestrian Safety

Pedestrian injuries are the leading cause of death in children aged 4 to 8, with the peak at age 6. Each year approximately 1,100 pedestrians ages 0 to 14 years are killed in traffic accidents. In addition, approximately 200 are killed in non-traffic locations such as private driveways, parking lots, and farms. One-year-old children are at highest risk. Annually, more than 80,000 children are treated in emergency rooms from injuries sustained in traffic accidents, many of whom require admission to hospitals.

Because of the tremendous force involved and the lack of protective structures surrounding pedestrians, severe multiple injuries are common. Case-fatality rates are very high when head injuries are present and are particularly high for children. Rates of death and serious injury are about twice as high in boys as in girls, and are especially high in urban and low-income areas.

Children are struck by cars when they dart into traffic, especially where parked cars obscure them from the driver's view, cross the street in front of school buses, and walk or crawl near motor vehicles in yards and driveways. Injuries are concentrated in the after-school hours from 3:00 to 7:00 P.M. During the hour after sunset, when visibility is poor, pedestrian deaths are especially likely.

Prevention requires separating children from vehicular traffic, making it easier for children and cars to see one another, slowing traffic in areas where children are apt to be crossing the street, supervising children until they are old enough to make reliable decisions regarding street crossing, and training those old enough to cross alone.

For elderly persons, poor night vision and reduced physical abilities may increase the risk of pedestrian accidents. These people should wear brightly colored clothing or clothing that contains retroreflective materials to increase nighttime visibility.

Motor Vehicles

Human error accounts for more than 80% of all accidents, including motor-vehicle accidents. The term frequently used to describe the causes of these accidents is "improper driving." This includes actions such as speeding, failure to yield right-of-way, driving left of center, incorrect passing, and following too closely.

Speed is considered to be the major factor in over 25% of all fatal motor vehicle accidents. Included in these statistics are fatalities resulting from operators driving too fast for road conditions, not necessarily exceeding posted speed limits. Even so, speed is definitely a factor. An estimated 2,000 to 4,000 lives were saved annually during the years when the 55-mph speed limit was in force. There is concern that recent laws that allow states to establish speed limits will lead to increased fatalities on our highways.

Nearly 20% of the annual motor-vehicle fatalities involve three types of right-of-way errors: failure to yield, not stopping at a stop sign, and disregarding a signal. Failure to yield accounts for the greatest percentage of these accidents. Defensive driving is the best approach to take in preventing right-of-way accidents. The driver should not assume that the other driver will follow the rules of the road.

The most important factor in fatal motor-vehicle accidents is alcohol. Annually, more than half of the motor-vehicle deaths in the United States are alcohol-related. Statistical estimates from the NHTSA indicate that two in five Americans will be involved in an alcohol-related crash at some point in their lives. Use of drugs and other chemical agents that impair driving ability also play a role in motor-vehicle accidents, particularly when drugs are combined with alcohol use.

Law enforcement personnel and organizations such as Mothers Against Drunk Driving (MADD) have worked closely with legislators and citizens to develop better ways to educate the public about the hazards of drinking and driving.

Environmental factors, both natural and manmade, account for less than 5% of vehicle accidents. When these factors are combined with some degree of human error, however, they become a significant factor in 27% of accidents. Natural environmental factors such as rain, snow, wind, fog, and ice cannot be directly controlled or prevented, but they can be modified to some extent through roadway design. Also, drivers must be educated about the risks associated with driving in adverse weather conditions.

Another factor that must be considered in motor-vehicle crashes is vehicle design. Improvements in vehicle characteristics and components such as braking, steering, mirrors, tires, seatbelts and airbags, and vehicle lighting enable the driver to handle the vehicle more safely and efficiently. Motor vehicles are safer for occupants than motor vehicles manufactured prior to 1966, in part because of the publication of Ralph Nader's book *Unsafe at Any Speed*. Nader described numerous hazards to occupants that have been addressed through improved design. As a consequence, vehicles are safer.

Passenger restraints, including seatbelts, reduce the risk of injury in the event of a motor-vehicle crash by protecting the passenger from impact with components of the vehicle's interior. Investigations by the NHTSA and other organizations have indicated that the life-saving effectiveness of lap and shoulder belts, when they are worn, is about 50%. Despite the benefits of safety belts and their presence in practically all passenger vehicles, many Americans do not use them regularly. Some studies indicate that almost half of U.S. motorists do not wear seatbelts.

In efforts to reduce injuries and fatalities in motor-vehicle crashes, many states have passed mandatory safety belt laws. Also, passive restraints or airbags now are installed in most new passenger vehicles. This should provide greater protection to occupants, especially the driver and front-seat passenger.

Although motor-vehicle accidents, the leading cause of accidental deaths, have declined in recent years, much more must be done in the future. Data indicate that too many drivers are driving while impaired, too many drivers exceed safe speeds, too many drivers fail to wear a seatbelt, and too many drivers fail to yield the right-of-way and commit other driving errors.

SUMMARY

Unintentional injuries constitute a continuing public health problem in the United States. Americans are at risk in their homes, on the highways, at work, and while engaging in recreational activities. Much has been learned about the actual causes of accidents through the application of epidemiological sciences to the study of accidents and through other research techniques. Research findings have led to reduction of injuries and fatalities in many categories of accidents.

Although the home environment is, indeed, an unsafe environment, this environment can be made safer for family and invited guests by better understanding the dynamics of home accidents. Adults must assume responsibility for making the home environment safe for members of the family who are at greatest risk: children and older adults.

Many popular recreational activities are extremely dangerous. Young, inexperienced persons seem to be at highest risk and should be supervised closely. Using proper equipment and avoiding alco-

hol while participating in recreational activities will reduce the risk of injury. Application of the 10 strategies for injury prevention and control presented in this chapter, along with application of the three E's of environmental safety (education, engineering, and enforcement) will help to make the country safer for all citizens.

KEY TERMS

Epidemiology, p. 232

Injury, p. 232

National Electronic Injury Surveillance System (NEISS), p. 234

Unintentional injury, p. 232

Years of potential life lost (YPLL), p. 232

REFERENCES

Berger, Lawrence R. 1985, Nov./Dec. Childhood injuries. *Public Health Reports.* 100, no. 6:572–574.

Bever, David L. 1992. *Safety: A Personal Focus*, 3rd ed. Mosby Yearbook, St. Louis.

Brobeck, Stephen, and Anne C. Averyt. 1983. *The Product Safety Book: The Ultimate Consumer Guide to Product Hazards*. E.P. Dutton, New York.

Centers for Disease Control and Prevention, U.S. Department of Health and Human Services. 1993, May. *Injury Control in the 1990's: A National Plan for Action*, Atlanta.

————. 1995. Injuries associated with use of snowmobiles—New Hampshire, 1989–92. *Morbidity and Mortality Weekly Report*, 44, no. 1:1–3.

————. 1994. Deaths resulting from residential fires—United States, 1991. *Morbidity and Mortality Weekly Report*. 43, no. 49:901–904.

————. 1994. Deaths resulting from firearm and motor vehicle-related injuries—United States, 1968–1991. *Morbidity and Mortality Weekly Report*. 43, no. 3:37–41.

————. 1993. Carbon monoxide poisoning—Weld County, Colorado, 1993. *Morbidity and Mortality Weekly Report* 43, no. 42:765–767.

————. 1993. Unintentional carbon monoxide poisoning following a winter storm—Washington, January 1993. *Morbidity and Mortality Weekly Report*, 42, no. 6:109–111.

————. 1992. Suction-drain injury in a public wading pool—North Carolina, 1991. *Morbidity and Mortality Weekly Report*. 41, no. 19:333–335.

———. 1991. Child passenger restraint use and motor vehicle-related fatalities among children—United States. *Morbidity and Mortality Weekly Report*. 40, no. 34.

———. 1990. Child drownings and near drownings—Maricopa County, Arizona, 1988 and 1989. *Morbidity and Mortality Weekly Report*. 39 no. 26:441–442.

———. 1990. Years of potential life lost before ages 65 and 85—United States, 1987 and 1988. *Morbidity and Mortality Weekly Report*. 39, no. 2:20–21.

Chemical Manufacturers Association, Simple steps to improve safety in the home. 1992, May. *Chemecology*:2–3.

Christoffel, Tom, and Katherine Christoffel. 1989, March. The Consumer Product Safety Commission's Opposition to consumer product safety: Lessons for public health advocates. *American Journal of Public Health*. 79:336–339.

Committee on Trauma Research, Commission on Life Sciences, National Research Council, and the Institute of Medicine. 1985. *Injury in America: A Continuing Public Health Problem*, National Academy Press, Washington, DC.

Gordon, John E. 1949, April. The epidemiology of accidents. *American Journal of Public Health*. 39, no. 4:504–515.

Governor's Task Force on Injury Prevention and Control. 1989, Oct. *Injury in North Carolina*. Raleigh, NC.

Iskrant, Albert P. and Paul Joilet. 1968. *Accidents and Homicide*. Harvard University Press, Cambridge, MA.

Moore, Jill D., and Luanne W. Gardner. 1994, Winter. Saving children's lives: Preventing childhood injuries. *North Carolina Public Health Forum*, 3, no. 1:10–16.

National Safety Council. 1993. *Accident Facts*, 1993 ed. Itasca, IL.

Rice, Dorothy P., Ellen J. Mackenzie, and Associates. 1989. *Cost of injury in the United States: A report to Congress*. Centers for Disease Control, Atlanta.

South Carolina Department of Health and Environmental Control. *South Carolina Plants May Poison*. Columbia, SC.

U.S. Consumer Product Safety Commission. 1992, Jan/Dec. Baby walker-related injuries. *NEISS Data Highlights*, 16.

U.S. Consumer Product Safety Commission. 1991, Jan/Dec. Power mower related injuries 1983–1990. *NEISS Data Highlights*, 15.

U.S. Consumer Product Safety Commission. 1990, Jan/Dec. Head injuries. *NEISS Data Highlights*, 14.

———. 1985. *Protect Someone You Love From Burns*. Washington, DC.

U.S. Department of Health and Human Services, Centers for Disease Control and Prevention. 1991, Oct. *Preventing Lead Poisoning in Young Children*. Atlanta.

Waller, Julian A. 1985, Nov./Dec. The epidemiologic basis for injury prevention. *Public Health Reports*. 100, no. 6:575–576.

———. 1980. Injury as a public health problem. In *Maxcy-Roseneu Public Health and Preventive Medicine*, 11th ed. Appleton-Century-Crofts, New York.

Wiant, Chris. 1993, Feb. Injuries are no accident. *Journal of Environmental Health*, 55, no. 4:36.

Wilson, Modena H.; Susan P. Baker, Stephen P. Teret, Susan Shock, and James Garbarino, 1991. *Saving Children: A Guide to Injury Prevention*. Oxford University Press, New York.

14

AIR QUALITY

L. Fleming Fallon, Jr., M.D., Dr. P.H.

Bowling Green State University

OBJECTIVES

■ Identify the components of air.

■ Identify and differentiate important air pollutants.

■ Discuss the historical origins of air pollution.

■ Discuss the sources of air pollution and describe methods used to control air pollutants.

■ Identify the causes and effects of acid precipitation.

■ Identify and describe human diseases associated with exposure to elevated levels of air pollution.

■ List the primary national laws that control and reduce air pollution.

■ Identify the causes that deplete the ozone layer and the overall impact on human health.

■ Recognize the impact of deforestation on air quality and the environment.

■ Calculate a community pollution standard index.

A person may survive for many days without food, or for a few days without water. Air is more immediately essential. Without air, a person can hardly exist long enough to walk 100 feet. The air that humans require is an odorless, colorless mixture of natural gases. It is composed of nitrogen (approximately 78%) and oxygen (21%). The remainder is mostly argon (0.93%) and carbon dioxide (0.032%) with traces of neon, helium, ozone, xenon, hydrogen, methane, and krypton. Local conditions determine the amount of water vapor. When anything else is added, the air becomes polluted.

HISTORICAL PERSPECTIVE

Until the 19th century and the Industrial Revolution, air pollution was not a widespread problem because pollution was readily diluted in the atmosphere. It did not build up over densely populated areas. When humans began to burn fuel (primarily wood and coal) in large quantities to convert water into steam to drive turbines, they started to create problems with air pollution. Smokestacks brought new wealth to industrialized nations. The grimy effluents that were belched out became the true price of the newly acquired affluence. Industrialization raised the standard of living for many while lowering the visibility for all and causing disease among all groups in society. People sought affluence without regard for the effluent created as a by-product of creating wealth. Only after air pollution disasters were clearly linked with adverse events that caused multiple deaths, did people become concerned about air pollution.

As an example, consider the following highly publicized event. During the last week of October 1948, a high concentration of smog from Pittsburgh settled down over the air surrounding Donora, Pennsylvania, and the surrounding area. At a London Public Health Congress, Harold Antoine Des Voeuy had coined the word **smog** to describe such highly polluted air. The smog that encompassed Donora on the morning of Wednesday, October 27, so reduced visibility that the streetlights came on and local people got lost. On Saturday morning, the first death occurred. The deaths continued until, by Sunday night, 19 people had died. One additional person became ill and died a week later.

Four years later, an air pollution episode in London stalled the city for five days. The thick yellow smog was so dense that people walked with handkerchiefs over their noses. Visibility was reduced to 12 feet. People walked into each other, and only the blind knew where they were going. The death of 4,000 people in London is attributed to the air pollution that covered the city in December of the same year. These deaths, attributed to the smog, were far in excess of the number typically expected to occur during that time of year.

New York City also has had episodes of severe air pollution. The worst occurred in 1965 and caused the death of an estimated 400 people. Air pollution episodes are not confined to large cities or locations downwind from large cities. In Belgium, the secluded Meuse Valley underwent an air pollution episode in 1930 that resulted in 63 deaths and 6,000 illnesses. These and other pollution disasters are listed in Table 14.1. The episodes in the table are examples of cases where the "dumping ground" (the atmosphere) could not disperse the materials being emitted from natural and man-made sources. As populations grew, power demands to operate

■ **TABLE 14.1** ■

AIR POLLUTION DISASTERS SINCE 1930 WITH THEIR ASSOCIATED DEATH RATES

Date	Location	Excess mortality (total less expected deaths)
1930	Meuse Valley, Belgium	63
1948	Donora Valley, PA	20
1950	Poza Rica, Mexico	22
1952	London, England	4,000
1953	New York, NY	250
1956	London, England	1,000
1957	London, England	700–800
1962	London, England	700
1963	New York, NY	200–400
1966	New York, NY	168

machinery, provide transportation, heat homes and other buildings, prepare food, and the like increased. The capacity of the atmosphere to dilute or disperse the pollutants was exceeded. A series of air pollution disasters was the result.

In Copperhill and Ducktown, Tennessee, coal was used to smelt copper ore. The coal contained high concentrations of sulfur. Over the years, so much high-sulfur coal was burned that sulfur dioxide (SO_2) was deposited in high concentrations in the local area. When sulfate combines with water, sulfuric acid (H_2SO_4) is formed. The pollution coming from the smokestacks and falling out around the smelting plant killed trees, grass and most other forms of vegetation.

In time, the pollution spread to Georgia. In reaction, the Georgia legislature contacted the U.S. Public Health Service, the controlling federal agency at the time. Noting that Tennessee did not have a right to pollute Georgia, the Public Health Service ordered Tennessee to stop the polluting activities. When the state of Tennessee ordered industry to cease polluting the atmosphere, industry sought relief in the courts. Along with others, this court case ultimately led to the passage of the initial Clean Air Act in 1963. The national air pollution program is based on a 1970 revision of the 1963 law. The Clean Air Act was again extensively amended in 1990.

Eventually, the smelter started looking for ways to stop or reduce the pollution. It began removing SO_2 from stack emissions and converting it into sulfuric acid under controlled conditions. This product was sold at a profit.

••••••••••••••

SOURCES OF AIR POLLUTION

Some *natural* sources of air pollution include forest fires, dust storms, and volcanic eruptions. Plants such as ragweed contaminate the air with pollen. Decaying leaves and other forms of vegetation release gases that contribute to air pollution and cause haze.

Anthropogenic air pollution, contamination produced by humans, may also adversely affect human health. Some sources of anthropogenic air pollution include smoke from chimneys; gases from septic tanks and house sewer system vents; odors from cooking food; and fumes, gases, vapors and particles released from paint, household cleaners, hair sprays, and the like. *Industrial pollution* is created by the release of gases, vapors and fumes from industries that manufacture automobiles, clothing, cleaners, chemicals, plastics, furniture and other products people purchase.

Air pollutants are created in *agriculture* when food is grown, stored, or processed. For example, crop yields are increased when insecticides and herbicides are used to control pests. At the same time, the insecticides and herbicides add to the burden of air pollution.

Transportation contributes to the problem of pollution. Internal combustion engines are significant sources of many air pollutants. Some experts assert that transportation accounts for approximately 50% of all air pollution. Carbon monoxide (CO) is a major source of air pollution generated by transportation. In 1983, 70% of the nonnatural emissions of carbon monoxide were from highway vehicles. Catalytic converters presently installed on most automobiles have significantly reduced CO emissions.

CO is the result of incomplete combustion of fuel. In contrast, complete combustion produces carbon dioxide (CO_2). Nitrogen oxides and hydrocarbons are additional by-products of the combus-

tion of petroleum products. Under the influence of sunlight, they undergo chemical reactions to produce **photochemical smog**, a major problem in urban areas.

Energy use and production are the major contributors to deterioration of ambient air quality. When coal or wood is burned to produce electricity or heat, the combustion process releases air pollutants: CO, CO_2, SO_2, nitrogen oxides (NOx), heat and particulate matter, depending on the fuel. Of particular importance are NOx and SO_2. These gasses combine with water to form acid rain. Sulfur dioxide gas is emitted into air by burning oil and coal that contain sulfur impurities. In the United States, 15% of SO_2 emissions is from industrial plants and 68% is from coal and oil-burning electric power-generating stations. Refuse is often burned to generate heat as electricity. This process, called waste-heat recovery, also generates a small percentage of air pollution.

••••••••••••••

EFFECTS OF AIR POLLUTION

Health Effects

Epidemiological studies have indicated that high levels of air pollutants contribute to or cause many serious respiratory conditions. A Harvard study estimated that as many as 60,000 people die annually from exposure to **particulate air pollution**. A phenomenon called **thermal inversion** traps pollutants beneath a layer of cool air so that pollutants cannot rise and disperse (Figure 14.1). Experts estimate that up to 30 million Americans with chronic respiratory problems are regularly exposed to harmful levels of smog that worsen their illnesses. Some of these respiratory conditions include the following:

1. *Asthma*. Particulates can irritate bronchial passages, leading to severe difficulties in breathing. Asthma is a growing public health problem worldwide. From 1983 to 1993, its prevalence in the United States increased 34%, according to the National Institutes of Health. In Australia, the incidence among children was one in five, a doubling of the

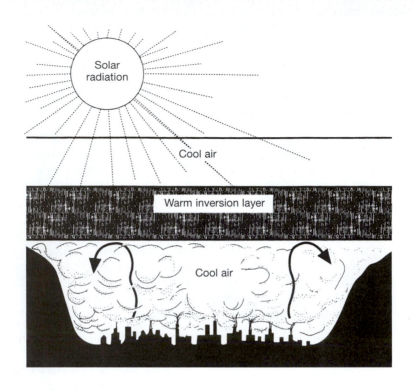

FIGURE 14.1 Thermal inversion.

rate in less than in 20 years. Persons living in urban areas, especially those with high levels of air pollutants, seem to be the most affected. SO_2 has also been linked to asthma. Indoor air pollution is also a significant contributor to this problem.

2. *Chronic bronchitis.* This occurs when an excessive amount of mucus is produced in the bronchi, which results in a lasting cough. There seems to be a significant correlation between death rates from chronic bronchitis and SO_2 concentrations. Sulfur dioxide may irritate the nasopharynx (mucous membrane) and the bronchi by forming sulfuric acid in situ. Repeated exposure to high levels of SO_2 over time may cause the body to produce excessive mucus as a defense. Chronic bronchi-

tis is also associated with cigarette smoking, a significant source of air pollution.

3. *Pulmonary emphysema.* This condition is characterized by weakening of the walls of the alveoli, the tiny air sacs in the lungs. As the disease progresses, their walls disintegrate and the alveoli coalesce in much the same manner as soap bubbles. Alveoli become enlarged and lose their resilience. Shortness of breath is a primary symptom. Nitrogen dioxide has been identified as one of the air pollutants that may contribute to emphysema. Heat from cigarette smoking also causes emphysema.

Lung cancer and heart disorders also may be caused or exacerbated by exposure to air pollutants.

CHARACTERISTICS OF SOME AIR POLLUTANTS

Name	Formula	Properties of Importance	Significance as Air Pollutant
Sulfur dioxide	SO_2	Colorless gas, intense choking odor, somewhat soluble in water to form sulfurous acid (H^2SOA_3)	Damage to vegetation, property, and health
Hydrogen sulfide	H_2S	Rotten egg odor at low concentrations, odorless at high concentrations	Highly toxic
Nitric oxide	NO	Colorless gas	Produced during high-temperature, high-pressure combustion. Oxidizes to NO_2.
Nitrogen dioxide	NO_2	Colored gas, used as carrier	Relatively inert. Not greatly produced in combustion.
Carbon monoxide	CO	Colorless and odorless	Product of incomplete combustion. Poisonous.
Carbon dioxide	CO_2	Colorless and ordorless	Formed during complete combustion. Possible effects in producing changes in global climate.
Ozone	O_3	Highly reactive	Damage to vegetation and property. Produced mainly during the formation of photochemical smog.

Other Effects

Sulfur dioxide, carbon monoxide, nitrogen oxides, and other contaminants not only adversely affect human health, but they also affect property. Some pollutants damage vegetation, thus affecting the landscape. Near Los Angeles, smog is destroying pine trees around the city. Some forms of air pollution directly damage leaves of crops and trees when these gases enter leaf pores (stomata). Chronic exposure to air pollutants, including NOx, SO_2, and ozone breaks down the waxy coating of leaves. This promotes excessive water loss and damage from disease, pests, drought, and frost. In addition, acid deposition can leach vital plant nutrients such as calcium from the soil and kill essential microorganisms such as decomposers.

Each year air pollutants cause millions of dollars in damage to various personal items. Exposure to ozone causes rubber to crack and lose its tensile strength. Sulfur dioxide is responsible for loss of strength and surface deterioration of leather and other natural fabrics. Pollutants can cause corrosion, erosion, discoloration, and soiling of stone, metals, paint, paper, and glass. Table 14.2 summarizes the significant impact of some air pollutants.

AIR POLLUTION CONTROL

In general, pollution control methods are approached from two aspects: input and output. Input control concentrates on preventing or reducing the severity of the problem, whereas output control treats symptoms after the fact, by attempting to remove pollutants after they have left a source of combustion. Ideally, this will occur before they enter the environment.

Input Control

Some **input control** methods for reducing the amount of pollution before it reaches the environment. This is a form of primary prevention and is less expensive than trying to clean up after pollution has been discharged into the environment. Examples of input control methods include the following:

1. Control population growth.

2. Reduce the demand for energy.

3. Recycle resources and prevent the discharge of metals and chemicals into the environment.

4. Encourage repair of products rather than supporting remove-and-replace practices.

5. Find new, nonpolluting sources of energy (e.g., wind, hydroelectric, tidal, and solar energy).

6. Reduce dependency upon fossil fuels.

7. Emphasize quality in products (e.g., cars) so they will last longer.

8. Enhance fuel-dependent units such as gas engines.

9. Reduce dependency upon conveniences and the desire for affluence.

10. Reduce dependency upon electricity by reducing the use of electric appliances. Electric toothbrushes, knives, and can openers may be convenient. They accomplish tasks that are easily and simply performed by hand.

Output Control

Strong emphasis on input control methods reduces the need for **output control**. This is also less expensive than relying on output controls. Some examples of output controls include the following practices:

1. Support improved methods of emission control.

2. Remove pollutants after combustion by using scrubbers and electrostatic precipitators.

3. Find ways to convert pollutants to usable resources and develop markets for any resulting products.

4. Develop new methods of removing pollutants from emissions.

5. Improve catalytic conversion in automobiles.

6. Add lime and other materials to raise the pH of lakes, streams, and soils damaged by acid rain.

Because air pollution affects health, crops, buildings, and the natural environment, efforts are made to reduce air pollution. **Catalytic converters** are used to improve the combustion efficiency of petroleum products so as to reduce the amount of carbon monoxide, nitric oxides, and hydrocarbons that enter the air. Fuel-efficient motor vehicles not only save energy but also emit fewer pollutants in their exhaust. Catalytic converters are expensive and best suited to mobile sources of emissions: motor vehicles.

Coal can be modified to reduce pollution. Sulfur dioxide can be removed and the coal can be converted into gas (**gasification**). Both of these steps reduce the amount of sulfur dioxide entering the air. This is especially important during thermal inversions. Coal that is naturally low in sulfur is being preferentially burned to help lower the SO_2 in the air. This practice, however, can hurt the economy in coal-mining areas that have coal with a higher sulfur content.

The bag house method was used for years by grain mills, cement factories, and the like. It utilizes fabric bags to capture particles in the air. This method works like a large vacuum cleaner. Electric utilities have tried to apply the bag house method to reduce air pollution in large power-generating plants. Their success in removing particulate matter has been minimal. This method is relatively inexpensive.

Contemporary emission control efforts concentrate on two components of the settling chamber in a combustion apparatus: the afterburner, which requires a high temperature to ignite and burn particles, and the electrostatic precipitator. First used in 1925 to control fly ash, the **electrostatic precipitator** now is applied widely in the United States. Operation consists of attaching electric charges to particles as they enter a smokestack. This is achieved using a high-voltage grid to give particles an electrical charge. Higher in the smokestack, the charged particles are attracted and adhere to charged metal plates called collection electrodes. The collected particles that do not pollute the air are intermittently removed from the plates. Electrostatic precipitation is more expensive than other methods of removing particles.

Legislation

Four years after the London air pollution episode of 1952, Great Britain passed its Clean Air Act. It tried to improve air quality by banning the burning of soft coal in homes and industries. Londoners were unhappy at first. However, after seeing changes in air quality, they welcomed the absence of the thick, yellow smog that had caused some 4,000 deaths.

Federal statutory law addressing air pollution began in the United States with the 1963 Clean Air Act. The scope of this legislation was expanded with the 1967 Air Quality Act. Although these laws provided broad clean air goals and money for air research, they did not provide for air pollution control throughout the entire United States. In 1970, the Clean Air Act was amended to encompass the entire United States. The U.S. Environmental Protection Agency was created to promulgate the 1970 amendments.

In accordance with a 1977 amendment to the Clean Air Act, the Environmental Protection Agency (EPA) and the Council on Environmental Quality, along with other agencies, developed a Pollutant Standard Index (PSI). The PSI is a national air-monitoring network using a uniform air quality index. The EPA believed it was necessary to devise a method of conveying air quality data to the public in a way that would give people a good understanding of how daily levels of air pollution might be affecting their health. Details of the PSI are provided in Table 14.3.

■ TABLE 14.3 ■

POLLUTANT STANDARD INDEX

Index Value	Health Effect Descriptor	General Health Effects	Cautionary Statements
0–50	Good	None	None
51–100	Moderate	Minimal	None
101–200	Unhealthful	Mild aggravation of symptoms in susceptible persons, with some similar symptoms among members of a healthy population.	Persons with existing heart or respiratory ailments should reduce physical exertion and outdoor activity.
201–300	Very unhealthful	Significant aggravation of symptoms and decreased exercise tolerance in persons with heart or lung disease with widespread symptoms in the healthy population.	Elderly and persons with existing heart or lung disease should stay indoors and avoid physical exertion and outdoor activity.
301–400	Hazardous	Premature onset of certain diseases in addition to significant aggravation of symptoms and decreased exercise tolerance in healthy persons.	Elderly and persons with existing diseases should stay indoors and avoid physical exertion. General population should avoid outdoor activity.
401–500	Hazardous	Premature death of ill and elderly persons. Healthy people will Experience adverse symptoms that affect their normal activities.	All persons should remain indoors, keeping windows and doors closed. All persons should minimize physical exertion and avoid traffic.

NATIONAL AMBIENT AIR QUALITY STANDARDS (NAAQS) (AS OF JULY 2000)

POLLUTANT	PRIMARY (HEALTH-RELATED) STANDARD LEVEL		SECONDARY (WELFARE-RELATED) STANDARD LEVEL	
	Averaging Time	Concentration	Averaging Time	Concentration
PM_{10}[b]	Annual Arithmetic Mean	50 $\mu g/m^3$	Same as primary	
	24-hour	150 $\mu g/m^3$	Same as primary	
$PM_{2.5}$	Annual Arithmetic Mean[c]	15 $\mu g/m^3$	Same as primary	
	24-hour[c]	65 $\mu g/m^3$	Same as primary	
SO_2	Annual Arithmetic Mean	0.03 ppm (80 $\mu g/m^3$)[a]	3-hour	0.50 ppm (1300 $\mu g/m^3$)
	24-hour	0.14 ppm (365 $\mu g/m^3$)		
CO	8-hour	9 ppm (10$\mu g/m^3$)	No secondary standard	
	1-hour	35 ppm (40 $\mu g/m^3$)	No secondary standard	
NO_2	Annual Arithmetic Mean	0.053 ppm (100 $\mu g/m^3$)	Same as primary	
O_3	1 Hour Average	0.12 ppm (235 $\mu g/m^3$)	Same as primary	
	8 Hour Average[c]	0.08 ppm (157 $\mu g/m^3$)	Same as primary	
Pb	Maximum Quarterly Average	1.5 $\mu g/m^3$	Same as primary	

a. The value in parentheses is an approximately equivalent concentration; the standard is in the first units shown.

b. Until July 1, 1987, total suspended particulate matter (TSP) was the indicator pollutant for the particulate matter standards. In 1987, The EPA adopted the PM_{10} standard (particles less than ten micrometers [μm] in diameter). Until attainment status of all Air Quality Control regions for PM_{10} is determined, and new plans are submitted and approved, many State Implementation Plans (SIPs) will continue to address TSP. The PM_{10} annual standard is attained when the expected annual arithmetic mean concentration is less than or equal to 50 $\mu g/m^3$. The PM_{10} 24-hour standard is attained when the expected number of days per calendar year above 150 $\mu g/m^3$ is less than or equal to one.

c. The ozone 8-hour standard and the PM 2.5 standards are included for information only. A 1999 federal court ruling blocked implementation of these standards, which EPA proposed in 1997. EPA has asked the U.S. Supreme Court to reconsider that decision.

Source: <http://www.epa.gov/airs/criteria.html> (July 10, 2000)

The Clean Air Act was most recently revised in 1990. Under this legislation, most enforcement power is concentrated at the federal level and is delegated to the states by the EPA. The states must demonstrate to the EPA that they can clean up the air to the levels required by the National Ambient Air Quality Standards (NAAQS), given in Table 14.4. The main intent of NAAQS is to protect public health and welfare. Air quality levels are determined as those implement the intent of the NAAQS. The states must have an Air Quality Implementation Plan (AQIP), containing all of the state's regulations governing air pollution control, including local regulations within the state. The EPA must approve each state's AQIP. Once approved, it has the force of federal law.

ACID PRECIPITATION

All rainfall is somewhat acidic. Decomposing organic matter, the movement of the sea, and volcanic eruptions all contribute to accumulation of acidic chemicals in the atmosphere. The primary natural source of acidity is atmospheric carbon dioxide. Man-made pollutants accelerate the acidification of rainfall. Emissions of sulfur dioxide (SO_2) and nitrogen oxides (NOx) are transformed into acids when they react with water in the atmosphere. The deposition of acid, more commonly called acid rain, is a misleading term because these acids and acid-forming substances are deposited not only in rain but also in snow, sleet, fog, and dew.

Acid precipitation has become a worldwide problem, first in the Scandinavian countries, then in the northeastern United States and southeastern Canada, then Europe, Japan, and Taiwan. Studies are revealing that what was considered pure rainwater is now highly acidic. This precipitation is the product of sulfur oxides (SOx) and nitrogen oxides (NOx) produced in the burning process combining with water. **Sulfur oxides** come from burning coal and other fuels that contain sulfur. Under certain conditions, the sulfur oxides convert to sulfuric acid in the atmosphere and return to earth in precipitation. **Nitrogen oxides** are produced from the high-temperature combustion of fossil fuels, such as in cars, in which the nitric oxides are converted to nitrogen dioxide (NO_2), which further oxidizes and dissolves in water droplets to form nitric acid. Acid precipitation lowers the pH of soil, lakes, rivers, and other natural resources after precipitation such as rain, snow, dew, or fog. In the northeastern United States, the basis for most of the acid precipitation is sulfuric acid coming from coal-fueled power plants located primarily along the Ohio River. Prevailing winds blowing from the southwest to the northeast carry the sulfuric acid to the northeastern United States and Canada (Figure 14.2).

Only precipitation that has a pH of 5.6 and below is considered to be acidic. In some parts of the world, the acidity of rainfall has fallen well below 5.6. In the northeastern United States, for example, the average pH of rainfall is 4.6. Rainfall with a pH of 4.0 is not unusual. This is 1,000 times more acidic than distilled water, which has a pH of 7.0. Figure 14.3 compares acid rain to other products in terms of pH.

The extent of damage caused by acid deposition in an area depends on several factors. For ex-

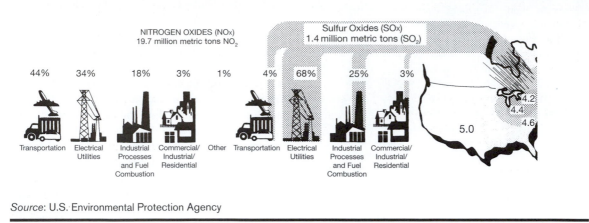

Source: U.S. Environmental Protection Agency

FIGURE 14.2 Precursors of acid precipitation in northeastern United States.

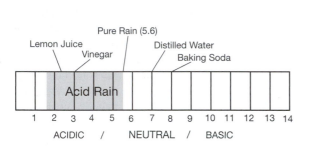

The pH scale ranges from 0 to 14. A value of 7.0 is neutral. Readings below 7.0 are acidic; readings above 7.0 are alkaline. The more pH decreases below 7.0, the more acidity increases.

Because the pH scale is logarithmic, there is a tenfold difference between one number and the one next to it. Therefore, a drop in pH from 6.0 to 5.0 represents a ten-fold increase in acidity, and a drop from 6.0 to 4.0 represents a hundred-fold increase.

Source: U.S. Environmental Protection Agency

FIGURE 14.3 Comparative pH of acid precipitation.

ample, an area with acid-neutralizing compounds in the soil does not develop problems as quickly as an area without the neutralizing compounds.

Aquatic ecosystems display the effects of acid precipitation more clearly than nonaquatic ecosystems. Precipitated acids lower the pH, creating an unfavorable environment for aquatic life. When exposed to acidic water, female fish, frogs, salamanders, and other creatures fail to produce eggs or may produce eggs that do not develop in a normal manner. Some scientists believe that acidic water kills fish and other aquatic life. They cite as evidence, some lakes that have been found to be highly acidic and lifeless in areas of high acid deposition.

The effect of acid precipitation on land, crops, forest, and other vegetation is not known with certainty. Some believe that "dieback" (unexplained death of whole sections of once-thriving forest) is caused by acid precipitation. Present concerns have been expressed in regard to trees dying in Germany and in the Appalachian Mountains of the United States. Many experts feel that foliage death is due to the demise of nitrogen-extracting microorganisms in soil that are highly sensitive to changes in soil pH. When these organisms die, nitrogen is no longer made available for plants. As a result, they also die.

The effect, if any, of acid precipitation on human health is not known. Other than the destruction of mucosal tissue in lungs, the effects of inhaling air that contains sulfur dioxide and nitrogen oxides are not known at this time. This is an issue of toxicology: the effect of exposure to any chemical is dependent on the duration and extent of exposure. The truth may be that, at present levels of understanding, acid precipitation is not harmful to human health. Future research may change this conclusion.

Recalling that prevention is cheaper than repair, some methods of controlling acid precipitation include the following:

1. Reduce population growth, and thus the number of people driving cars and needing energy. Prevent unwanted pregnancies and restrict immigration.

2. Reduce the demand for electricity and other forms of energy.

3. Use energy more efficiently. Over 50% of energy used in the United States each year is wasted. Use energy-efficient heat pumps to provide space heating rather than burning oil.

4. Reduce the need for energy by emphasizing recycling and conservation and by de-emphasizing material competition.

5. Design better and more efficient automobiles, heating units, and coal- and oil-fueled power plants.

6. Plant trees and other plants that remove carbon dioxide and produce more oxygen for better burning.

7. Reduce the need to travel by using communication methods such as telephones, faxes, and e-mail.

8. Engage in carpooling to work, school, and other trips, whenever possible.

9. Shift from fossil fuels to a mix of energy sources such as solar, tidal, nuclear, geo-thermal, hydroelectric, refuse, and biomass energy.

10. Convert coal to gaseous fuel or a liquid to remove sulfur and to reduce emissions of sulfur oxides from burning solid coal.

11. Shift to low-sulfur coal (less than 1%) for power plants, homes, and the like. Convert high-sulfur coal to gasoline.

12. Remove sulfur from coal, even if expensive, rather than pay high prices for foreign oil.

13. Increase the efficiency of scrubbers and electrostatic precipitators.

···············

THE GREENHOUSE EFFECT

The earth's temperature remains relatively constant because a significant fraction of the solar energy that impacts the earth's atmosphere is radiated back into space. Since the 1800s, however, the energy is not being radiated to the extent that it once was. More is being retained in the atmosphere and the earth has been undergoing a warming trend. This warming is due to increased carbon dioxide, water vapor, and other substances in the air.

The industrial age began with the discovery that the energy in coal could be used to convert water into steam. In turn, the steam can be used to drive the shaft of a motor or turbine. This newly mobile source of power could then be used to power trains, boats, and machinery in factories. The development of electricity accelerated the burning of fuels as sources of energy. When fossil fuels, initially coal and later oil, are burned, they emit carbon dioxide. Worldwide energy demands have become so great that carbon dioxide is now being produced in huge quantities.

Two methods are available to remove carbon dioxide (CO_2) from the atmosphere. Green plants break down carbon dioxide during the process of photosynthesis. Carbon dioxide gas that dissolves in the ocean may be converted to dolomite (calcium magnesium carbonate).

The capacity of these two systems is severely limited. As humans destroy forests by cutting wood without planting new trees and pollute oceans by dumping substances into them, the need for carbon dioxide from the air decreases. At the same time, the world is producing ever-increasing amounts of carbon dioxide each year as the population grows. Thus, more carbon dioxide remains in the atmosphere each year. Studies reveal that about half of the carbon dioxide presently emitted into the air remains there.

The sun radiates heat into space in every direction. Some solar energy has been reaching earth ever since its genesis. This radiation is either reflected back into space or absorbed by the earth itself. **Ozone** (O_3) in the upper atmosphere absorbs some of the ultraviolet light, X-ray, and gamma radiation in the short-wavelength range and prevents it from reaching the earth's surface. Approximately half of the incoming energy reaches vegetation, seas, snow-covered land, and ice-covered seas that can reflect it back into space. At atmospheric levels lower than the **ozone layer**, dust particles suspended in the air, clouds, and the earth's surface reflect about 3% of the incoming radiation back into space. About one-fifth of solar energy is absorbed by water droplets, water vapor, and dust in the air.

Because burning fossil fuels in automobiles, coal-fired electric plants and other generators produces both carbon dioxide and water vapor, more of these gases are remaining in the atmosphere each year. Research has shown that water vapor and carbon dioxide absorb radiation. Hence, more and more radiation is being absorbed and trapped in the atmosphere. This causes an increase in the earth's temperature, termed the **greenhouse effect**. A greenhouse lets in sunlight through its glass. The light warms the inside, and the glass prevents the heat from escaping. Like the glass, carbon dioxide and water vapor in the atmosphere absorb the long-wavelength heat radiated by the earth.

The greenhouse effect causes much concern because of the possible repercussions of **global warming**. A National Academy of Sciences committee of experts estimated that a global temperature increase of 3°C would occur with a doubling of the carbon dioxide content of the atmosphere. A normal sample of air contains approximately 0.03% or 320 ppm of CO_2. According to the committee, the carbon dioxide level increased by 10% to 12% in the century following 1880. The effect was an increase of 0.4°C in the mean global temperature. The temperature increase resulted in melting of some of the polar ice caps and glaciers. The global ocean level increased by 5.4 inches (14 cm) in that time span.

Seventy atmospheric scientists of the National Academy of Sciences issued a report in 1983. Based on computer models of atmospheric processes, they warned that a doubling of the 1980 carbon dioxide levels in the atmosphere would raise the average global atmosphere temperature between 1.5°C and 4.5°C (2.7°F and 8.1°F). Further, the temperature increase at the earth's polar regions might be two to three times these levels. A 1985 model of the earth's atmosphere suggested that global warming from carbon dioxide buildup might only be half as great as the earlier projections because denser, wetter clouds containing more carbon dioxide should reflect more sunlight into space. Other studies, however, have speculated that dozens of other gases such as chlorofluorocarbons (CFCs) found in trace amounts in the atmosphere could produce a global warming at least as great as that caused by carbon dioxide alone.

There are two effects of global warming that are potentially very harmful. The distribution of rainfall and snowfall over much of the earth can change. Such changes may mean that the world's major food-growing regions (such as those in much of the United States) will shift northward into areas of Canada and other higher latitude areas where the soils tend to be poorer and less productive. Second, glaciers and ice fields in polar regions might melt, causing a projected rise in the average sea level of about 8 feet (2.4 meters) by 2100. If this occurs, there is a high probability that coastal cities and industrial areas will be flooded.

·················

CHLOROFLUOROCARBONS AND OZONE LAYER DEPLETION

Chlorofluorocarbons (CFCs) have become suspect in depletion of the ozone layer. Thomas Midgley developed CFCs in 1930 to replace the poisonous ammonia used in refrigerators during the 1920s. CFCs were considered safe because they did not react with other substances or break down easily. Although CFCs did not break down below the stratosphere, their inventor did not see their reaction in the stratosphere.

Chlorofluorocarbons contain chlorine. At altitudes of 10 to 20 miles in the atmosphere, chlorine is released when the molecular bonds of CFCs break down. Once released, the free chlorine interacts with ozone (O_3) to form elemental oxygen gas (O_2), which has no sun-blocking properties.

Some researchers suspect that bromine also destroys the ozone layer. A study of bromine levels in the Arctic by Walter W. Berg, a scientist for the National Center for Atmospheric Research, and other scientists found a substantial amount of bromine in the Arctic atmosphere. These scientists reported bromine levels that were 10 times higher than normal and about the same level found in other, heavily polluted environments. Berg suggested that the two major contributors to depletion of the ozone layer are red algae and long-range man-made air pollution (CFCs). Red algae produce large quantities of bromine-contaminated compounds in the water under the Arctic ice. Other scientists agree that the major source of bromine is marine in origin but question the mechanism for releasing the bromine into the atmosphere. The significance of the bromine is believed to be its synergism with the chlorine chains, which could aid in destruction of the ozone layer at lower altitudes in the stratosphere and under dark conditions, the opposite of reactions involving chlorine.

Early in 1989, scientists were surprised that the ozone layer above the Antarctic had become significantly thinner. David Hofman of the University of Wyoming discovered this fact by conducting tests with balloon-borne instruments. The Antarctic ozone "hole" in 1989 was almost twice the area of the Antarctic continent. It has since increased slightly in size.

The Arctic ozone layer also has been studied. Scientists from Norway concluded that weather conditions over the Arctic are too dark for chlorine to destroy the ozone layer. They say, however, that destruction may come later because of an increase in sunlight. These scientists concluded that polar stratospheric clouds, in conjunction with sunlight, promote chemical reactions that turn pollutants into ozone-depleting chemicals.

The major concern with depletion of the ozone layer is that the increase in ultraviolet light will reach the surface of the earth, increasing the incidence of skin cancer and cataracts. Such rises have recently been reported in New Zealand and Australia. Ozone depletion could also affect plants and the food chain in some as-yet-undetermined manner. Despite all of the research, experts disagree as to the severity of ozone depletion. Additional research must be conducted to understand all dimensions of the problem.

At present, chlorofluorocarbons are thought to be the main cause of ozone layer depletion. Chlorofluorocarbons are propellants used in products such as hair spray and bathroom cleaners that are sold in aerosol containers. They were also used in refrigeration units in appliances and air conditioners. Chlorofluorocarbons are also minor by-products from the production of foam coffee cups, egg cartons, furniture cushions, and building insulation. Hospi-

tals use a nonflammable gas made of chlorofluorocarbons for sterilization of medical equipment. In the United States and much of the industrialized world, most of the applications using chlorofluorocarbons have been discontinued since 2000.

By far the main focus of research seems to be developing a new form of CFCs that will not harm the environment, especially the ozone layer. After years of denying the adverse effects of CFCs, manufacturers now recognize the problem. They have begun using CFC replacements as well as curbing CFC production. Manufacturers of foam food containers also are involved in researching substitute compounds.

According to many researchers, the best answer to the ozone problem is a new breed of CFCs that are less likely to harm the environment. One alternative compound, HCFC-22 or chlorodifluoromethane, is already on the market. It is 95% less destructive to the ozone layer than standard CFCs. Although it costs up to 50% more than its predecessors, HCFC-22 is gaining popularity as a coolant for commercial and residential air-conditioning systems. In December 1987, the Food and Drug Administration approved HCFC-22 for use in containers used by the fast-food industry.

One drawback to HCFC-22 is that it is less versatile than many of the ozone-depleting CFCs. It is an inferior substitute for building insulation and for use in automobile air-conditioning systems. It has less desirable insulating qualities and a high boiling point. It also requires higher pressure to operate in air-conditioning systems.

Chemical companies have developed other alternative CFCs. These have caused problems in the waste products they give off during the manufacturing process. Years of toxicity testing are necessary before these compounds can be commercially marketed.

The National Aeronautics and Space Administration, the National Oceanic and Atmospheric Administration, the Federal Aviation Administration, the World Meteorological Organization, and the United Nations Environment Program have studied ozone depletion using ground-based and satellite instrumentation. They concluded that between 1969 and 1986, the decline in annual average levels of ozone was from 1.7% to 3% in the Northern

Hemisphere. They also found losses of 95% between altitudes of 9 and 12 miles.

·················

DEFORESTATION EFFECTS

Although they may seem peaceful, forests are places of intense activity. Countless animals, plants, and microorganisms grow and reproduce there. In the process, they filter the air and water, regulate stream flow, store water, and reduce soil erosion. Removing trees changes the ecology in several ways. For example, if even a small plot of tropical forest is cut, the temperature of the region fluctuates from extremely high during the day to cool temperatures at night.

Deforestation can change weather patterns as it has in Panama. Rainfall in areas where deforestation occurred 50 years ago has decreased by 1 cm every year (50 cm for the 50 years) compared to adjacent uncleared land. Forest soil filters polluted rainfall and cleanses it before the water reenters the surface or groundwater supply. Forest vegetation and soil also purify the air. Many environmental pollutants adhere to leaves and branches and are removed. Environmental pollutants are also removed by leaves, detoxified by microorganisms, and taken up by plant roots. Hence, air is cleaner when it leaves the forest than when it enters.

Desertification is a problem related to deforestation. When trees are removed and the land is overgrazed or cultivated, it affects the ecosystem. That is evidenced by the drought that killed tens of thousands of people in the Sahel region of Africa in the early 1970s. In many developing countries, desertification is accelerated by deforestation when wood is burned for fuel and the land is overused. This is evidenced around Khartoum, Sudan, where the native acacia tree no longer grows.

Soil erosion and flooding are direct results of deforestation. Where clear-cutting of trees (cutting everything) occurs, soil erosion often follows. Also, when all of the trees are cut, more water runs off the land and flooding ensues. This happens because trees that once retained water on their trunks, limbs, and leaves are no longer there to hold water during peak runoff after a rain. Some of the water retained on the trees before they were cut reentered the hydrologic cycle by evaporation, thus not adding to

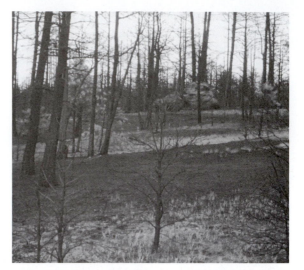

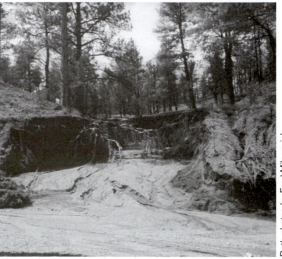

Both photos by Fred Milenovich

It takes years to restore a forest after a forest fire. With fewer trees, erosion is the result.

the peak flow and contributing to floods. Forests also act as sponges, soaking up rainfall during wet weather and releasing it during dry weather.

Plants use carbon dioxide and give off oxygen. Another effect of deforestation is the loss of the oxygen-generating "factories" of photosynthesis. By depleting the forest, the ability to remove carbon dioxide from the environment is reduced. This is a serious contemporary problem as the need for oxygen is increasing.

SUMMARY

Health effects of air pollution can be serious, including asthma, chronic bronchitis, pulmonary emphysema, lung cancer, and heart disorders. Air pollution has been classified by its major sources. Examples of *natural* sources of air pollution are forest fires, dust storms, and volcanic eruptions, as well as pollen-laden plants that irritate mucous membranes. *Anthropogenic* air pollution is produced by humans and includes sources such as smoke, paint vapors and particles, and gases from septic tanks and house sewer systems.

Industrial pollution is created wherever industry releases gases, vapors, fumes, and the like from the manufacture of cars, plastics, clothing, furniture, and other products. *Agricultural* pollutants are created where food is grown, particularly when insecticides and herbicides are used. *Transportation* is a major contributor to air pollution, accounting for approximately half of all air pollution. The use of catalytic converters in automobiles has drastically reduced carbon monoxide pollution from emissions. A final source is *energy* use and production, notably the generation of electricity.

Some important air quality phenomena are acid precipitation, desertification and deforestation, the greenhouse effect, and ozone layer depletion. A recent 10-year study by the EPA suggests that urban air quality is improving. The study reported the following findings for the United States:

- Smog (ground-level ozone) has been reduced by 12%.
- Lead levels in the air have decreased by 89%.
- Sulfur dioxide levels have declined by 26%.
- Carbon monoxide levels have been reduced by 37%.
- Nitrogen dioxide levels have dropped by 12%.
- Particulate levels have decreased by 20%.

In other parts of the world, air pollution levels remain significantly higher than in the United States. This is especially true in urban areas. Many developing countries lack the resources to clean up their environments.

The findings reported above are encouraging and should motivate Americans to continue to make improvements that will protect the health of millions who live, work, and play in areas where air pollutant levels are still too high.

KEY TERMS

Anthropogenic air pollution, p. 249

Catalytic converter, p. 252

Chlorofluorocarbons, p. 258

Deforestation, p. 260

Desertification, p. 260

Electrostatic precipitator, p. 252

Gasification, p. 252

Global warming, p. 258

Greenhouse effect, p. 258

Input control, p. 252

Nitrogen oxides, p. 255

Output control, p. 252

Ozone, p. 257

Ozone layer, p. 258

Particulate air, pollution, p. 249

Photochemical smog, p. 249

Smog, p. 248

Sulfur oxides, p. 255

Thermal inversion, p. 249

REFERENCES

Alvarez-Cohen, Lisa, and William W. Nazaroff. 2000. *Environmental Engineering Science.* John Wiley & Sons, New York.

Doyle, Jack. 2000. *Taken for a Ride: Detroit's Big Three and the Politics of Air Pollution.* Four Walls, Eight Windows, New York.

Ellerman, A. D., P. L. Joskow, R. Schmalensee, J. P. Montero, and E. M. Bailey. 2000. *Markets for Clean Air: The U.S. Acid Rain Program.* Cambridge University Press, New York.

Godish, Thad. 1997. Air Quality, 3rd ed. Lewis Publishers, Boca Raton, FL.

Harrop, Owen. 2001. *Air Quality Assessment and Management: A Practical Guide.* E & F N Spon, London.

Lenz, Hans P. and Christian Cozzarrini. 1999. *Emissions and Air Quality.* Society of Automotive Engineers, Warrendale, PA.

Liu, David H. and Bela G. Liptbak. 1999. *Air Pollution.* Lewis Publishers, Boca Raton, FL.

MacMillan, Donald. 2000. *Smoke Wars: Anaconda Copper, Montana Air Pollution, and the Courts, 1890–1924.* Missoula, MT, Montana Historical Society.

Sokhi, Ranjeet S. 1998. *Urban Air Quality: Monitoring and Modeling.* Kluwer Academic Publishers, Boston, MA.

Turco, Richard P. 2001. *Earth Under Siege: From Air Pollution to Global Change,* 2nd ed. Oxford University Press, New York.

15

OCCUPATIONAL HEALTH

Carolyn Hester Harvey, Ph.D.

Eastern Kentucky University

OBJECTIVES

- Discuss the issues surrounding the need for occupational health and safety.

- Identify the rules, regulations, and federal organizations that implement and enforce these regulations.

- Identify and discuss the occupational health team members, their duties, and their roles in today's society.

- Discuss various types of occupational diseases associated with microbial exposure, their occurrence, treatment, and control.

- Identify chemical and physical hazards in the environment, their sources, impact on the exposed population, and methods of reduction.

HISTORY OF OCCUPATIONAL HYGIENE

Occupational health is the science of protecting man's health through control of the work environment. Man and his environment are indivisible. It is assumed that man moves through his environment and molds it to his desires; however, it may be more productive to think of the environment and man as moving through and changing each other simultaneously.

For centuries, employers and employees have recognized the need for health and safety in the workplace. As early as the 4th century, B.C., lead toxicity in the mining industry was recognized and recorded by Hippocrates. During the 1st century, A.D., Pliny the Elder, a Roman scholar, made reference to the dangers inherent in dealing with zinc and sulfur and described a bladder-derived protective mask to be used by laborers subjected to large amounts of dust or lead fumes. In the 2nd century, Galen, a Greek physician, wrote volumes on anatomy and pathology. Galen recognized the dangers of acid mists to copper miners but did not attempt to solve the problem. In 1473, Ulrich Ellenbog's pamphlet was published in which he described the symptoms of industrial poisoning from lead and mercury with suggested preventive measures. Georgius Agricola, a German scholar, published *De Re Metallica* in 1556. Agricola's book discussed mining, smelting, and refining accidents and descriptions of what we refer to today as "trench foot" and silicosis as well as suggestions for mine ventilation and protective masks for miners. It was translated into English in 1912. In 1567, Paracelsus described respiratory diseases among miners with an excellent description of mercury poisoning. He is remembered as the "Father of Toxicology" and stated, "All substances are poisons with sufficient dose."

In 1713, Bernardo Ramazzini wrote the first book that could be considered a complete treatise on occupational diseases, *De Morbis Artificum Diatriba* (*Diseases of Workers*). He described scores of occupations, their hazards, and resulting diseases. He recommended doctors who treated workers to ask "of what trade he is?" Ramazzini is considered the "Father of Industrial Medicine."

In the late 18th century, Percival Pott described scrotum cancer in chimney sweepers and attributed it to coal soot and lack of hygiene. In the early 19th century, Charles Thrackrah authored the first book on occupational diseases to be published in England and Benjamin W. McCready wrote the book, *On the Influence of Trades, Professions, and Occupations in the United States, in the Production of Disease*, which is generally recognized as the first work on occupational medicine published in the United States. The first legislation regulating conditions in factories was the British Factory and Workshops Act of 1802, which required ventilation in workplaces.

In the early years of the 20th century, Dr. Alice Hamilton published her book, *Exploring the Dangerous Trades*, after working in Illinois on a commission to survey the extent of occupational health problems in that state. She was one of the first American specialists in the field of occupational disease and generally is considered to be the founder of occupational medicine in the United States. In 1910, she began to study the ill effects of dangerous trades. Her famed Illinois survey investigated the health conditions in the lead industry. The problems she found among felt-hat and lead industry workers were shocking. In completing her study, she remarked that "the health effects of new chemicals used in industry were determined by using the workers as guinea pigs." Dr. Hamilton's emphasis on evaluation and control of exposures by applying engineering controls to process technology had a powerful impact on the development of the field of industrial hygiene in the United States. In 1913, the first formal governmental program, the New York Department of Labor's Division of Industrial Hygiene, was established. In 1914, the Office of Industrial Hygiene and Sanitation was formed in the USPHS and subsequently underwent much reorganization before becoming NIOSH in 1971. The Social Security Act of 1935 made federal resources available to states to aid in developing industrial hygiene programs. It was the passage of the Walsh-Healey Public Contracts Act in 1936 that initiated the federal safety and health activities in general industry.

· · · · · · · · · · · · · · ·

THE NEED FOR OCCUPATIONAL HEALTH AND SAFETY

After 1950, a movement began that would eventually develop into Public Law 91-596, the Occupational Safety and Health Act (OSHAct) of 1970. After years of government neglect, the first comprehensive federal health and safety law was proposed under President Lyndon Johnson in 1968. Industry initially united and defeated the bill, but during the late 1960s and early 1970s, Congress enacted four safety and health laws that had a significant impact on industrial hygiene activities in the United States, including the Federal Metal and Nonmetallic Mine Safety Act of 1966, the Federal Coal Mine Health and Safety Act of 1969, the Occupational Safety and Health Act of 1970, and the Federal Mine Safety and Health Act of 1977. Support for these new laws developed over time from sources such as individual congressmen and senators (Senators Williams and Steiger for OSHAct), professionals in the occupational health and health promotion fields, labor unions, foundations, and researchers in the discipline.

Prior to enactment of these laws, governmental regulations of safety and health matters had been largely the concern of state agencies. There was little uniformity of application of codes and standards from one state to another, and almost no enforcement proceedings were lodged against violators of those standards. Some states spent as much as $2.70

per worker, and others spent less than one cent per worker. The federal government had only limited safety and health standards for its contractors. Most federal programs focused only on specific occupations such as railroad workers, longshoremen, federally contracted construction workers and service suppliers, atomic energy workers, and miners. Enforcement of federal safety and health laws was the responsibility of the Bureau of Labor Standards in the U.S. Department of Labor. Although there were thousands of federal contractors, inspection and enforcement activities were extremely limited because of inadequate funding and insufficient staff. Regulations of the OSHAct of 1970 signaled an important shift in governmental involvement in the area of occupational health promotion. The OSHAct moved the focus of employers from treatment-oriented medicine to preventive measures—a strategy deemed necessary to reduce occupational disease.

The OSHAct guaranteed a safe and healthful workplace to all people, recognized the rights of workers, and gave workers the protection of the U.S. government. The act required employers to furnish each employee a place of employment free from recognized hazards that caused or were likely to cause death or serious physical harm to employees and to comply with occupational safety and health standards instituted under the act. The act also granted employees the right to be notified by their employers when they were exposed to toxic materials or harmful physical agents, the right to file confidential complaints with the Occupational Safety and Health Administration regarding unsafe conditions, and the right not to be discriminated against by the employer for exercising any rights granted by the Act. It called for inspection of the workplace without prior notice to a company and allowed a representative of the workers to accompany the inspector on the tour. The act carried fines for violations and required employers to maintain records of work-related deaths, injuries, and illnesses, as well as exposure to toxic materials and harmful agents. The records were required to be available to the workers and the government. The OSHAct required employees to comply with occupational safety and health standards and all rules issued by the act that were applicable to employees' actions and conduct.

OSHA

The OSHAct also provided for the formation of the Department of Labor's Occupational Safety and Health Administration (OSHA). OSHA was charged with setting standards for safety and health in the workplace and with maintaining compliance with these standards. OSHA also was given the authority to set and enforce regulations for workplace safety and health through civil penalties. OSHA allowed any worker to register a complaint and call for an inspection, while protecting the worker from discrimination for using provisions of the OSHAct.

NIOSH

In addition to creating OSHA, the Occupational Safety and Health Act of 1970 resulted in establishment of the Department of Health and Human Services' National Institute for Occupational Safety and Health (NIOSH). The act authorized NIOSH to conduct research and identify industrial hazards, as well as to promote occupational safety and health through education and the dissemination of information. Since its creation, NIOSH has researched and published many important criteria documents for industrial exposure, as well as describing risks and protective measures. Industrial situations that NIOSH has studied include occupational exposure to coke oven emissions, asbestos, arsenic, mercury, vinyl chloride, benzene, and a number of organic solvents. Passage of the OSHAct and creation of NIOSH represents tremendous progress in the history of occupational safety and health.

Meticulous attention to and support of occupational health programs benefit private enterprises. Labor turnover, absenteeism, and liability compensation for occupational illness and injury are three sources of significant financial loss to business and industry. Industrial health programs are important in decreasing the monetary costs associated with these factors. Healthy workers are more capable, productive, and dependable than unhealthy workers. Occupational health programs also benefit the employee and the community. For employees and their dependents, occupational health programs facilitate sustained earnings, lower personal health care costs, increase and extend productivity, and increase job satisfaction and security. In the community, occupational health programs increase prosperity, reduce welfare costs, decrease incidents of labor unrest, and support higher-quality community medical and public health services.

········

THE OCCUPATIONAL HEALTH TEAM

The development of occupational health and industrial hygiene programs in the United States originated in factories, manufacturing plants, and mills and remained exclusive to these industries for many years. Today, occupational health and industrial hygiene programs are found in every type of industry. Members of the occupational health and industrial hygiene team employed by an industry are responsible for operation of the program and delivery of medical care in the workplace.

In general, the occupational health and industrial hygiene program is designed to protect workers from illness and injury on the job, either by law, regulation, or contract. The definition of occupational medicine by the Council on Industrial Health of the American Medical Association is as follows: Occupational medicine deals with the restoration and conservation of health in relation to work, the working environment, and maximum efficiency. It involves prevention, recognition, and treatment of occupational disabilities and requires the application of special techniques in the fields of rehabilitation, environmental hygiene, toxicology, sanitation, and human relations.

A good industrial health program is designed primarily for the benefit of the workers, although employers often gain substantially from the program as well. The Council on Industrial Health of the American Medical Association lists the objectives of an occupational health program as:

1. To protect individuals against health hazards in their work environment;

2. To ensure and facilitate the suitable placement of individuals according to their physical capacities and their emotional makeup in work that they can perform with an acceptable degree of efficiency and without endan-

gering their own health and safety or that of their fellow employees; and

3. To encourage personal health maintenance.

The Council on Industrial Health further describes the following services that the occupational health team of an industry should provide:

1. Regular appraisal of plant sanitation

2. Periodic inspection for occupational disease hazards

3. Adoption and maintenance of adequate control measures

4. Provision of first aid and emergency services

5. Prompt and early treatment for all illnesses resulting from occupational exposure

6. Referral to the family physician of individuals with conditions requiring attention and cooperation between the patient and the physician to remedy the condition

7. Uniform recording of absenteeism from all types of disability

8. Unbiased health appraisals of all workers

9. Access to rehabilitation services within industry

10. Availability of a beneficial health education program

The number and character of workers engaged in the occupational health and industrial hygiene program in a given industry vary with the number of employees, type of industry, demands of the workers, and philosophy of the management. Like any other major management function, safety and health management requires a defined chain of command, ending with an individual who is accountable at the level of president or vice president. Very small plants often make provisions only for first aid, or for a physician to be called in the case of an emergency. Medium-size plants or companies often employ a full-time occupational health nurse who administers routine care. Larger industries may have facilities including an infirmary, eye and dental clinics, X-ray and laboratory services, along with the appropriate number of physicians and technical support staff these facilities require. Large occupational medical staffs usually are supplemented by the work of industrial hygienists, safety professionals, and industrial health educators who work together to ensure a workplace that promotes optimum health, safety, and productivity of those who work there.

Occupational Health Nurse

Central to most occupational health programs is the **occupational health nurse**. The role of the occupational health nurse varies with the needs of the employers for whom the nurse works. In the past, the occupational health nurse was primarily a first-aid giver. This role has changed during the last decades. Today the occupational health nurse is responsible for the care of illnesses and injuries occurring at the workplace. For workers who require additional or specialized care, the occupational health nurse must provide referrals to appropriate qualified physicians. The nurse must be knowledgeable in the areas of preventive and rehabilitative health. If the industry does not employ an industrial health educator, the occupational health nurse often is responsible for counseling and providing health and safety education. The responsibility for maintaining complex occupational health record systems often rests with the occupational health nurse, in addition to the routine duties of assisting the occupational physician with workers' physical examinations and health screening tests.

Occupational Physician

Most industries do not require the services of an **occupational physician** full-time, but, rather, arrange for physicians' services on a contractual basis. The occupational physician may maintain regularly scheduled hours on certain days at the company clinic or may provide care from his or her office. The occupational health physician typically performs pre-employment physicals on prospective employees, treats work-related injuries and illnesses, supervises drug screening, and determines the presence and extent of workers' disability for the company and various government agencies.

Industrial Hygienist

Industrial hygiene activities are defined as the anticipation, recognition, evaluation, and control of environmental factors that have an adverse effect on the health and efficiency of employees. The **industrial hygienist** assesses and recommends methodology for controlling environmental hazards and toxic substances such as dusts, gases, vapors, and fumes; physical agents such as excessive noise, heat, and radiation; biological hazards such as blood-borne pathogens; and other job-related stresses such as repetitive motion or other ergonomic stresses. In the past, only the larger corporations typically employed industrial hygienists, but in recent years even small companies employ or contract the services of an industrial hygienist.

Responsibilities of the industrial hygienist include the following:

- Direct the industrial hygiene program.
- Examine the work environment and environs.
- Study work operations and processes, and obtain full details of the nature of the work, materials, and equipment used, products and byproducts, number and sex of employees, and hours of work.
- Make appropriate measurements to determine the magnitude of exposure or nuisance to workers.
- Study and test biological materials, such as blood and urine, by chemical and physical means, when such examination will aid in determining the extent of exposure.
- Interpret results of the examination of the work environment and environs in terms of ability to impair health, nature of health impairment, workers' efficiency, and community nuisance and/or damage, and present specific conclusions to appropriate interested parties such as management and health officials.
- Make specific decisions as to the need for, or effectiveness of, control measures, and, when necessary, advise as to the procedures that will be suitable and effective for both the environment and environs.

- Prepare rules, regulations, standards, and procedures for the healthful conduct of work and the prevention of nuisance in the community.

- Present expert testimony before courts of law, hearing boards, workers compensation commissions, regulatory agencies, and legally appointed investigative bodies covering all matters pertaining to industrial hygiene.

- Prepare appropriate text for labels and precautionary information for materials and products to be used by workers and the public.

- Conduct programs for the education of workers and the public on how to prevent occupational disease and community nuisance.

- Conduct epidemiological studies among workers and industries to discover possibilities of the presence of occupational disease, and establish or improve threshold limit values or standards as guides for maintaining of health and efficiency.

- Conduct research to advance knowledge concerning the effects of occupation upon health and means of preventing occupational health impairment, community air pollution, noise, nuisance, and related problems.

Safety Engineer

The level of education and training of the **safety engineer** traditionally has varied greatly, from technicians who performed simple control procedures to the personnel manager responsible for completing accident reports and other forms required by government agencies and insurance companies. Today, the safety engineer commonly possesses a master's or even a doctoral degree and has the responsibility of developing complex systems for the analysis and control of occupational hazards. The safety engineer in an industry with diversified processes must be a generalist. He or she must be knowledgeable in a wide range of technical, legal, and administrative areas. The safety engineer is concerned not only with preventing accidents but also with hazard control systems based on environmental and human factor analysis. According to the American Society of Safety Engineers

(ASSE), the major functions of the safety engineer are the following:

- Identifying and appraising accident- and loss-producing conditions and practices and evaluating the severity of the accident problem;

- Developing accident prevention and loss control methods, procedures, and programs;

- Communicating accident- and loss-control information to those directly involved;

- Measuring and evaluating the effectiveness of the accident- and loss-control system and the modifications needed to achieve optimum results.

The safety engineer and associated staff usually are responsible for executing the following safety functions:

- Ensure that federal, state, and local safety laws, regulations, codes, and rules are observed.

- Ensure that OSHA record-keeping and reporting requirements are met.

- Assist management in preparing safety policies and ensure that they are carried out.

- Monitor all activities where accidents could occur that would cause injury to personnel, damage to equipment or facilities, or loss of materials.

- Cease any operation or activity that constitutes an imminent hazard to personnel or could result in loss of equipment or facilities.

- Establish liaison and working arrangements with other activities involved in accident prevention, such as plant security officers, fire prevention workers, and medical personnel.

- Assist in the formation of safety committees and direct their activities.

- Review and approve the safety aspects of plant facility designs and of equipment procured.

- Assure that hazardous areas and dangerous equipment are posted according to standards.

- Control selection and use of hazard monitoring, personal protective and emergency equipment.

- Conduct safety training of personnel at all levels.
- Investigate accidents and hazardous conditions, and prepare necessary reports.
- Disseminate information on safety to all employees.
- Accompany inspectors from governmental agencies and insurance companies at the plant.
- Establish procedures for hazardous operations.
- Make on-site reviews of activities and determine their potential for accidents.
- Inspect emergency supplies.
- Maintain all records relating to safety activities.

Industrial Health Educator

The **industrial health educator** is a recent addition to the occupational health care team. In small industries the occupational health nurse may counsel and educate workers concerning health and safety in the workplace. In other companies, the safety engineer may have the role of health and safety training and education. As government and other agencies increase their scrutiny and documentation requirements of health and safety practices and controls in industry, the occupational health nurse and safety engineer have less and less time to educate employees effectively in the areas of health and safety practices. The industrial health educator may possess a bachelor's, master's, or doctoral degree, and is qualified to execute the following responsibilities:

- Educate workers and the public in the prevention of occupational diseases and back injury, dermatitis, and others.
- Counsel workers concerning job-related stress, sexual harassment, drug abuse, and other problems that could affect their job performance and productivity.
- Conduct epidemiological studies, surveys, and audits to determine the prevalence of certain occupational diseases and illnesses among workers, as well as health and safety attitudes of workers.

- Prepare appropriate text for labels and precautionary information for materials and products to be used by workers and the public.
- Conduct research to advance knowledge concerning the effects of certain occupations upon health, and determine the means of preventing occupational health impairment.

· · · · · · · · · · · · · · · ·

OCCUPATIONAL DISEASES

Biological Hazards

Biological agents generally represent fewer hazardous exposures than those of a physical or chemical nature. Certain occupations, however, allow a significant number of exposures. These occupations include laboratory, research, and hospital personnel, as well as physicians, veterinarians, and people involved with food and food processing, plants, and animals. Miners and farmers also are at a greater risk than most other workers because of their contact with the soil, which may harbor potentially hazardous biological agents.

Biological hazards, also known as **biohazards**, are living organisms that are infectious agents and represent a potential risk to human or animal health. The five types of biological agents that may produce infection in humans are: bacteria, viruses, rickettsiae, fungi, and parasites. Transmission of biohazardous agents may occur through inhalation, injection, ingestion, or physical contact. Whether a person exposed to the biohazardous agent will contract the disease depends on a number of factors, including the number of organisms, the virulence of the organisms, and the person's resistance to the organism. Biohazardous agents may be both synergistic and additive. For this reason, a person exposed to a combination of stresses, such as those of a physical or chemical nature, is more likely to be susceptible to the biohazard and thus contract the disease.

Classification of Biological Hazards

Identification and classification of biohazards are essential to determine the appropriate means of control to prevent infections. The U.S. Public Health Service (USPHS) and the U.S. Department of Agriculture (USDA) contributed to development of standard classifications for evaluating the hazards represented by a variety of biohazardous agents. The standard provides a means of describing minimal safety conditions. The standard defines four classes of biohazardous agents and a fifth class representing animal pathogens that are excluded from the United States by law. Agents comprising Class 1 are less hazardous than those of Class 2, and so on. The standard provides only for the minimum safety conditions considered necessary. The five classes of agents are as follows:

Class 1 Agents of no or minimal hazard under ordinary conditions of handling that can be handled safely without special apparatus or equipment, using techniques generally acceptable for nonpathogenic materials. Class 1 includes all bacterial, fungal, viral, rickettsial, chlamydial, and parasitic agents not included in higher classes.

Class 2 Includes agents that may produce disease of varying degrees of severity through accidental inoculation, injection, or other means of cutaneous penetration but that usually can be contained adequately and safely by ordinary laboratory techniques.

Class 3 Agents involving special hazards or agents derived from outside the United States that require a USDA permit for importation unless they are specified for higher classification. Class 3 includes pathogens that require special conditions for containment.

Class 4 Agents that require the most stringent conditions for containment because they are extremely hazardous to personnel or may cause serious epidemic disease. Class 4 requires special conditions for containment.

Class 5 Foreign animal pathogens that are excluded from the United States by law or whose entry is restricted by USDA administrative policy.

BACTERIAL AGENTS

Bacteria are simple, single-cell organisms visible only under the microscope. They multiply by fission or simple division into two parts. Bacteria include *cocci*, which are round and resemble a string of beads, the *rod-shaped bacilli*, and the *corkscrew-shaped spirilla*. Some bacteria are disease causing, or pathogenic; others are harmless or even useful. Neglected minor wounds and abrasions in which the integrity of the skin surface is compromised usually cause occupationally induced bacterial infections. Mixed bacteria typically cause these infections, but staphylococci and streptococci most often are the primary offending organisms.

RICKETTSIAL AND CHLAMYDIAL AGENTS

The rod-shaped or coccoid rickettsiae are bacterial in nature but smaller in size. As obligate parasites, they rely on their hosts to provide everything they need for growth, reproduction, and even survival. Because rickettsiae can survive only within living cells, these microbes are associated with and transmitted to people via blood-sucking arthropods such as fleas, ticks, and lice. Typhus and Rocky Mountain spotted fever are transmitted by rickettsiae. Chlamydiae, bacterial in nature, also are obligate parasites. As intracellular microorganisms, they are distinguished from rickettsiae by their smaller size and their more complicated method of reproduction. Chlamydiae usually are transmitted in the air and gain access to the body through the respiratory system. Chlamydiae occur as two species, both of which are pathogenic to humans. The primary source of human infection is birds.

VIRAL AGENTS

Viruses are noncellular, parasitic pathogens that are smaller than bacteria, rickettsiae, or chlamydiae. In fact, they are the smallest organism known and can be seen only with the aid of an electron microscope. Viruses are obligate parasites that are neither living nor nonliving, but require association with a living cell to grow, reproduce, and function. Occupationally acquired viral diseases are likely to include animal respiratory viruses, poxviruses, enteroviruses, and arboviruses. Infections may be acquired from the vector or from handling animals or animal products. Laboratory-acquired infections may result from working with the infectious agent, from accidents, animals, clinical or autopsy specimens, from aerosols, or from glassware. In hospitals, viral transmission may occur among patients and staff.

FUNGAL AGENTS

Fungi are a phylum of plants derived from algae, of which more than 70,000 species are known. All fungi lack chlorophyll and other pigment. Because they are incapable of synthesizing protein or other organic material from simple compounds, fungi are considered parasitic or saprophytic. Occupationally acquired fungal disease is not significant and is confined mainly to farmers, animal handlers, and other outdoor workers. Diagnosis of fungal diseases is made by microscopic identification of the fungus with cultural confirmation. Fungal diseases may be classified according to their effects, which may be systemic, subcutaneous, superficial (such as ringworm or athlete's foot), or hypersensitivity effects. Hypersensitivity effects usually are attributable to fungal antigens inhaled with dusts and usually involve pneumonitis with symptoms similar to asthma.

PARASITIC AGENTS

Although microbes such as bacteria and viruses can be parasitic, the classification of parasitic agents generally includes not the microbes but, instead, the parasitic organisms that are either a plant or an animal. Parasites live advantageously in or on another organism to whose welfare they contribute nothing. Protozoa, metazoa (helminths), and arthropods typically cause infections of occupational significance. Malaria and other blood and gastrointestinal disorders are caused by protozoa. Helminths are responsible for the transmission of schistosomiasis and hookworm. Mites and chiggers are arthropods and may cause simple dermatoses or may act as vectors or hosts for other non-arthropod parasites. A parasitic disease is any disease resulting from the invasion of the body by parasitic agents. Depending on the virulence of the parasite and resistance of the host, the host may or may not contract the disease.

Control of Biohazards

The effects of biological hazardous agents often are subtle and develop after a lag time. An agent representing a biological hazard may be invisible, odorless, and tasteless. For this reason, workers often are not cognizant that they are being exposed. In addition, when an infection does develop, its origin may be difficult to determine. In light of these characteristics of biohazardous agents, education and training are required to increase awareness of the need for control of biological hazardous agents. Because of the serious potential risks of biohazards, effective biohazard control is essential.

The biological hazard control program usually consists of analyzing biohazards, developing safety regulations, training and educating personnel, inspecting and enforcing safety rules, reporting and investigating accidents properly, and funding programs adequately to carry them out to completion.

The primary emphasis of biohazard control should be at the source of potential contamination. Control practices usually include a health surveillance program, standardized work procedures, education of employees, and environmental control procedures. The primary goal of biohazard control is to prevent illnesses in the worker. Control efforts may be difficult because the results of exposure to a biohazard typically are not clinically evident for a considerable time. Unintended exposure to biohazards often stems from poor working habits of the employees.

Management's role in the control of biohazards is to educate employees about the potential risks of the substances with which they are dealing. Although the degree of hazard to the employee depends primarily upon the biological agent itself and its conditions of use, employees should receive proper instruction concerning the hazards to which they will be exposed each time they work with a biohazardous substance. The employees should assume that every biological agent to which they are exposed presents a hazard and, for this reason, they should exercise every precaution available to them when handling any biohazardous substance.

All new employees should receive a pre-employment physical examination to establish a baseline reference. Workers currently employed by or transferred to the biohazardous area also should receive regular physical examinations. Workers exposed to biohazards include those handling potentially oncogenic, biological, or toxic chemical materials, those responsible for cleaning laboratory glassware, handling experimental animals or their tissues, and those who perform janitorial duties.

The current health status of employees should be considered when working with biohazards, as a worker may become more susceptible to infection or harm as a result of change in health status, such as in the case of pregnancy.

Workers likely to be exposed to biohazards should be vaccinated if a satisfactory vaccine exists. The efficiency of vaccines in preventing infection in workers may be less than that of the general population because the worker may receive a higher dose of the infectious microorganisms than the general public would. In addition, the worker may be subject to exposure by a different route than normally would be expected in the general population.

Management should establish and implement an environmental control and personnel safety program that includes biological safety. A safety manual with written safety policies concerning biohazards should be made available to all personnel likely to be exposed. The manual should cover general safe practices and procedures. Also, specific procedures for each department's employees should be made available to workers.

To further control exposure to biological hazards, no person should be admitted to a biohazardous area unless he or she is assigned specifically to work within that area. Eating, drinking, smoking, and gum chewing should be prohibited in areas where work with infectious agents is conducted. Employees who work with biohazardous material should be required to carefully wash and disinfect their hands before and after eating or smoking. All unnecessary materials and equipment should be restricted from the biohazardous area.

Employees and visitors entering biohazardous areas should be required to wear protective clothing commensurate with the level of risk involved. Protective clothing should not be worn outside the work area. The OSHAct required universal biohazard symbol should be used to identify all restricted biohazardous areas. All storage spaces, incubators, refrigerators, and other equipment associated with biohazardous materials also should bear this symbol. All surfaces likely to come in contact with the infectious agent areas should be disinfected with a suitable germicide.

Appropriate precautions should be exercised to reduce the risks associated with processes such as centrifugation, grinding, and other processes likely to generate aerosols. Contaminated wastes should be decontaminated before disposal. Before incineration or autoclaving, dry contaminated wastes should be collected in impermeable bags and sealed. Heat or chemicals should be used to decontaminate wet wastes before discharging them into the sanitary system. For biohazard control to be effective, all personnel involved with biohazards must work together to reduce the amount of potential health hazard by following and enforcing the recommended procedures and guidelines.

Chemical Hazards

Each year more than 5,000 new chemicals are developed, many of which will be used in the workplace. Most chemical substances have the potential to cause injury or illness of the worker who handles them. Chemicals that are not inherently toxic still may pose a potential hazard because of their potential for fire or explosion. Only small amounts of highly toxic substances such as cyanide, arsenic, mercury, and beryllium compounds can produce significant harm. All materials can be relatively safe if the proper precautions are taken while handling them.

The three primary routes by which chemical substances can enter the body are inhalation, absorption through the skin, and ingestion. A less common route of entry is by injection with sharp objects, compressed air, or pressurized liquid.

1. *Inhalation.* The surface area of the lungs ranges from 300 square feet at rest to about 1,000 square feet during inspiration. This allows inhaled chemicals to be absorbed rapidly into the bloodstream and distributed throughout the entire body. Approximately 90% of all industrial poisonings, other than dermatitis, are attributable to inhalation. Although many air contaminants are absorbed and distributed throughout the body, several remain in the lungs and cause pulmonary inflammation and subsequent scarring, also known by the names of anthracosis, byssinosis, siderosis, silicosis, and asbestosis.

2. *Absorption.* Absorption of toxic chemicals through the skin usually is slower than in-

halation. If the integrity of the skin has been compromised, however, absorption can be rapid. Some chemicals are absorbed readily through the skin and hair follicles. Although the skin has an outer coating of sebum, sweat and keratin that provides a small amount of protection, this coating is washed away easily with soap and water, as well as many organic solvents and bases. Chemicals readily absorbed through the skin include benzene, toluene, nitroglyceride, tetraethyl (organic), lead, mercury, and arsenic. Absorption is facilitated in hot environments and when body oils have been removed by degreasers and solvents. Contact dermatitis accounts for 30% of all worker compensation cases and occupational diseases.

3. *Ingestion*. Chemical substances generally are not ingested intentionally by workers, but accidental ingestion may occur by eating, smoking, or drinking in areas where toxic chemicals exist. Most chemicals are easily absorbed into the bloodstream during digestion. Careful washing before eating and drinking is required to prevent unintentional ingestion of toxic substances. Lead and arsenic are two of the more toxic substances ingested.

Contaminants

Excluding dermatitis, inhalation of air contaminants is the leading cause of occupational diseases. Chemical hazards exist as air contaminants in the following forms:

Mist.   A mist is composed of liquid droplets suspended in air and is formed by condensation in a gas to a liquid or by dispersing liquid into tiny particles. Dispersion can be accomplished by various processes, including sparging, foaming, and spraying. Chromic, hydrochloric, hydrofluoric, nitric, and sulfuric acids often are used in a diluted form in pickling, cleaning, and electroplating operations. These acids frequently are sprayed, causing mists to form. When inhaled, all acid mists are dangerous lung irritants. Adequate ventilation around these operations is necessary to remove any toxic mists that develop, and personal protective equipment, such as appropriate respirators, should be worn wherever acid mists are found.

Vapor.   Vapors are the gaseous forms of substances that exist normally as liquids or solids at room temperature and pressure. Vapors generally are present wherever their liquid sources are found. Vapors may be present when using organic solvents, paint thinner, cleaners, and other agents. To determine the relative amount of vapor present and, thus, the severity of a vapor hazard, the vapor pressure of the liquid must be known. The higher the vapor pressure, the greater is the amount of vapors released from a liquid. Vapors generally gain entrance to the body through inhalation, and through skin absorption to a lesser extent. Many vapors present fire and explosion hazards, necessitating that each vapor be evaluated on an individual basis to determine the hazard it presents and to determine its appropriate handling, storage, disposal, and emergency procedures.

Gases.   Gases are fluids that take the shape of whatever container is available to them. Gases diffuse and can be converted to a liquid or solid state by increasing the pressure and decreasing the temperature. Gases typically are produced by arc welding, combustion, and other chemical reactions. Each gas has a unique action on lung tissue. Some gases do not harm the lung tissue but, rather, dissolve in the blood and exert toxic effects in some other area of the body. Carbon monoxide, a toxic gas, is an example of this mode of action. It is commonly found in industry and is responsible for more deaths by asphyxiation than any other gas. Carbon monoxide most often is produced by incomplete combustion of petroleum products in internal combustion engines. Some gases produce adverse reactions directly on the lung tissue. Phosgene gas, for example, is a highly irritating gas that causes fluid to form in the lungs so the individual literally drowns.

Smoke.   Smokes are produced by the incomplete combustion of organic materials such as wood, coal and petroleum products. Smoke consists of particles smaller than 0.1 micron, which are smaller in size than dust particles. Smoke generally contains gases, droplets, and dry particles.

Dust. Dusts are solid particles produced by crushing, grinding, drilling, and otherwise handling materials. Dust particles range in size from 0.1 micron to 25 microns. Those from 0.5 to 5 microns settle deep in the lung and cause most dust-induced illnesses. Larger dust particles usually are filtered by hairs in the nose, pharynx, throat, or bronchi before gaining access to or reaching the alveoli of the lung. Dust is either organic or inorganic. *Organic* dust is a product of living material, such as grain. *Inorganic* dusts originate from nonliving matter, such as minerals and metals. Some dust-induced diseases, such as anthracosis and silicosis, may manifest themselves only after years of exposure. Other dust-induced illnesses, such as those caused by toxic metal exposure from lead and manganese, appear in only days to weeks. Allergic reactions from dust may occur in seconds.

Fumes. Fumes are solid particles created by condensation of a substance from a gaseous state. Fumes generally occur after a molten metal changes from a liquid to a vapor or gas and is condensed in the air. This process usually produces oxides when the vaporized metal reacts with the air. All metal fumes and dusts are irritating, but some cause much more serious harm than simple irritation when inhaled. Fumes and dusts are produced in operations such as smelting, grinding, and welding. Metals creating a health hazard include antimony, arsenic, beryllium, cadmium, chromium, copper, iron, cobalt, lead, mercury, selenium, tellurium, thallium, and manganese. To keep fumes at a minimum, good housekeeping must be practiced, and all employees with significant exposures should be included in a surveillance program that includes monitoring blood and urine for metal levels.

Aerosol. Aerosols are liquid droplets or solid particles that remain dispersed in the air for a prolonged period of time. When deposited in the lungs, aerosols may produce rapid local tissue damage, some slower tissue reactions, eventual disease, or only physical blocking. Some toxic aerosols do not affect the lung tissue locally but are transferred from the lungs into the bloodstream, where they are distributed to other organs. Asbestos fibers may be considered an aerosol, causing fibrotic growth in the alveolar tissue, clogging the ducts, or limiting the effective area of the alveolar lining.

Absorption. Chemical hazards arise from high concentrations of mists, vapors, gases, or solids in the form of dusts or fumes in the air. In addition to the hazard of inhalation, many of these materials act as skin irritants or may be toxic by absorption through the skin. Organic and inorganic chemicals are the major sources of occupational dermatoses. Most chemical agents are classified as primary irritants.

Primary irritants are likely to evoke adverse reactions in *all* people. These chemical substances react on contact, dissolving a portion of the skin. The result may range from complete destruction of the skin to burning or inflammation, depending on the concentration of the chemical and the duration of exposure to the skin. Many primary irritants damage skin because they are water-soluble. Even the water-insoluble compounds, of which many are solvents, react with the lipids in the skin. The exact mechanism of primary skin irritation is not completely understood. About 80% of all occupational dermatoses are caused by primary irritants. Most inorganic and organic acids act as primary irritants. Certain inorganic alkalis, such as ammonium hydroxide and sodium hydroxide, are primary skin irritants. Metallic salts, especially the arsenicals, chromates, mercurials, nickel sulphate, and zinc chloride, product solvents, representing a large number of substances, irritate the skin because of their solvent properties. Because the skin irritation generally is confined to the area of direct contact, dermatitis caused by a primary irritant is referred to as contact dermatitis. Although a contact dermatitis can be severe, it should not recur as long as the infected person avoids contact with the irritant. This may be accomplished either by a job reassignment or through the use of protective gear that prevents skin contact with the offending substance.

CONTROL OF AIRBORNE CHEMICAL HAZARDS

Because chemical hazards often are airborne, control of air contamination should receive priority. Some common control methods include the following:

1. *Substitution or replacement.* Replacing toxic substances with innocuous substitutes is often possible. Many harmless chemical substitutes perform as well as harmful agents and at a fraction of the original hazard potential.

2. *Isolation of operation.* Isolating the hazard-generating process within an enclosure prevents contamination of the surrounding clean areas. This method includes mechanization or automation of the process so employees are not exposed to the hazards the process generates.

3. *Elimination or reduction of employee exposure.* A work area generating significant amounts of contaminated air is isolated from other working areas. The isolated areas have self-closing doors, no windows, and a slightly negative pressure to prevent contamination of the general work area. When possible, employees are restricted from this hazardous area to minimize exposures.

4. *Local exhaust.* Air contaminants are captured at their sources and removed from the area by using hoods and fans. Local exhaust can be used effectively to rid workers' air of dust, fumes, and vapors.

5. **Ventilation**. A general ventilation system typically is not sufficient to control airborne contaminants that represent significant health hazards. In the case of numerous, widely distributed, and low-toxicity sources of contamination throughout a building, general ventilation is helpful. General ventilation includes opening windows and doors and operating fans.

6. *Wetting methods.* Wetting is especially useful with dust hazards. Wetting reduces or eliminates the amount of dust generated. Cutting, drilling, grinding, and other operations are all rendered less hazardous by wetting control methods.

7. *Housekeeping.* Air contaminants often can be effectively controlled or eliminated by good housekeeping practices, which include sealing stored solvents, wiping up spills, and removing dust as it accumulates.

8. *Personal protective equipment.* Respirators are effective in reducing the hazard associated with airborne contaminants. The type of respirator must be appropriate for the hazard involved. To be effective, respirators must be properly fitted, maintained, and worn. Other protective equipment may include clothing, gloves, boots, and coveralls.

9. *Control of occupational skin disease.* Almost all chemical substances represent a hazard to the skin. Control of occupational skin disease begins with the worker's recognition of those substances related to his or her job that cause skin irritations. Proper precautions should be taken to minimize exposure. Where possible, less irritating or nonirritating chemicals should be substituted. Enclosures, temperature controls, automated handling devices, exhaust hoods, and process changes all are engineering controls that can reduce exposure to irritating substances.

10. *Detailed and accurate labeling* of known irritant chemicals and *strictly enforced standard practices* for their handling and use are effective control methods. Employers should alert and educate employees about the hazards associated with chemicals the employees use, in addition to the precautions to be taken in their use. Employees can effectively use personal protective equipment, such as gloves and special clothing, to avoid or minimize exposure to skin irritants. For each chemical, employees should use the appropriate protective gear, as some chemicals degrade or dissolve protective gloves and clothing. To provide additional protection to the skin, employees can use barrier creams and ointments with gloves and protective clothing, but they should remove the ointments after the job is completed.

Physical Hazards

Physical hazards include excessive levels of electromagnetic and ionizing radiation, noise and vibration, and extremes of temperature and pressure.

RADIATION

More and more industry relies upon radiation for many processes, including nondestructive testing of welds, fastening and other internal structures, medical diagnoses and treatment, examination of packages and baggage, and use in radioactive gauges in quality control. Ionizing radiation consists of alpha, beta, and neutron particles, and X-rays and gamma rays. Each of these may cause injury by producing ionization of the cellular components, leading to functional changes in body tissues. The body's tissues differ in their sensitivity and biological responses to ionizing radiation. The injury resulting from radiation exposure is dependent on (a) time and (b) intensity of exposure. The greater the length of time a worker is exposed to a radiation source, the greater is the injury that can result. The intensity of a dose depends on the strength of the source, distance from the source, and presence and amount of any shielding. Radiation effects generated during a massive single exposure are acute and can produce both immediate and delayed effects on the body. Low but repeated radiation exposures are chronic and generally have delayed effects. Acute exposures typically are caused by accidents.

Chronic exposures generally are the result of unrecognized hazardous conditions. The most common way to prevent workers' overexposure to radiation is to closely monitor exposure to radiation. Employers use film badges, film rings, or pocket dosimeters to monitor ionizing radiation exposure. Pocket dosimeters are preferable as they give a continuous reading of ionizing radiation present. Film badges must be removed and processed to determine the dose of ionizing radiation received, thus giving the employee no warning of overexposure. In addition to careful monitoring of radiation exposure, employers should observe the following precautionary measures against ionizing radiation:

1. Permit only qualified personnel to operate and handle any equipment or material that produces ionizing radiation.

2. Prepare and post in the worksite operating and emergency procedures for radiation safety.

3. Restrict access to areas in which equipment or materials produce ionizing radiation.

4. Require personnel entering areas where ionizing radiation is present to wear protective clothing and equipment.

5. Ban the use of edible materials, cosmetics, and cigarettes in areas where ionizing radiation is used.

6. Develop clean-up techniques and procedures for every area using any radioactive material.

NOISE POLLUTION

Noise is defined as unwanted sound. Fourteen million workers in the United States are exposed to hazardous noise. Noise is one pollutant that dissipates when generated, but the effects may linger until death. According to some authorities, the world noise level is increasing by 1 decibel per year. Noise can be an indoor problem or a community concern.

Indoor noise consists of sound generated by the electric home can opener, mixer, electric knife, air conditioner fan, radio, television, food blender, garbage grinder, and vacuum cleaner. In offices, the telephone, computer, copier, and whining air conditioner or fan generate noise. Industry has numerous sources of noise, such as engine blades, belts, wheels, and abrasive devices.

Among the various sources of community noise are trucks, cars, airplanes, tractors, helicopters, and motorcycles. As if those are not enough, we produce off-road bikes, snowmobiles, motor boats, and race cars. At construction and demolition sites vehicles and tools create noise. For example, bulldozers, earth movers, concrete breakers (jackhammers), power saws, pile drivers, pumps and motors, and pneumatic riveters all produce high levels of noise. Power lawnmowers, weed eaters, and other home and garden tools generate noise in addition to banging garbage cans, barking dogs and racing three wheelers. In addition, on holidays we shoot firecrackers to make noise. A hundred years ago people thought horses, mooing cows, and crowing chickens were too noisy!

To determine levels of noise, a sound level meter or a noise meter measures sound pressure in **decibels (dB)**. In a noise survey, levels are expressed on a logarithmic scale. Thus, 80 dB is 10 times as loud as 70 dB and 90 dB is 100 times as loud as 70 dB, 100 dB is 1,000 times as loud as 70 dB, etc.

Exposure to noise levels greater than 85 dB for lengthy periods can result in hearing loss. The hear-

■ TABLE 15.1 ■

RATINGS OF COMMON NOISE SOURCES

Response criteria	dBA	Sound source
Painful noise	150	
	140	Aircraft carrier deck
Limited amplified speech	130	
	120	Jet aircraft flyover
Maximum vocal effort	110	Discotheque (rock band) Chainsaw Riveting machine
Very annoying	100	Motorcycle
Hearing damage (8 hours)	90	Heavy truck Power lawnmower Snowmobile
Annoying	80	Heavy traffic (50 ft)
Telephone use difficult	70	Freeway traffic (50 ft) Dishwasher
Intrusive	60	Conversational speech (3 ft)
Quiet	50	Business office
	40	Average residence
Very quiet	30	Library
	20	Broadcast studio
Just audible	10	
Threshold hearing	0	

Source: *Environmental Quality,* First Annual Report of the Council on Environment Quality

ing loss depends on how loud the noise is and the length of time it is heard. Table 15.1 gives ratings for some common sources of noise.

If noise did not harm the body, it would not be considered an environmental health issue. Vern Knudren from the University of California, Los Angeles, said, "Noise, like smog, is a slow agent of death." It can cause psychological, psychophysical, and physiological damage.

1. Loud noises affect the body psychologically in several ways. Hearing a neighbor's televi-sion when trying to sleep or a loud radio while studying is not only an invasion of one's privacy but also a source of tension, anxiety, and anger. These reactions could lead to a loss of temper, culminating in quar-rels, fights, and even homicide.

2. The psychophysical effect pertains to com-munication interface, such as speech. Particu-larly loud or unsettling speech can trigger in-voluntary or voluntary reactions, such as stress or overreaction, which prevent the body from relaxing and disturb rest. Noise also may prevent a person from hearing warning signals, thereby precipitating an accident.

3. Loud noises affect the body physiologically in several ways. Generally, hearing loss, the major problem associated with noise, is at-tributable to the irreversible damage to the inner ear.

Noise causes headaches, gastric ulcers, poor circulation, irregular heartbeat, and stomach spasms. When subjected to loud noises, adrenaline is pumped into the bloodstream, which in turn causes the heart to beat faster and the metabolism rate to increase. As the heart beats faster, the blood vessels constrict (in the brain they dilate, or ex-pand). This causes blood pressure to rise and the heart to work harder, which can precipitate heart problems. Noise causes the ciliary muscles in the eye to tear and the pupil of the eye to dilate, permit-ting unwanted light (glare) to enter. This glare often causes accidents in noisy environments.

Any one or a combination of these factors can lead to reduced job performance, increased absen-teeism and accident rates, poor morale, high labor turnover, and increased workers' compensation claims.

Because noise is potentially harmful to the human body, employers should control it. Noise control includes reducing the source, putting dis-tance between the person and the source, and filter-ing out or attenuating the noise.

1. Employees reduce noise at its *source* by using quieter machines, appliances, auto mufflers, and tires. By using fewer power tools and appliances and by maintaining

vehicles and equipment, employees can cut down on noise. Jet aircraft engines can be designed to reduce the noise at the point of its generation. Garbage cans and lids can be quieted by special design. Noise can be reduced by controlling the volume of television sets, radios, and juke boxes.

2. Planning and zoning can increase the dis*tance* and thus reduce the amount of noise reaching people. Locating nursing homes, hospitals, schools, and homes away from noisy industry, airports, and other noise-generating sources such as interstate highways can help to put some distance between people and noise.

3. If it is impossible to reduce the noise or to put distance between you and the noise, the noise can be attenuated by filtering. Ear muffs and acoustic materials such as glass can prevent sound from entering houses. The purpose of soundproofing buildings where people live, work, and recreate is to attenuate noise. Sound can be absorbed by earth mounds, walls of concrete, and or stonework as barriers, and dense rows of trees along highways. It is better, however, to prevent the noise if possible.

TEMPERATURE EXTREMES

Evaluation of the hazards represented by temperature extremes include length of exposure, nature of the work, wind speed, humidity, and the worker's physical condition. Extreme low temperatures may cause tissue damage from hypothermia and frostbite with little warning. Frostbite results from prolonged and severe constriction of the blood vessels at temperatures below 32°F. Severe cold injuries such as those of deep frostbite generally are irreversible, and amputation of the affected body part may be necessary. Continued exposure to extreme cold may cause death.

Heat stress consists of the body's natural responses to stresses brought on by excess heat. Heat stress taxes the cardiovascular system, and can cause cramps, heat exhaustion, heat stroke, and even death. The same degree of exposure to excessive heat may produce different effects depending on the susceptibility of the worker exposed.

Extremes in temperature affect work performance. The extent to which performance is lowered depends on the intensity of heat or coldness, duration of the exposure period, tasks conducted during exposure, physical condition of the worker exposed, and the presence or absence of other stressors.

Control of temperature extremes includes continuous monitoring of the temperatures to which workers are exposed. Employers should provide outdoor workers, such as construction and agricultural workers, with adequate shelter from the heat and cold. Workers in hot environments should have unlimited access to cool water and should be allowed frequent breaks to drink. Employers should provide appropriate clothing and protective gear. For extremely low temperatures they should provide suitable coats, gloves, hats, and boots. For extremely high temperatures, appropriate clothing should be cotton, lightweight, and permeable for air flow.

Employers should limit their employees' exposure to temperature extremes and carefully monitor employees who are exposed to high and low temperatures. Employees should use the buddy system when they enter extremely cold or hot areas, as loss of consciousness can occur almost immediately. Employers should implement a work-rest schedule to reduce stress peaks and to schedule strenuous work for the appropriate time of day based on temperature. Where possible, mechanical heating or cooling of the environment is effective in controlling extremes in temperature.

....

INDUSTRIAL TOXICOLOGY

Toxicology is the science that studies poisonous and toxic substances and their mechanisms and effects on living organisms. In and out of the workplace, everyone is exposed to a tremendous array of chemical substances. Most of these chemicals do not present a hazard under ordinary circumstances, but all substances have the potential to cause harm at some sufficiently high level of exposure. Philippus Paracelsus stated, "No substance is a poison by itself. It is the dose that makes a substance a poison." How a material is used is the major determinant of its hazard potential. Any substance contacting or entering the body will have adverse effects at some excessive level of exposure. The potentially fatal condition known as water toxicity demonstrates that excessive intake of a substance as innocuous as water can be harmful. By the same token, the body can tolerate any substance without harmful effect at some lower exposure. No substance can be labeled absolutely as toxic or nontoxic.

Toxicity generally is considered the ability of a substance to produce an undesirable physiologic effect when the chemical has reached a sufficient concentration at a specific site in the body. A **toxic effect** is any noxious effect or undesirable disturbance of the body's physiologic function, whether reversible or irreversible. The toxicity of any chemical depends upon the degree of exposure. The **industrial toxicologist** is responsible for defining quantitatively the level of exposure at which harm occurs. The toxicologist also prescribes precautionary measures and exposure limitations so that normal, recommended use of a chemical substance does not result in excessive exposure and subsequent harm. A material is considered toxic if it demonstrates the potential to induce cancer, to produce long-term disease or bodily injury, to affect health adversely, to produce acute discomfort, or to endanger human or animal life through exposure via the respiratory tract, skin, eyes, mouth, or other routes.

The National Institute of Occupational Safety and Health (NIOSH) has listed more than 12,000 toxic materials that meet these criteria, and new chemicals are being introduced into industry at the alarming rate of approximately 500 a year. At this rate, the likelihood of proper experimentation and testing of these materials for toxic properties being conducted is questionable.

The factors that contribute to determining the degree of hazard a toxin may pose are the route of entry, dosage, and physiological state of the worker at the time of exposure and environmental variables. Toxins vary in their degree of harm within the same person, depending upon the time of day he or she is exposed. Genetic factors and other interacting toxins and stressors also influence an individual's sensitivity to the chemical substance. Many chemical agents are nonselective in their actions on tissues or cells, exerting harmful effects on all living matter. Other chemical agents act only on specific cells.

Harmful effects include local and systemic damage.

1. *Local effects* usually involve injury at the point of contact with the chemical substance: the skin, eyes and mucous membranes of the upper respiratory tract.

2. A toxicant can cause injury *systemically* only after it is absorbed by the organism and distributed to the internal organs of the body.

Common routes of entry into the body are ingestion, injection, skin absorption, and inhalation. The nature and intensity of chemical effects on an organism depend not only on the administered dose but also on other physiologic factors including absorption, distribution, binding, and excretion of the chemical substance in the body.

The extent to which a chemical substance should be controlled depends on the severity of its effect on the body and its established dose-response relationship. The dose-response relationship indicates how a biological organism's response to a toxic substance changes as its exposure to a substance increases. For example, a small amount of carbon monoxide causes drowsiness, whereas a larger dose can be fatal. A dose-response curve relates percent mortality to dose administered. In determining a dose-response relationship, it is assumed that a threshold exposure exists below which no harmful effect occurs. Toxicologists doubt that this threshold concept is valid for radiation damage and carcinogenesis. Radiation damage and the initiation of cancer may exhibit a zero threshold. This means that no dosage can be considered safe; even the most minute exposure has the potential to cause physiologic damage.

Exposure limits called **threshold limit values** (TLVs) have been developed by the American Conference of Governmental Industrial Hygienists and adopted as standards by the U.S. government. Threshold limit values are intended to be used only as guidelines in the control of occupational exposures. TLVs are not meant to protect every worker even though a safety factor is used subjectively to calculate the TLV so it usually is below the smallest level believed to cause any toxic effect. Strong evidence exists that the mechanisms for radiation damage and carcinogenesis are different from those for ordinary toxic effects. Because exposure to radiation and carcinogens, however small, has the potential to inflict permanent damage, the threshold below which no damage occurs is said to be zero.

·················

ENFORCEMENT OF LAWS

Prior to the passage of the Occupational Safety and Health Act (OSHAct) on December 29, 1970, governmental regulations regarding safety and health had been the responsibility of state agencies. One of the primary reasons for passage of the OSHAct was that the existing state programs were grossly inadequate and had little uniformity of application of codes and standards from one state to another. In any given state, almost no enforcement proceedings were undertaken against even blatant violators of those standards. In many instances, state safety codes and regulations were inadequate in their provisions and poorly enforced because of insufficient funding of the state programs. Inspectors and enforcement personnel were poorly trained and empowered to enforce the laws.

Although the OSHAct was created as a federal law, it permitted the states to regain sole authority to police occupational safety within its borders if they met specific conditions. A state desiring to regain control over regulation of its industries was required to submit a proposed plan indicating how it intended to execute a program that would be at least as effective as the federal one. The Secretary of Labor then would have to approve the plan and, if approved, the state would pay half of the cost of the approved program and the federal government would pay the other half. The Secretary of Labor is the principal administering officer of the OSHAct. Once the state gained control of the program, the U.S. Department of Labor was required to maintain surveillance over the state program for 3 years to ensure that the state executed its responsibilities properly.

Upon enactment of the OSHAct, a number of states objected to the extreme costs necessary to ensure that OSHAct requirements were carried out. These states declined to assume responsibility for enforcing the OSHAct and relinquished enforcement of the act to the federal government. The states that chose to regain control of enforcement of the OSHAct and standards developed their own enabling legislation and standards. The legislation and standards of the individual states are more stringent than those of the federal government in many cases.

The OSHAct describes responsibilities that employers and employees alike must carry out. Only the employers, however, can be penalized for failing to comply with the law. The employee is obligated to comply with occupational safety and health standards and all rules, regulations, and orders issued pursuant to the act that are applicable to his or her own actions and standards. The employee may file complaints of violations by his or her employer with the Department of Labor. The Department of Labor has the authority to inspect the establishment without notification. If an employee fails to adhere to the prescribed health and safety standards, even willfully, the employer may be cited for violation.

Occupational safety and health compliance officers may conduct inspections of any workplace without prior notification. Compliance officers must be admitted to the worksite, if denied entry, they may obtain a search warrant to enter the premises where they have the right to inspect the facilities and safety records. The following priorities may be used in making inspections.

1. An inspection will follow any accidental death or accident in which five or more workers are injured. According to the OSHAct, such an accident must be reported within 48 hours of its occurrence.

2. A worksite will be inspected if a report of an imminent hazard is received. The inspection will be conducted to determine if an imminent hazard indeed exists and to ensure that noted imminent hazards have been eliminated.

3. Industries that are themselves considered inherently hazardous will be inspected at frequencies and times established by the responsible Occupational Safety and Health Administration (OSHA) office.

4. Other industries will be inspected according to schedules to be established by OSHA offices.

If the compliance officer considers an industry in violation of the OSHA standards, he or she must issue a citation to the employer within 6 months of the violation. The citation will indicate a reasonable time for eliminating or abating the hazard. The four possible types of citations for OSHA standards violations are as follows:

1. *Imminent danger.* Any condition or practice that reasonably could be expected to cause death or serious physical harm immediately or before correction can be made through normal procedures.

2. *Serious violation.* Any condition or practice, means, method, operation, or process that has a substantial probability of causing deaths or serious physical harm.

3. *Nonserious violation.* Any condition in which an incident or occupational illness resulting from violation of a standard probably would not cause death or serious physical harm to workers. No permanent injury is likely to result from a nonserious violation.

4. *De minimus* (no penalty). Any condition in which a violation of standard has no immediate or direct relationship to the safety or health of the workers.

OSHA can request the employer to halt immediately any operation that represents an imminent danger. If the employer refuses to halt the operation, the compliance officer will notify employees of the hazard. The Department of Labor then may request a court to shut down the operation.

For any violation, the inspecting compliance officer may propose a penalty of up to $1,000 per day until the condition is corrected. These penalties are mandatory for serious violations. Serious violations can be assessed up to $7,000 per occurrence. Imposition of the penalties is optional in cases of nonserious violations. Willful or repeated violations each may be assessed a civil penalty of up to $70,000. If the death of an employee results from a willful violation, the employer may be punished by a fine of not more than $100,000, imprisonment of not more than 6 months, or both if he or she is convicted in a court of law. These penalties may be doubled upon subsequent convictions.

The Toxic Substances Control Act (TOSCA) of 1976 was designed to protect workers from chemical hazards. The act requires that sufficient appropriate data be developed on the health and environmental effects of chemicals. Development of these data and information is the responsibility of the chemical manufacturers and processors. The EPA is required to establish the standards to be used for testing chemicals. The chemical tested may be banned or regulated if the EPA considers test information to be insufficient or if the chemical would be widely distributed. The EPA is required to ban or restrict the use of any chemical substance representing an unreasonable risk of injury to health or the environment.

The OSHAct requires the Secretary of Health and Human Services to publish an annual toxic substances list with the purpose of identifying all known toxic substances in accordance with common definitions that may be used to describe toxicity. If a substance does not appear on the list, this does not indicate that it is nontoxic but that its effects may be unknown. A listing on the toxic substances list does indicate that the listed substance has the documented potential of being hazardous if misused.

OSHA is responsible for establishing permissible standards of potentially toxic substances in the workplace. Criteria documents are developed for each significant toxic substance. Criteria documents represent extremely thorough searches of the literature that summarize all significant work related to establishment of the desired standard. To aid OSHA in meeting its responsibility, the National Institute for Occupational Safety and Health (NIOSH) has been charged with developing criteria documents for chemical substances. In addition to OSHA, other federal government regulatory agencies have enforcement powers.

- *Mine Safety and Health Administration.* Established by the Secretary of the Interior in 1973, it is responsible for administering the enforcement provisions of the Federal Coal Mine Health and Safety Act of 1969 and the Federal Metal and Nonmetallic Mine Safety Act. The Federal Mine Safety and Health Amendments Act of 1977

(MSHA) transferred the authority for enforcement of mining safety and health from the Department of the Interior to the Department of Labor.

- *Nuclear Regulatory Commission (NRC).* Established as an independent regulatory agency under the provisions of the Energy Reorganization Act of 1974, the NRC now is responsible for all licensing and related regulatory functions formerly assigned to the Atomic Energy Commission. The NRC licenses and regulates the uses of nuclear energy to protect public health and safety and the environment. This is accomplished by licensing persons and companies to own and use nuclear materials and to build and operate nuclear reactors. The NRC develops regulations and sets standards for these types of licenses. It also inspects the activities of licensed persons and companies to ensure that they are not in violation of NRC's safety rules.

SUMMARY

The workplace—where people spend 8 to 12 hours of a 24-hour day for 30 years or more—should be safe and free of the biological, chemical, and physical agents of disease. These agents may be inhaled, injected, ingested, or transferred by physical contact. Biological hazards, called biohazards, are living organisms classified as bacteria, viruses, rickettsiae, fungi, and parasites. Chemical toxins are found in mist, vapor, gases, smoke, dust, fumes, and aerosol. Physical hazards include radiation, noise pollution, and temperature extremes.

To provide an environment conducive to good health, a variety of occupational specialists are required. These include the occupational health nurse, occupational physician, industrial hygienist, safety engineer, and industrial health educator.

Legislation has been enacted to promote workplace health and to establish agencies to oversee compliance. Foremost of these are the Public Health Service, a division of the Center for Disease Control and Prevention, and the Occupational Safety and Health Administration, which was created by the OSHAct and in charge of setting standards for safety in the workplace. The OSHAct also created the National Institute for Occupational Safety and Health (NIOSH) as a part of the Department of Health and Human Services to identify workplace hazards, to develop criteria documents, and to train the workers in the workplace.

KEY TERMS

Aerosol, p. 274

Biohazards, p. 269

Decibels (dB), p. 276

Dust, p. 274

Fumes, p. 274

Gases, p. 273

Industrial health educator, p. 269

Industrial hygienist, p. 267

Industrial toxicologist, p. 279

Mist, p. 273

Noise, p. 276

Occupational health nurse, p. 267

Occupational hygiene, p. 263

Occupational physician, p. 267

Primary irritants, p. 274

Safety engineer, p. 268

Smoke, p. 273

Threshold limit values (TLVs), p. 279

Toxic effects, p. 279

Toxicology, p. 278

Vapor, p. 273

Ventilation, p. 275

REFERENCES

Amdur, M.O., J. Doull, and C.D. Klassen, eds. 1991. *Casarett and Doull's Toxicology—The Basic Science of Poisons*, 4th ed. Pergamon Press, New York.

American Conference of Governmental Industrial Hygienist (ACGIH). 1999. *TLVs and BEIs—Threshold Limit Values for Chemical Substances and Physical Agents—Biological Exposure Indices*. Cincinnati, OH.

Ashford, N. A. 1976. *Crisis in the Workplace: Occupational Disease and Injury*. MIT Press, Cambridge, MA.

Bird, E. E., and G. L. Germain. 1985. *Practical Loss Control Leadership*. Institute Publishing, Loganville.

Brandt, A. D. 1947. *Industrial Health Engineering*. Chapman and Hall Ltd., London.

Brown, H. V. 1965. "This history of industrial hygiene: a review with special reference to silicosis." *American Industrial Hygiene Association Journal*, 26:212–226.

Chapter 15

Cralley, L. J. 1996. "Industrial Hygiene in the U.S. Public Health Service (1914–1968)." *Applied Occupational Environmental Hygiene*, 11:147–155.

Daubenspeck, G. W. 1974. *Occupational Health Hazards*. Exposition Press, New York.

DiNardi, S. J. 1995. *Calculation Methods for Industrial Hygiene*. Van Nostrand Reinhold, New York.

DiNardi, S. R., ed. 1998. *The Occupational Environment—Its Evaluation and Control*. American Industrial Hygiene Association, Fairfax, VA.

Everly, G. S., and R. H. L. Feldman. 1985. *Occupational Health Promotion*. John Wiley and Sons, New York.

Felton, J. S. 1994. "History." *Occupational Health & Safety*, 2nd ed., J. LaDou, ed. National Safety Council, Istasca, IL.

Goldwater, L. J. 1985. "Historical Highlights in Occupational Medicine." *Readings and Perspectives in Medicine, Booklet 9*. Duke University Medical Center, Durham, NC.

Hamilton, A. 1943. *Exploring the Dangerous Trades*. Little, Brown, Boston.

Hammer, W. 1976. *Occupational Safety Management and Engineering*. Prentice Hall, Englewood, NJ.

Hanlon, J.J. 1964. *Principles of Public Health*. C.X. Mosby, St. Louis.

Johnstone, R. T., and S. E. Miller. 1961. *Occupational Diseases and Industrial Medicine*. W. B. Saunders, Philadelphia.

Key, M. M., A. E Henschel, J. Butler, R.N. Ligo, I. R. Tabershaw, and L. Ede. 1977. *Occupational Diseases*. U.S. Department of Health, Education and Welfare, Washington, DC.

Kohn, J. P., M. A. Friend, and C. A. Winterberger. 1996. *Fundamentals of Occupational Safety and Health*. Government Institutes, Rockville, MD.

Kryter, K. D. 1984. *Physiological, Psychological and Social Effects of Noise*. NASA Scientific and Technical Information, Washington, DC.

LaGrega, Michael D., Philip L. Buckingham, Jeffrey C. Evans, and Environmental Resources Management Group. 1994. *Hazardous Waste Management*. McGraw-Hill, Hightstown, NJ.

Loomis, T. A. 1978. *Essentials of Toxicology*. 3rd ed. Lea & Febiger, Philadelphia.

LaDou, J., ed. 1994. *Occupational Health & Safety*, 2nd Ed. National Safety Council, Itasca, IL.

Luxon, G. G. 1984. "A History of Industrial Hygiene." *American Industrial Hygiene Journal*, 45:731–739.

McReady, B. W. 1837. *On the Influence of Trades, Professions and Occupations in the United States in Production of Disease* (translations of the Medical Society of New York, vol. III). Medical Society of the State of New York, Albany, NY.

National Safety Council. 1996. *Fundamentals of Industrial Hygiene*, 4th ed. Chicago.

Occupational Safety and Health Act. 1970. Public Law 91–596. Section 2193, 91st Congress, December 29, 1970.

Patty, F. A. 1978. "Industrial Hygiene: Retrospect and Prospect." *Patty's Industrial Hygiene and Toxicology*, vol.1, 3rd ed. John Wiley & Sons, New York.

Perkins, Jimmy L. 1997. *Modern Industrial Hygiene*. Van Nostrand Reinhold, New York.

Ramazzini, B. 1964. *Diseases of Workers*. Hafner Publishing Co., New York.

Roberts, J. M. 1976. *OSHA Compliance Manual*. Teston Publishing, Virginia.

Rose, V. E. 1988. "The Development of Occupational Hygiene in the United States—A History." *Annals of American Conference of Governmental Industrial Hygiene*, 15:5–8.

Stellman, J. M., and S. M. Daum. 1971. *Work is Dangerous to Your Health*. Pantheon Books, New York.

U.S. Environmental Protection Agency. 1971. *Noise from Construction Equipment and Operations, Building Equipment and Home Appliances*. Government Printing Office, Washington, DC.

16

ENVIRONMENTAL PLANNING

Steve Konkel, Ph.D.

Eastern Kentucky University

- Define planning in operational terms, as it is practiced by planners.
- Understand why we need to establish baselines in environmental health for sound planning.
- Understand examples of problems encountered in solid waste management and in developing a vector control program.
- Identify why trends in globalization and communication technology increasingly affect environmental planning.
- Discuss the limitations of environmental laws due to the lack of an integrating environmental statute.
- List the ten steps that make up a planning process and explain how these planning steps can also be consolidated into six major elements.
- Discuss potential human health impacts from inadequate planning and the lack of infrastructure.
- Discuss how haphazard growth creates resource allocation problems
- Understand why identifying values, interests, and expectations (VIE) is essential to strategic planning and key to understanding interested party, or "stakeholder," views and positions.
- Understand why environmental policy, programs, procedures, and rules and regulations are all essential to environmental regulation and management.
- Understand why identifying agency roles, responsibilities, and jurisdictional boundaries are essential to creating effective governmental agency and consultant performance.
- Develop approaches incorporating sound scientific and technical information.
- Identify alternatives to litigation for conflict resolution in environmental health decision making.
- Identify the roles risk analysis plays in prioritizing goals and budgets.
- Explain how risk management measures can assist in development of a preventative approach, rather than a treatment approach, to environmental health.

INTRODUCTION

There are three essential components of all planning and these are as follows:

1. *Where you are now*. It is essential that you know where you are now in regard to the subject that you are planning. This is one of the most frequent mistakes made in the development of plans. Knowledge of present conditions and challenges in regard to the plan are essential to justifying the funds appropriated to the program for which the plan has been implemented. Food inspection programs amply demonstrate this point. Federal, state, and local authorities carry out complex programs. Few would argue that such programs are essential, since they pay for themselves many times over. However, since baseline data do not exist to mark where we started, and the major successes are in prevention of the wide variety of diseases discussed in Chapter 11, environmental health professionals cannot effectively provide the taxpayer with the overall benefits derived from these programs.

2. *Where you want to be*. This process is defined as the **vision** in strategic planning or as the desired outcome in planning environmental health and other programs.

3. *Charting a path to get from where you are now to where you want to be*. This part of the planning and **implementation** process involves linking an organization's values and vision through **assessments** of its strengths, weaknesses, opportunities, threats, and the design of strategies to address the key issues facing the organization. This complex but linear process is described in detail in "Participatory Planning" (Beck and Konkel, 1999). It is important to involve *all* constituencies with "stakes" in the outcome, in order to establish ownership and accountability for the plan. Recent events reinforce the observation that "It takes many people to build a bridge, but only a few to destroy it."

Our understanding of the importance of healthy ecosystems and the impact of people on the natural and the built environment continues to grow. The need for **stewardship** to preserve, protect, and enhance the natural environment and promote healthy populations is increasingly seen as a universal responsibility of environmental health and safety (EHS) professionals. At the same time, we have seen an unprecedented growth and sophistication in technology, from semiconductors and aircraft engines to emerging biotechnology products, pharmaceuticals, and health care technologies. Technological developments affect the food we eat, how we communicate, how we work and play, and our quality of life.

Despite technological advances, we face the dilemma of earlier civilizations:

- "How do we create a sustainable and high quality of life given an ever-growing population?"
- How do we regulate economic activity in order to achieve profitability while reducing adverse impact and enhancing environmental stewardship?

In the environmental health field our colleagues and the general public constantly struggle with acquiring the resources to implement environmental health policies, programs, and projects that will make us better off. As taxpayers, we often seek efficient and equitable solutions to the wide array of problems we encounter. As professionals we must increasingly compete for limited funds aimed at improving the health status of populations and efficiency of industrial operations. The author argues herein that sound planning is essential if we are to accomplish our shared environmental health goals. Many accepted societal goals are listed in a "big-picture" planning guidance document titled "Healthy People 2010" (see "An Example of a Planning Framework—Healthy People 2010" herein).

In this opening section of the Environmental Planning chapter, key planning terms are defined. The author also takes seriously the charge of EHS professionals: to make a difference in people's lives today and to achieve a brighter future. We must be willing to balance various factors and harness the power of science and technology. In the long run education may be the key to helping people make the small choices that add up to improvements in environmental quality. We trust that this book helps students take the first steps. As the recent bioterrorism events amply demonstrate, not planning is simply not an option. We need to solve the right problems in a way that works. Unfortunately, September 11, 2001 is a day marked in infamy; its events and the loss of lives remind us across the globe of the importance of managing risks and making investments to preserve the freedoms and way of life that we enjoy.

Environmental planning provides tools and mechanisms to better understand ourselves and the individual and collective choices we have. We all play a role in developing the physical and social fabric of communities. Risk analysis and managing risky decisions help us identify risk factors, draw priorities, and allocate resources. In addressing risky decisions, we need to use sound science and technical information. We need to assess alternatives and find ways to mitigate or avoid adverse consequences of development. We need to find constructive ways to manage conflict, rather than a "winner takes all" approach. The alternative of neglecting to plan or identifying appropriate risks often leads to unanticipated and undesirable health outcomes, poor use of resources, and a waste of time and energy.

In this chapter there is an underlying premise that most individuals plan. Environmental planning has to do with the advance thinking that we do that relates to the built and natural environment, the presence of nature and wildlife, and promoting human health and welfare. In today's specialized work world, it is not enough to know how to plan projects to be on time, on budget, and to specifications. One also has to be able to acquire scientific knowledge and technical expertise as needed—a new requirement for "technological literacy." So, for example, a biotechnology planner would have to understand the impact of pesticides on the environment, and how altering the genetic makeup of plants might impact the soil, insects, and flora and fauna. Using pesticides or pharmaceuticals on the farm can leave residual levels of chemicals in the

products, from grains to chickens, and there is much controversy today regarding consumer fears about the potential effects of consuming these genetically altered plants and animals on humans. How we resolve these issues will govern the food quality we enjoy and count on for human sustenance. There will also be profound affects on the world we live in, as economic activity and environmental impacts result from these choices.

·················
THE NEED FOR PLANNING

Primitive people did little, if any, planning. They reacted to events, rather than acting proactively and thinking reflectively about their experiences. If it rained, then they found shelter. If they were hungry, they hunted for food. Later, early humans planned for rain by building shelters. They planted gardens and cultivated crops in order to supplement and eventually to largely supplant hunting for subsistence. They learned ways to preserve food and make it safe for human consumption. Native Alaskans still depend on "living off the land" through **subsistence** activity. Modern communities are constantly evolving, learning to use new communication and transportation technologies, such as hand-held global positioning systems and the latest jet airplanes, while also importing traditions and ways from other cultures. These developments guide planners in understanding the importance of values in seeking improvements in the health and quality of life of populations.

Early civilizations did not plan environmental programs. Their needs were often met in a much more spontaneous manner. They did not plan water supply and water treatment programs, sewage disposal programs, nor their housing. Often they were mobile and moved according to the seasons and the productivity of hunting grounds. They often reacted to immediate needs. Even in places that were heavily impacted by migration and industrialization, environmental health gains did not come easy, nor were health hazards always recognized as they are today.

Places like London, England, attracted new urban residents seeking jobs and more money than was available in rural areas dependent on farming.

Although rural workers realized opportunities associated with migration, the urban places that they moved to were often unable to accommodate their needs for housing, clean water, sewage systems, and other necessities. This often led to poor living conditions, especially in urbanizing areas where large populations settled. Action was taken only after outbreaks of disease, epidemics, suffering, and death. For example, early 19th century Liverpool, England, had little, if any, planning. There was no planning for water supply, sewers, housing, smoke control, or occupational health; there was no city planning either. Statistics reflect starkly the seriousness of these oversights. In Liverpool the life expectancy for the wealthy in the early 1840s was a mere 36 years old, as cited in Edwin Chadwick's 1842 report, "A Report on the Sanitary Condition of the Laboring Population of Great Britain and on the Means of Its Improvement." Chadwick also estimated 22 years life expectancy for the middle class and a mere 16 years for the laboring classes. It is insightful to view health and disease in places like London over the period from 1750 to the present (see Rotberg et al., 2000). Edwin Chadwick effectively documented one of the primary results of haphazard growth and crowding—a lack of proper planning for infrastructure and its related impacts on the health and life span of urban residents.

In the United States we tend to take clean water, sewage disposal, clean air, and many other amenities for granted today. However, there are many areas of the country where we have aging or inadequate infrastructure, such as leaking water supply aqueducts, and sewage treatment plants that cannot fully treat human waste, especially when they become overloaded with **combined sewer overflows (CSOs)**. Aquifers and wells have been contaminated, community water supplies have been lost, and we still have places where human waste is sent via "straight pipes" directly into streams without sufficient treatment. Urbanization and the need for planning are linked, but rural residents also benefit from planning.

Environmental planning evolved because of epidemics, or, in other words, disease arising from the environmental conditions of overcrowding, particularly in major cities. Planning is needed for orderly, healthy, and economic social growth.

Amenities like libraries and the urban design created by scores of individual structures affect our community livability, just as investments in clean water and safe food supplies improve our health and well-being. Urban planners concern themselves with how transportation systems, buildings, land uses, and natural amenities combine to create a high quality of life in cities and population centers. An urban designer or planner is to city architecture and cultural experiences what an architect is to an individual building: a system thinker focused on physical, environmental, and sociocultural factors affecting how civilization works. *Rural by Design* (Brabec et al., 1994) and articles on the new urbanism (e.g., Lockwood, 2001) explore solutions for the commonly identified problem of urban sprawl.

The benefits of planning are obvious everywhere in the country. Farmers plan their crops; business people plan their marketing and sales; architects plan buildings; and politicians plan their campaigns. Investment counselors plan for investments; health planners plan health programs; dentists plan corrective measures for dental health; and students plan curricula and careers. Civic groups engage in planning for civic activity; doctors plan courses for patient recovery; lawyers plan their advocacy for cases and achieving justice through the legal system. Everyone plans, but many may not see it as a formal activity, as well as an "art form." Good planners consider uncertainties and make contingency plans. The alternative to planning is really an acceptance of the "no action" or let's see approach; it by definition is planning because it endorses the existing value structure and results, which may not hold up to future scrutiny. Wise decisions usually incorporate sound scientific and technical information.

We all plan budgets, trips, weekends, weddings, vacations, and family activities. Many advocate that a great need in the 21st century is for family planning, and the author is certainly in agreement with those who see profound impacts over time of increased human populations on social, economic, and natural environments.

While planning is a part of our daily lives, good or bad environmental planning can greatly affect the quality of our entire lives. Good planning utilizes systems thinking—so, for example, land uses reflect decisions regarding emergency services, transportation, housing, natural systems, infrastructure, and the impacts of development on people. Peoples' quality of life is determined by the interaction of all of these factors and the myriad of decisions with environmental implications made by individuals, organizations, and agencies. Haphazard, unplanned growth is often the product of decisions of individuals who do not account for the cumulative impact of these decisions on the welfare of the community as a whole. Traffic gridlock is just one manifestation of the lack of proper attention to infrastructure planning, design, funding, program development, and implementation. Failure to plan can be seen as planning to fail. Inadequate plans carry social/individual costs.

....

DEFINITIONS AND TYPES OF PLANNING

Planning is defined as organizing a way of getting from here to there, or where we are now and where we want to go. It is a means to ends. In developing hundreds of strategic plans for organizations and agencies, we first explore values and create a vision for the future—then we assess where we are now, and chart a path to the future (Beck and Konkel, 1999). This avoids "parachuting into a minefield and deciding where to take the first step." This is one of the most common mistakes people make when planning. Developing a course of action is the essence of the process of making and carrying out plans. Good planners identify and navigate obstacles; they are politically aware and astute communicators. Planners develop goals, policies, and procedures for a social or economic or governmental unit; for example, a church, a business, or an environmental protection or transportation agency of state or federal government.

A **goal** may be defined as "the end towards which the effort is directed." We all have a goal of wanting to earn a sufficient amount of money to assist in having a good quality of life. To some, a good quality of life can be achieved by owning a few acres, with a house, fish pond, cat, dog, horse, spouse, and children. To others, a good quality of life means owning several cars, TV sets, a house,

boat, business, and other material goods. Regardless of how we define quality of life, we realize that none of us can reach this goal without good health in an environment that supports the pursuit of life, human liberty, and happiness. Life is about the journey, and not a destination. Goals help set the direction and the intensity of the journey.

In **strategic planning**, a distinction is usually made between the strategic plan (the fabric of which contains a vision, mission statement, goals, and an outline of strategies) and program or **tactical planning**. The latter entails defining milestones, designates who will do what and when, and how the accomplishments of tasks contributes to achievement of goals (Beck and Konkel, 1999). Another point concerning the "language" that planners use is important here: some consider goals to be targets that can be reset to higher levels, whereas **objectives** are usually considered by planners and public administrators to be "measurable." Some business texts reverse this distinction, considering "objectives" equivalent to goals and making goals the measurable, operational part of implementation. The overall goal of a recreation program is to maintain or improve health, while individual objectives may be to reduce disease, to augment health by increasing exercise, and to reduce the number of accidental injuries, which originate in recreational areas.

A **policy** can be defined as "a plan of action, guidelines, or a managerial tool for identifying and setting expectations given resource assets and limitations." It would be poor policy to promote what you cannot accomplish. A sound energy policy should balance the need for electricity generation and fuel production, such as natural gas and oil, with implementing conservation and efficiency programs. One should explicitly consider the impacts of development of energy supplies on the natural environment, pollution, human health implications, and the effect on social and economic systems. Sound complex? No wonder this has proven to be a controversial and challenging charge!

A **policywonk** is an individual who, by studying, assessing, evaluating, and making recommendations on policies, has a key practical role in the public policy arena. This term, which was invented by analysts and those interested in governmental policies, acknowledges that one must follow issues to understand the implications of alternative courses of action.

A **procedure** is a way of going forward, a way or method of doing things. For example, the procedure for starting a car is to get in, turn the ignition on, put the car into gear for forward or backward motion, and steer as one drives the vehicle.

There are multiple types of planning that are extremely relevant to environmental specialists and environmental health professionals. Selected types of these are noted below:

- **Project planning** has been widely used over the years. A good example is Boulder Dam in Colorado, which generates electricity. Complexity of planning varies greatly. For example, planning and sizing an air duct system for the heating, ventilating, and air-conditioning system in a house is only a portion of house design and building. Another example of project planning is planning for orbiting satellites for communications purposes. This planning involves physics, chemistry, geography, geology, engineering, astronomy, and economics. Project planning for buildings addresses site-specific impacts, as well as financial, economic, timing, scheduling, and user requirements.

- **Comprehensive planning** is a term that has different connotations. On a personal level, it describes the ultimate state in a person's endeavor to perform, a major achievement that shapes the environment or one's future. For a city and its surrounding region, it aims to integrate various natural and socioeconomic systems to produce a pleasing quality of life. **Zoning**, a means of designating allowable land uses (residential, commercial, and industrial, and their intensity, e.g., single-family versus up to six apartment units) is often used as a means of implementing policies and procedures in accordance with a comprehensive plan. This planning helps guide decisions on expanding infrastructure, such as water, sewers, and electricity.

- **Urban planning** is the planning of human habitats, reinforcing positive linkages and relationships with natural systems while minimizing constraints from pollution and other environmental factors. The relationship of individual buildings, infrastructure, and sociocultural systems is the challenge of the architect, planners, and developers tackling urban design issues. Faneuil Hall, on the Boston waterfront, is a development created by James Rouse's Baltimore-based company that demonstrates a successful waterfront development concept of mixed land uses by design of a pedestrian-oriented environment with cafes, street theater, and open-air markets.

- **Public health planning** usually is seen as including three arenas: environmental health, community health, and personal health promotion, including mental health. How bioterrorism and other developments like the hole in the ozone layer affect public health are pushing the boundaries of this **paradigm**, or "mental model." Health planners plot courses of action to protect, promote, and enhance people's health. Healthy People 2000 and Healthy People 2010 are examples of the efforts of diverse coalitions to chart the goals and a viable path.

- **Environmental health planning** is planning a course of action to protect, promote, and preserve people's health by envisioning, designing, and implementing programs to control environmental factors. These factors are identified, and authors suggest various means for preservation, conservation, prevention, management, and control of them, in individual chapters of this book. **Program planning** must identify the values, interests, and expectations of various interested parties who want to have a say in the role and authority of governmental agencies in setting policy and implementing regulations.

THE PLANNING PROCESS

Historically, environmental planners have had to deal with challenges such as which agency has jurisdiction over a particular issue or permitting situation, the multimedia nature of **pollution** (air, land, and water), and fragmented efforts of various stakeholders or interested parties to maximize their interests. Environmental planning has been piecemeal, since, for example, using scrubbers to remove sulfur from coal air emissions then creates ash, which has to be properly managed. The environment should be planned as a series of systems whenever possible, rather than as categorical areas. Pollution prevention is an example of an area where planning industrial processes avoids environmental releases of toxic materials and the associated cleanup and health effects liability. Another example is climate, a system that affects us all. The climate determines whether land is suitable for crops grown for food, cotton, tobacco, and so on, and thus can support the demands of human populations. The climate also determines if disease-producing insects, such as flies and mosquitoes, will inhabit an area, as many times in the past flies and mosquitoes have influenced human habitation. Hence, climate is a factor to be considered in environmental health planning. Other environmental factors that affect the environmental health of populations include terrain, rainfall, wildlife, transportation, and sociocultural characteristics of populations. The latter include religion, age, gender, family structure, ethnic background, and socioeconomic level.

Ten-Step Planning Process

The planning process consists of ten steps:

1. Identify the problem.
2. Analysis.
3. Set goals (targets, outcomes).
4. Set objectives.
5. Develop alternative solutions.
6. Test alternatives.
7. Make modifications to mitigate adverse consequences and promote positive aspects of the plan.
8. Select the best solution.
9. Implement the plan (sometimes called tactical planning).
10. Conduct **program evaluation**—measuring progress towards goals and objectives.

Another approach to planning consolidates these into just six steps.

Six-Step Method of Planning

1. Examine the situation and its "context."[1]
2. Set goals, or targets.
3. Set measurable objectives
4. Design the program.[2]
5. Implement the program.
6. Conduct program evaluation.

Examine the Situation and Its "Context"

Before developing a new environmental health program or modifying an ongoing one, it is necessary to get a complete picture of the situation. One needs to know the size, nature, and context of the problem. A planner needs information concerning planned activities for public and environmental health problem areas, available physical and human resources, and information about the population being served. Successful planners also require information about an area's geography, weather, and man-made features (infrastructure such as water and sewer lines, highways, electricity and energy sources, as well as housing, proximate land uses, and industrial plants). **Geographic information systems**, also known as GIS, are increasingly used to organize and map massive amounts of data, which can be layered or overlaid to yield insight into how cities and regions work. Planners often benefit from proactive strategies to involve the public in the development of values, mission statements, visioning, and goal setting (see Beck and Konkel, 1999). Various agencies have data and analyses relevant to the information needs of planners. Developing current conditions (a baseline) and evaluating trends and uncertainties to make forecasts is part of the "art" in the planning profession.

---

[1](1) **Examine the situation and its "context"** combines steps (1) and (2) from the ten-step process.

[2](4) **Design the program** incorporates steps (5) Develop alternative solutions, (6) Test alternatives, (7) Make modifications to mitigate adverse consequences and promote positive aspects of the plan, and (8) Selecting the best solution from the ten-step process.

There are numerous examples of development issues that affect public health and welfare. For example, in Kentucky, there are currently many proposals to develop coal-fired power plants to supplement electricity supplies. Whereas the environmental health and impacts on air, land, and water are primarily local and regional impacts, the mining and burning of coal increasingly takes place in a regional context, where electricity can be moved across state lines. In fact, **electricity deregulation** policies often mandate not only access to an electricity grid, but also sharing the burdens of upgrades. Policies for deregulation of electricity in states like California can affect prices paid for coal and prices paid for electricity in other regions and at other locations. Bond prices in New York can affect prices paid for reclamation bonds in Kentucky. **Spot prices**, prices paid for delivery of a good on a short-term basis, may be driven by changes in prices for related commodities. Project developers need to pay attention to these types of linkages. We are increasingly affected by developments outside our local counties, in other parts of the state, in other states, in Canada and Mexico, and even globally.

Set Goals

A clear statement of goals is essential to the development of a program. Goals should be broad targets and not be "beyond the pale." Sometimes when goals are attained earlier than expected then they are set at even higher levels.

Set Objectives

Objectives should be clearly stated and measurable. Some professions tend to have objectives as the "higher order" and goals as means of meeting the objectives. Though this convention can be confusing, it can work if it is used with consistency. If one sets a personal goal of receiving a master's degree in public health, specializing in environmental health, objectives could include taking the courses in the curriculum, obtaining and excelling in work internships with various employers, and finding a great job once one attains the degree. This does not preclude resetting the goal to add more diverse work experience, undertaking a Ph.D. degree, obtaining more training, or setting new professional goals.

Design the Program

In this step, the planner should brainstorm, create, and mold an integrated set of activities, procedures, and resources that make attainment of the goals and objectives possible. This may result in a completely new program, or a modified version of an existing program. The program should be described in detail, with its requirements—including such elements as full-time equivalents (FTEs) of labor, money, facilities, and equipment.

Implement the Program

In this phase, the planned program is put into action. This means committing the necessary materials, equipment, personnel, and technology. Shortages of materials, changes in requirements previously specified, lack of equipment, unqualified personnel, and unavailability of technology often challenge a planner in this phase. Sometimes general economic conditions change the premises upon which estimates were made, so inflation or recession in the economy may limit what can be done without additional project resources.

Evaluate the Program

Evaluations of what is expected and deviations in plans can lead to adjustments. These may be able to compensate for situation changes, poor assumptions, estimate errors, inflation, and unanticipated changes in program operations. Every year or two it is wise for planners to reconsider the problem for which the program was planned. Continuous monitoring is an asset for a successful program. It is useful to design alternative approaches to assist in meeting overall goals. Evaluation involves measurement of progress toward the goals and objectives identified for the program. Planning is a dynamic rather than a static process. In many cases it is art as well as science, an ability to deliver on time, on budget, and to specifications the desired programmatic results.

STYLES OF REGULATION

Collaborative Planning in the Regulatory Environment

The federal Environmental Protection Agency (EPA) and the Occupational Health and Safety Administration (OSHA) need strategic plans, policies, and programs to avoid the polarization with industry and common public perceptions as always being painted as the "bad guys," enforcing regulations against "bad actors." OSHA has developed a **Voluntary Protection Program (VPP)** in which the agency assists companies in identifying and correcting problems without the traditional inspection, violation, fines, and negotiation parts of the cycle. The National Academy of Public Administrators (NAPA, 1995; also see Appendix 1) has criticized the federal EPA for the way it has set priorities and the results it has achieved given its mission and resources. This may be changing. For example, the EPA is working with 27 companies to test or develop innovative management strategies in order to achieve better results than what would be achieved under current law in "**Project XL**." In rulemaking, a multimedia environmental rule that the EPA recently issued for the pulp and paper industry allows companies to delay compliance with more stringent water pollution control requirements if they commit to installing more advanced technologies.

Another example of the EPA working with industry to solve environmental pollution problems is the Common Sense Initiative, which aims at cutting toxic emissions 75% compared to 1992. In the metal-finishing industry, firms obtain regulatory relief and other benefits in exchange for going beyond compliance. This affects 11,000 metal-finishing shops nationwide.

CASE STUDY I—SOLID WASTE

Now that we have discussed the planning process, let's look at a hypothetical example.

The Solid Waste Situation in a County

In a rural county in a mountainous state, one-half of the county is not served by solid waste collection. Houses are located on average one-fourth of a mile apart in an area predominantly used for farming. Since it is not economically feasible for the poor county to provide house-to-house solid waste collection, the waste often finds its way into streams and into open pit dumps throughout the area. The improperly disposed waste serves as a breeding place for rats, roaches, flies, and other insects. In addition, the county and residents are degrading the environment by polluting the water, land, and air, and open pit burning and backyard incineration of the refuse is commonplace.

The state has recognized that the improper disposal of food, household trash, paint, and other wastes has possible impact on the health of communities, to say nothing of the tourism dollars lost because of unsightly, illegal dumps. The legislature and the governor have been debating the issue of what to do statewide. Currently there is controversy and gridlock in the senate over whether to put a container deposit on certain beverages, and how to pay for cleanup of illegal dumps. Some federal grants may be available for cleaning up the worst of the trash dumps. Without new legislation or container deposits, however, it is expected that the problem of illegal dumps will continue to plague the Commonwealth.

The Goal

The goal for the program is to protect and enhance the health and welfare of community residents by collecting and properly disposing of solid waste in order to reduce insect and other vector-borne disease, while improving environmental and ecological conditions in a cost-effective manner.

Objectives

- To reduce diseases spread by insects and rodents.
- To enhance environmental and ecological conditions by removing open dumps (which are illegal); and to discourage creation of new ones.
- To reduce the amount of waste that finds its way into streams.
- To reduce air pollution by stopping the burning of trash by individual homeowners.
- To reduce litter and the blight of illegal dumps.
- To reduce stream and groundwater pollution.
- To provide an economical system for homeowners to dispose of their trash.

The Program

The distance between houses makes it economically infeasible to provide house-to-house collection, as mentioned earlier. Therefore providing refuse receptacles, the "green box" method of utilizing a central receiving area, is the method of choice selected by the county planner. At central locations in the rural parts of the county, the county, using its local property tax receipts for funds, will provide 20 cubic yard bulk refuse receptacles. In the event that this source of revenue is "tapped out," a small assessment ($ per thousand dollars assessed value for land and improvements) may be added to the local taxes. This is a decision that must be made by the local decision maker; in this case, the judge executive makes the decision.

The planner has done some checking with other municipalities and engineers in surrounding jurisdictions and has determined that the county should provide five locations for the green box refuse receptacles according to population and other factors. Citizens will bring their refuse and dump it into the containers. The county has also evaluated whether these areas can also be used to collect recyclable materials presorted by residents, such as newspaper, cans, and clear and colored glass. Buyers have been found for the recyclables. The county will collect and dispose of the refuse from the central sites twice a week and hire two people to monitor the five storage areas as well as purchase a front loader compactor-type collection truck to collect the refuse and transport it to the county sanitary landfill.

Implementation

The county will hire two people to monitor the five receiving sites and will build a shelter at each site to be used in monitoring activities. The county will purchase a garbage truck and will hire the driver. The county will purchase the bulk refuse receptacles and will place them at the five sites along with the recyclable collection bins. Community residents will bring their refuse to the five sites. Trucks will transport the waste to the county landfill.

Program Evaluation

The program can be evaluated by the following:

- Determining the reduction of waste in streams and associated benefits of improved water quality.
- Determining the reduction of waste in open dumps.
- Determining the reduction of waste treated in backyard incinerators, and the associated environmental burden on air quality.
- Determining the improvements in the general appearance of the areas of the county newly served by solid waste disposal services.
- Determining the reduction of rats and insects and the prevalence of the diseases that they spread.

CASE STUDY II—TICK-BORNE TYPHUS

The control of tick-borne typhus (formerly Rocky Mountain Spotted Fever) is another good example for planning programs with environmental health benefits.

The Situation

Tick-borne typhus is a disease that was first a problem in the Rocky Mountains, but now is a threat to the majority of the United States. In recent years it has been of much concern in the Appalachian Mountains, particularly in the southern parts. The wood tick, borne by dogs and other like animals, spreads the disease. It is caused by a rickettsial organism. Since the organism can be transovarially transmitted from the mother to the offspring, it is more of a threat than other tick and insect-borne diseases. In many related diseases, the vector must bite a host that possesses the causative agent before it can spread the disease. However, tick-borne typhus needs no such agent, only vector and victim. Since tick-borne typhus can be transovarially transmitted and because ticks are difficult to control (it is not possible to spray the total country to eradicate ticks), it is therefore a greater threat than

malaria, for example, where we can drain water bodies and standing pools, and use chemicals and fish to kill the larvae and pupa. Since it is also a threat to farmers, hunters, campers, and anyone who walks outdoors in grass, weeds, and woods, health departments should have a planned program for preventing tick-borne typhus.

The Goal

The goal is to enhance the public's health by reducing their chances of suffering or dying from tick-borne typhus.

The Objectives

The objectives are the following:

- To prevent loss of time from work.
- To prevent the need to spend money for medical care.
- To prevent the risk of dying from tick-borne typhus.
- To prevent people from having to curb hiking, camping, and other outdoor activities that enhance their health.
- To reduce the chance of tick paralysis.

The Program

Since it is impractical to spray the countryside to control the tick, other measures must be utilized. The program has to be one of reducing the chances of human exposure to ticks. This can be accomplished by reducing hiking, camping activities, and other outdoor activities, that is, sports that are played on grass. But it is impractical to expect farmers, ranchers, gardeners, game wardens, and so on, to reduce their outside activities and it is not desirable to stop hiking and camping. It is also not feasible to immunize the total population.

Areas often used for outdoor sports should be surveyed for the prevalence of ticks. This can be done by pulling a cloth (sheet or similar-sized item) over a designated area. The ticks have a means of sensing heat (a warm-blooded animal and a new blood meal), thus as it is pulled along by a person, the tick latches onto the sheet as well as the clothes of the person pulling the cloth. Tick counts are made by simply turning the cloth over and counting the ticks in order to calculate the number of ticks per acre. This prevalence number can be used to determine if, after the survey, an area can be deemed suitable for outdoor activities. If the number of ticks is extremely high, the area may be sprayed.

Educating the public is necessary for reducing the cases of tick-borne typhus. Environmentalists working with the health educators in the health department and the members of the public health team should develop a program for educating the public. The risk communication messages should be broadcast through newspapers, television (e.g., "Kentucky Outdoors"), magazines ("Field and Stream," "Hunter's World") radio, and other means. The profiles of the tick-borne disease should describe how tick-borne typhus spreads, and how to prevent it, that is, socks over pants, shirt tails tucked in, tight cuffs, use of repellant, avoiding areas that surveys determine as having excessive numbers of ticks. The public should become aware of the need and procedure for detecting ticks after outdoor activities. Information concerning "hot spots" should be made available to the public by utilizing the news media as well as flyers and posting areas. The public should become aware of the times of the year when the ticks are most prevalent and present the greatest risk.

Implementation

The program should be implemented in the spring when the tick becomes active and when people start their outdoor activities. The implementation would include the following:

- Conduct tick surveys two weeks before activities to enhance options for controls.
- Spray camping, hiking, and playground areas periodically if they are highly infested.
- Prepare and release material for educating the general public, scout troops, and recreational area personnel (such as those who run state parks and local park facilities) on how to properly remove ticks. This can be done by cutting off the oxygen supply by completely covering the tick with cooking oil.

Program Evaluation

The program can be evaluated by doing the following:

- Assessing the reduction in the number of cases of tick-borne typhus through effective surveillance programs.
- Determining the reduction by repeating the survey procedure after spraying.

AN EXAMPLE OF A PLANNING FRAMEWORK—HEALTHY PEOPLE 2010

One of the challenges in public health has been to develop environmental health objectives. In order to meld environmental health programs and policies with associated objectives in public health as a whole, it is advantageous to take a look at "big-picture" issues and approaches. The Department of Health and Human Services (DHHS) has sponsored such an initiative, known as **Healthy People 2000**. There were earlier versions as well. This framework was updated (January 2000)—with the new edition known as **Healthy People 2010** representing both a planning process to set up a framework for planning as well as an evaluation process to measure success or progress toward goals.

The Healthy People 2000 Framework set national goals, which were developed to reduce premature mortality and preventable disease. Measurable objectives were developed to reduce lead poisoning, cardiovascular disease, asthma, diabetes, blood lead levels; the list is extensive and enlightening (Healthy People 2000, 1970). In this initiative there were 17 environmental health objectives, and environmental health was cast in a bigger picture view of environmental quality.

Healthy People 2010

The process of planning for preventing and controlling environmentally caused diseases has three distinct elements: establishing goals and objectives, programming, and continuous assessment.

Healthy People 2010 contains a set of health objectives for the nation to achieve over the first decade of the new century. It can be used by many different people, states, communities, professional organizations, and others to help them develop programs to improve health.

Healthy People 2010 builds on initiatives pursued over the past three decades. The 1979 Surgeon General's Report, Healthy People, and Healthy People 2000 both established national health objectives and served as the basis for the development of state and community plans. Like its predecessors, Healthy People 2010 was developed through a broad consultation process, built on the best scientific knowledge, and designed to measure programs over time.

Healthy People 2010 Overarching Goals

Goal 1: **Increase Quality and Years of Healthy Life**

The first goal of Healthy People 2010 is to help individuals of all ages increase life expectancy and improve their quality of life.

Goal 2: **Eliminate Health Disparities**

The second goal of Healthy People 2010 is to eliminate health disparities among different segments of the population. The segments of the population include: the indigent, racial minorities, children, and the elderly.

The Environmental Quality section indicators relevant to Environmental Health include 30 objectives relating to exposure media such as air, soil, and water. These issues are addressed through health promotion, health protection and preventive services, including environmental risk reduction programs. This area is one of the 10 leading Health Indicators for Healthy People 2010.

Additional Examples of EPA Collaborative Approaches

The **33/50 program** set ambitious goals to reduce toxic emissions 33% and 50% by 1992 and 1995, respectively. EPA recognized over 40 companies for their results.

A voluntary agreement between the EPA and car manufacturers is focused on offering less polluting vehicles in the northeast region of the United States and the District of Columbia for 2001 model year vehicles. Pollution reduction of up to 70% of previous emissions is one of the goals.

The EPA is also supporting cleanup of community "**brownfields**"—sites that can be (and are often) overlooked for development or redevelopment because of the presence of contamination and its associated liability. EPA has funded cleanup and restoration seed grants amounting to $24 million, provided technical assistance to 121 communities, and supported new tax incentives, which are estimated to have led to $300 million in investment and affected more than 5,000 communities. Reuse of these sites will reduce the real estate pressure on open space and "**greenfield**" areas—areas that are more rural in character and often require extensive investments in utilities and site access.

Although the EPA has offered more compliance assistance to industries affected by its rules and regulations, EPA also collected the largest fines (dollar amount) ever in 1997. EPA is attempting to move toward good faith efforts toward finding, disclosing, and fixing environmental problems. During 1997, 247 companies reported violations at more than 760 facilities. Clearly there is an enormous amount of work to do to improve the effectiveness and efficiency of protecting the environment and human health.

Time will tell if the initiatives profiled above will emerge as a catalyst in changing our "regulatory culture" in the United States. Clearly, not all nations have the legal and political approach to "**command-and-control**" regulation that we have adopted in the United States. International comparative studies bear this out (e.g., Vogel, 1986). It pays to have a more global than local perspective on developments in the regulatory arena because economic systems are interrelated. For example, some government agencies and firms are obtaining international certifications of their environmental and quality management systems—certifications such as the International Standards Organization (ISO 14000 series) and Quality Standards (9000 series). These certifications often have market share implications. It is also a fact of life that many corporations sell their products on more than one continent; and increasingly corporations will operate plants in more than one country. The North American Free Trade Agreement (NAFTA) and the continued integration efforts of the European Union (EU) suggest that the trends are moving to more, rather than less, globalization of economic and information activity.

· · · · · · · · · · · · · ·

NEED FOR INTEGRATION OF ENVIRONMENTAL STATUTES

The 1970s are often looked at as the "decade of the environment" in the sense that a plethora of environmental laws were passed, the EPA and OSHA were created as governmental agencies in 1970, and regulation of air quality, water quality, solid waste and toxic materials moved front and center. Earth Days began and were celebrated annually starting on April 22, 1970. Perhaps one of the more prescient and important statutes was Public Law 91–190, the National Environmental Policy Act of 1969 (signed into law by President Richard M. Nixon, January 1, 1970). It is known in common professional jargon simply as "NEPA." Senators Edmund Muskie (D-ME) and Henry M. "Scoop" Jackson (D-WA) championed this legislation in the U.S. Senate.

The procedural requirements of NEPA require not only an assessment by the appropriate federal officials or private-sector consultants of whether or not the project has significant environmental impacts—known as the **environmental assessment (EA)**—but in cases where an **environmental impact statement (EIS)** is written, there must be opportunities for public comment and provisions to address comments of the public and others, such as federal, state, and local government entities. This process can lead to substantive or substantial improvements by designing in mitigation measures, or ways to avoid incurring adverse impacts.

Environmental impact assessments and statements can identify impacts not readily apparent when projects are first developed. For example, the proposed 1984 Louisiana Exposition (Theme— "Fresh Water as a Source of Life") was to be sited in the "Warehouse District" along the Mississippi River waterfront in New Orleans. In a business-by-business survey, consultants doing the EIS discovered that over 1,750 jobs were within the boundaries to be fenced off for the duration of the six-month Exposition. Projected impacts included firms with these employees having to relocate; but also many firms going out of business with associated job losses. The discovery of the number of jobs and ability to renegotiate the fair "footprint" allowed the city of New Orleans to retain more than 1,000 jobs that otherwise would have been lost. Also, the projections of revenues and number of attendees received attention due to the EIS work performed for the U.S. Department of Commerce ("Social, Economic, and Urban Design Impacts of the Louisiana World Exposition," U.S. Dept. of Commerce, Bureau of International Expositions, 1982).

New fields have emerged from the impasses and conflicts generated by public policy decisions, such as siting locally unwanted (but regionally necessary) facilities. These fields supplement one of our oldest means in the United States of deciding—litigation before a judge or jury. Arbitration and mediated negotiation involve a third party who has a role in decision making or in helping the parties come to an agreement. When there is a responsibility for the third party to make a decision, and that decision is final (not appealable) then binding arbitration may meet the needs of all parties (as occurs in some major league baseball contracts).

Environmental policy is a tool to integrate economic, environmental, and energy impacts into planning for sustainable development. The ideal target is to figure out how populations can improve on individual and community quality of life; analogous to "living on the interest while not depleting the principal in financial terms." This is a tough balancing act considering intergenerational equity and the current pace of 90 million additional people added to the earth's population each year.

· · · · · · · · · · · · · ·

RISKY DECISIONS

Given politics and our individual differences and interests, it is the author's assertion that consensus-based and collaborative processes have an increasingly important role to play in environmental planning and education. Both involve listening and explicit attention to values, which tend to drive actions of interested parties in conflict situations. Joe Beck and the author argue in their publications that the values, interests, and expectations of stakeholders are the key to understanding their interests and positions in multiparty, multi-issue, disputes. This is not meant to imply that timing, availability of resources, enforcement effectiveness, and other factors are insignificant matters, whether the issues at hand are negotiated (as in negotiated rulemaking) or whether they are brought up in citizen's or agency lawsuits.

An example of a risky decision is the siting of a coal-fired or nuclear-powered generating station. Another example is selection of a technology to destroy stockpiles of mustard gas and nerve gas at eight locations within the continental United States. Conventional wisdom tends to place a premium on "knowing the facts"; we believe parties are selective in citing facts. One may even argue that the preconceived notions of parties tend to drive them to look for the science and scientific experts that support their view of what is important.

A favorite teacher and mentor of the author's once remarked "We all believe in the public interest to the extent that our private ox is not gored" (Professor Harvey Brooks, 1990, personal communication). Although enforcement and fines, injunctions and other penalties must be a part of governmental regulation of economic activity, the author believes that if people understand the implications of pollution on health they can take steps to solve problems, rather than become part of the problem or the perpetuation of the problem. Incentives can motivate behavior and practices.

Programs like the EPA's Project XL and the 33/50 program, as well as the National Academy of Public Administrators' review of the EPA, indicate that cooperative approaches have promise. Also, the Occupational Health and Safety Administration's VPP illustrates the value of moving toward more collaborative approaches to achieve improved results, over and above "compliance." These developments are overdue and encouraging, since industry brings substantial resources to the table and can often use innovation to solve problems.

In order to achieve better results in energy and environmental policy, we must find ways to incorporate sound scientific and technical judgments. Often litigation is costly, time-consuming, and the adversarial proceedings strain relationships that sometimes must survive differences of opinion as well as the different mission orientation of organizations and governmental agencies. Especially in multiparty, multi-issue disputes, alternatives to litigation can meet this overall purpose of using science and scientific experts in a productive manner. There are numerous examples of using **mediation** for **conflict resolution** in environmental health decision making (e.g. Konkel, 1987; Susskind and Ozawa, 1985). Pacific Northwest National Laboratory (PNNL) mediated a future use planning process among more than 20 federal, state, and local agencies, and three distinct Indian tribes in the mid-1990s to set guidelines for development of a Hanford future land use plan at the site managed by the U.S. Department of Energy.

Risk analysis can be used to identify risk factors. For example, studies have shown that diet, exercise, and smoking are risk factors affecting cardiovascular performance. There are many excellent texts on the use and techniques for **risk assessment** (e.g., Moeller, 1997, Chapter 16; Cohrssen and Covello, 1989; Also See "Risk Assessment in the Federal Government: Managing the Process," 1983). The probabilities and consequences of various actions and events are a very useful planning tool. Nevertheless, decisions are not made solely on the basis of engineering calculations and forecasts; social, economic, and political factors are of paramount importance in decisions regarding environmental health programs and policies.

SUMMARY

Environmental planning is a means of identifying where we want to go, where we are at the present time, and charting a path to achieve the envisioned outcomes. In the public health arena, environmental health planners focus on promotion of behaviors that enhance an individual's or community's health status, including quality of life as well as longevity. In this Chapter a ten-step planning process (and an abbreviated six-step process) show how one moves from identification of a problem through to the design of programmatic solutions that meet the values, interests, and expectations of interested parties, also known as "**stakeholders**." The process is iterative and dynamic.

The regulatory structure in which the Environmental Protection Agency and the Occupational Safety and Health Administration operate is largely based on "command and control" responses to public policy issues. There are many statutes and associated polices, programs, and rules and regulations that business must comply with in order to be in compliance with the law. There are evolving cooperative and collaborative programs that have promise as agencies and business work to achieve better results. EPA should use comparative risk analysis to help set program priorities and budgets. We are all responsible for stewardship of our natural resources and prevention of injury, illness, and disease in populations—by anticipating problems, setting priorities, preventing pollution, and solving the "right" problems.

KEY LAW ACRONYMS

CAA—Clean Air Act of 1970, 1990 amendments

CWA—Clean Water Act of 1972, 1977

EA—Environmental Assessment

EIS—Environmental Impact Statement

EPA—United States Environmental Protection Agency

FONSI—Finding of No Significant (Environmental) Impact

NEPA—National Environmental Policy Act of 1969

OSHA—Occupational Safety and Health Administration

OSHAct—Occupational Safety and Health Act of 1970

SWDA—Solid Waste Disposal Act of 1976

TSCA—Toxic Substances Control Act of 1976

KEY TERMS

APPENDIX 1

NAPA is the National Association of Public Administrators. The essence of their advice to the EPA is the following:

- Create stronger partnership with state agencies.
- Sector- and community-based approaches have value.
- Develop incentives to encourage better performance.
- Market-based forces should guide action.
- Create the infrastructure to managing in the information age.
- Support the public's right-to-know.
- New approaches to enforcement and compliance.
- Cut red tape and regulatory burdens.

REFERENCES

Beardsley, Daniel P. 1996. *Incentives for Environmental Improvement: An Assessment of Selected Innovative Programs in the States and Europe*. Prepared for Global Environmental Management Initiative. Prepared by Albers and Co., 11 DuPont Circle NW, Ste. 300, Washington, DC 20036. August.

Beck, Joe E., and R. Steven Konkel. 1999. "Participatory Planning." *Occupational Health and Safety Magazine*, 68, no. 8:97–103.

———. 2000. "Developing a Customer-First Attitude (But First, Does Anybody Know Who the Customers Are?)" *Occupational Health and Safety Magazine*, 69, no.3:20–23. March.

Brabec, Elizabeth A., et al. 1994. *Rural by Design*. American Planning Association, Chicago, IL.

Buck, Susan J. 1996. *Understanding Environmental Administration and Law*, 2nd ed. Island Press, Covelo, CA.

Capper, Stuart A., Peter M. Ginter, and Linda E. Swayne. 2002. *Public Health Leadership and Management: Cases and Context*. Sage Publications, Thousand Oaks, CA.

Carpenter, Susan L., and W. J. D. Kennedy. 2001. *Managing Public Disputes: A Practical Guide for Professionals in Government, Business, and Citizen's Groups*. Jossey-Bass (A Wiley Co.), San Francisco, CA.

Cohrssen, John J., and V. Covello. 1989. *Risk Assessment: A Guide to Principles and Methods for Analyzing Health and Environmental Risks*. National Technical Information Service, Springfield, VA.

Daly, Herman E., and Kenneth N. Townsend. 1993. *Valuing the Earth: Economics, Ecology, Ethics*. MIT Press, Cambridge, MA.

Davies, Terry, and Jan Mazurak. 1996. *Industry Incentives for Environmental Improvement: Evaluation of U.S. Federal Incentives*. Prepared by Resources for the Future, prepared for Global Environmental Management Initiative (GEMI).

Douglas, Mary, and Aaron Wildavsky. 1982. *Risk and Culture: An Essay on the Selection of Technological and Environmental Dangers*. U. of California Press, Berkeley, CA.

Forester, John. 1999. *The Deliberative Practitioner: Encouraging Participatory Planning Processes*. MIT Press, Cambridge, MA.

GEMI, 1090 Vermont Ave. NW, 3rd Flr., Washington, DC 20005. *gemi@worldweb.net http://www.gemi.org* (202)296–7449. EH&S excellence.

Hamilton, James T., and W. Kip Viscusi. 1999. *Calculating Risks? The Spatial and Political Dimensions of Hazardous Waste Policy*. MIT Press, Cambridge, MA.

Jain, R. K., L. V. Urban, G. S. Stacy, and H. E. Balbach. 1993. *Environmental Assessment*. McGraw-Hill, Inc., New York.

Konkel, R. Steven. 1987. "Risk Management in the United States: Three Case Studies"; "Dioxin Emissions and Trash-to-Energy Plants in New York City"; "Liquified Natural Gas: Spectre of a Marine Spill in Boston Harbor"; and "Carbaryl and the Gypsy Moth: A Massachusetts Pesticide Controversy," in *Environmental Impact Assessment Review*, 7, no. 1:37–76.

Konkel, R. Steven and Lawrence Susskind. 1989. *Risk Management: Developing a Research Agenda*. Proceedings of the MIT Faculty Seminar on Risk Management. Sponsored by the MIT Center for Technology, Policy, and Industrial Development (CTPID) and the Science, Technology, and Society Program. August.

McGregor, Gregor. 1994. *Environmental Law and Enforcement*. Lewis Publishers (CRC Press), Boca Raton, FL.

Moeller, Dade. 1997. *Environmental Health*. Harvard University Press, Cambridge, MA.

Moore, Gary S., ed. 2001. *Environmental Compliance: A Web-Enhanced Resource*. Lewis Publishers (CRC Press) Boca Raton, FL.

Murray, Christopher J., and Alan D. Lopez., eds. 1996. *The Global Burden of Disease*. Published by the Harvard School of Public Health on Behalf of the World Health Organization and the World Bank. Distributed by Harvard U. Press, Cambridge, MA.

National Academy of Public Administrators. 1995. *Setting Priorities, Getting Results: A New Direction for the Environmental Protection Agency*. A National Academy of Public Administration Report to Congress. Sherwood Fletcher Associates, Silver Spring, MD.

National Research Council. 1983. *Committee on the Institutional Means for Assessment of Risks to Public Health, Commission on Life Sciences*. National Academy Press, Washington, DC.

Pollard, Trip. 2001. "Greening the American Dream?" in *Planning*. American Planning Association, Chicago, IL. October, 10–15.

Rotberg, Robert I., ed. 2000. *Health and Disease in Human History*. MIT Press, Cambridge, MA.

Susskind, Larry, and Jeffrey Cruikshank. 1987. *Breaking the Impasse: Consensual Approaches to Resolving Public Disputes*. Basic Books, Inc., New York.

Susskind, L., and C. Ozawa. 1985. "Mediating Science-Intensive Policy Disputes." In *Journal of Policy Analysis and Management*, 5, no. 1:23–39.

U.S. Department of Commerce. 1982. "Social, Economic, and Urban Design Impacts of the 1984 World

Exposition." Prepared by Howard, Needles, Tammen, and Bergendoff. Prepared for the Bureau of International Expositions. U.S. Department of Commerce, Bureau of International Expositions, Washington, DC.

U.S. EPA. 1998. "The Changing Nature of Environmental and Public Health Protection: An Annual Report on Reinvention." U.S. Environmental Protection Agency, Washington, DC. March.

U.S. Dept. of Health and Human Services, Office of Disease Prevention and Health Promotion. Healthy People 2010. 2000. Special CD Conference Edition. Washington, D.C. Jan. 25, 2000. Also see *www.health.gov/healthypeople*.

Vogel, David. 1986. *National Styles of Regulation: Environmental Policy in Great Britain and the United States*. Cornell U. Press, Ithaca, NY.

Yosie, Terry F., and Timothy D. Herbst. 1996. *Corporate Environmental Health and Safety Practices in Transition: Management System Responses to Changing Public Expectations, Regulatory Requirements, and Incentives*. Prepared by Resources for the Future and E. Bruce Harrison, Ruder Finn, Inc. Prepared for Global Environmental Management Initiative. Sept.

17

PRINCIPLES OF ENVIRONMENTAL HEALTH ADMINISTRATION

Larry Gordon, M.S., M.P.H.

University of New Mexico

OBJECTIVES

- Understand the scope of environmental health and protection, and name at least 30 problems addressed.

- List at least 10 common program activities.

- List at least five important support services.

- Discuss why ecological considerations are important to environmental health and protection.

- Describe the mission of environmental health and protection agencies.

- Understand the importance of basing priorities and decisions on sound risk assessment and public health assessment.

- Explain risk communication and how it differs from public information.

- Identify at least 10 federal agencies that have major environmental health and protection responsibilities.

. . . .

INTRODUCTION

Public and scientific concern regarding the quality of the environment and related public health and ecological considerations continues to be intense. **Environmental health and protection** is expected and demanded by the public, the media, and political leaders, and are widely considered an entitlement.

Environmental health and protection services are integral components of the continuum of health services, and are essential precursors to the efficacy of the other components of the health services continuum. Other health continuum services include personal public health services (population-based disease prevention and health promotion), as well as health care (diagnosis, treatment, and/or rehabilitation of a patient under care on a one-on-one basis).

Environmental health and protection administration is as complex as the nature and causes of the problems, and involves both the public and private sectors. Program administration impacts the health of the public, the quality of the environment, and the economy. Program administration requires properly qualified personnel; an informed and supportive citizenry; environmental health and protection leadership; a sound scientific basis; the data necessary to measure and understand problems and trends; a number of vital support services; rational public and private sector policies and workable legislation; and budgets prioritized to deal with the more significant problems as determined by sound epidemiology, toxicology, risk assessment, and public health assessment, as well as public demands and expectations.

DEFINITION

Environmental health and protection is the art and science of protecting against environmental factors that may adversely impact human health or the ecological balances essential to long-term human health and environmental quality. Such factors include, but are not limited to air, food and water contaminants; radiation; toxic chemicals; wastes; disease vectors; safety hazards; and habitat alterations.

The term "environmental health *and* protection," rather than "environmental health" *or* "environmental protection," is being widely used. The separate terms have denoted programs based on organizational settings rather than logical or definable differences in programs, missions, or goals. Such distinctions are largely artificial, and have led to organizational confusion, undesirable programmatic gaps and overlaps, and separation of activities that share the common goal of protecting the public's health and enhancing environmental quality. In some cases, the separate terminologies have created divisive administrative barriers rather than building administrative bridges between the organizations involved in the common struggle for environmental quality.

ORGANIZATIONAL DIVERSITY

Environmental health, along with personal public health measures, has always been one of the two basic components of the field of public health.

At the federal level, most environmental health and protection programs are administered by agencies other than the U.S. Public Health Service. Among states, some 90% to 95% of environmental health and protection activities are administered by agencies other than state health departments.

At the state level, environmental health and protection expenditures and numbers of personnel approximate half of the field of public health, and is the largest single component of the field of public health.

A 1996 study conducted by Public Technology, Inc. indicates that, at the local level, increasing environmental health and protection responsibilities are being assigned to agencies other than local health departments.

VALUES AND BENEFITS

The values and benefits of environmental health and protection include the following:

- Enhanced economic status
- Enhanced productivity
- Enhanced educational achievement
- Less social problems
- A more livable environment
- Better quality of life
- Reduced disease and disability
- Reduced health care costs

SCOPE OF ENVIRONMENTAL HEALTH AND PROTECTION

The scope of environmental health and protection continues to expand and become more complex. Environmental health and protection administration is based on risk assessment, risk communication, and risk management applied to one or more of the following problems (a reasonably discrete environmental health and protection issue having an impact on human health, safety, or the quality of the environment):

Ambient air	Radon
Indoor air	Asbestos

Noise pollution

Radiation

Tanning parlors

Water pollution

Safe drinking water

Liquid wastes

Cross-connections

Eating and drinking establishments

Food wholesalers

Food retailers

Itinerant food establishments

Fish sanitation

Shellfish production and sanitation

Pure food control

Slaughterhouses

Poultry processing

Milk sanitation

Industrial hygiene and safety

Disaster planning and response

Healthful housing

Educational facilities

Temporary mass gatherings

Health care facilities

Day care facilities

Correctional facilities

Massage clinics

Body art establishments

Unintentional injuries

Bioterrorism

Swimming pools and spas

Beaches

Park and recreational areas

Solid wastes

Hazardous wastes

Toxic chemicals

Lead poisoning

Pesticides and herbicides

Migrant workers

Hazardous spills

Brownfields

Leaking storage tanks

Insects and rodents

Nuisances

Animal bites

Fertilizers

Weeds

Global warming

Stratospheric ozone depletion

Global toxification

Program activities to prevent or ameliorate the foregoing problems include:

Surveillance, sampling, monitoring

Regulation, including:

    Warnings

    Administrative hearings

    Permits

    Grading

    Compliance schedules

    Variances

    Injunctions

    Administrative and judicial penalties

    Embargoes

    Environmental impact requirements

    Court preparation/testifying

Inspection

Complaint response

Consultation

Networking and community involvement

Pollution prevention

Plan and design review

Economic and social incentives

Public information and education

Problem prioritization

Public policy development and implementation

Program marketing

Strategic planning

Planning for prevention of environmental health problems through effective involvement during the planning, design and implementation stages of:

Energy production and utilization

Land use

Transportation systems

Resource development and consumption, and

Product and facility design

Support services for the foregoing include the following :

Epidemiology

Laboratory

Legal

Geographic information systems

Personnel training

Information technology

Research

. . . .

ECOLOGICAL CONSIDERATIONS

Public health personnel have traditionally justified, designed, and administered environmental programs based narrowly on public health issues. But as environmental problems, priorities, public perception and involvement, goals, and public policy have evolved, ecological considerations have become increasingly important. Whatever long-term health threats exist, the public and public policy leaders also know that pollution kills fish, limits visibility, creates foul stenches, ruins lakes and rivers, degrades recreational areas, and endangers plant and animal life.

The report of the U.S. Environmental Protection Agency's Science Advisory Board, *Reducing Risk: Setting Priorities and Strategies for Environmental Protection,* states:

> . . . there is no doubt that over time the quality of human life declines as the quality of natural ecosystems declines . . . over the past 20 years and especially over the past decade, EPA has paid too little attention to natural ecosystems. The Agency has considered the protection of public health to be its primary mission, and it has been less concerned about risks posed to ecosystems . . . EPA's response to human health risks as compared to ecological risks is inappropriate, because, in the real world, there is little distinction between the two. Over the long term, ecological degradation either directly or indirectly degrades human health and the economy . . . human health and welfare ultimately rely upon the life support systems and natural resources provided by healthy ecosystems.

MISSION

Environmental health and protection agencies should have missions of administering services in such a manner as to protect the health of the public and the quality of the environment.

Additionally, environmental health and protection administrators should stimulate interest in related areas in which they may not have primary responsibility. For example, it may be desirable to support and promote such environmental health and protection-related activities as long-range community planning, recycling programs, zoning ordinances, plumbing codes, building codes, solid waste systems, economic development, energy conservation, land-use, and transportation systems.

Agencies such as agriculture departments have obvious and appropriate missions of promoting and protecting specific industries or segments of public interest. Conflicts of interest occur when missions are mixed, thereby resulting in the familiar "fox in the henhouse" syndrome. Such conflicts of interest result in the public being defrauded rather than receiving the protection they deserve. If environmental health and protection administrators do not articulate and adhere to a mission of protecting the health of the public and the quality of the environment, they may end up inadvertently protecting or promoting the interests of those they are charged with regulating.

GOAL

The goal of environmental health and protection is to ensure an environment that will provide optimal public health and safety, ecological well-being, and quality of life for this and future generations.

We do not live in a risk-free society or environment. Therefore, the goal for many environmental health and protection program administration is not always "zero-risk." The pursuit of zero-risk as a standard or goal is frequently unnecessary, economically impractical, and frequently unattainable, and may create unfounded public concern when zero-risk is not attained. The pursuit of zero-risk as a goal for one issue may also preclude resource availability to deal with other priorities.

RISK ASSESSMENT

The public is barraged with "catastrophe-of-the-week" information regarding environmental risk coupled with a paucity of critical scientific inquiry. Administrators should recognize that there would be many times the actual morbidity and mortality if all the predicted catastrophes were factual. And finally, administrators must be scientifically critical, routinely questioning existing policies, standards and regulations, as well as proposals to ensure that all measures reflect valid priorities and needs.

Considering the serious differences in perceived priorities between scientists and those of the public and political leaders, **risk assessment** must be considered an administrative issue to be understood and practiced by all interests involved in protecting the health of the public and the quality of the environment.

The U.S. Environmental Protection Agency's Science Advisory Board has defined risk assessment as the process by which the form, dimension, and characteristics of risk are estimated. Utilizing sound scientific principles to assess risk is vital to communicating risk, recommending priorities, designing and administering risk management programs, requesting funds, and evaluating control efforts. However, the results of risk assessment models may vary considerably depending on the assumptions, data, and models utilized. Serious debate continues over the validity of risk assessment models and methods. Such differences may be confusing to public policymakers, and may create a credibility gap concerning risk assessment as a useful process.

Many agencies have developed models that utilize the following risk assessment components:

- Hazard identification to determine the health, ecological, economic, or quality of life effects of a substance, activity, or problem.

- Exposure assessment to evaluate the routes, media, magnitudes, time and duration of actual or anticipated exposure, and of anticipated exposures, as well as the number of people, species, and/or areas exposed.

- Amount or dose-response assessment to estimate the relationship between the amount of the substance and the incidence of adverse effects.

- Risk characterization to estimate the probable incidence of an adverse effect under various conditions of exposure, including a description of the uncertainties involved.

Public policymakers and environmental health and protection administrators have always utilized risk assessment informally and even intuitively. Utilizing risk assessment mathematical models has been a comparatively recent development. Whenever a decision or recommendation has been made to develop a policy or manage an environmental problem based on available information, a risk assessment has been performed. Frequently, environmental health and protection administrators must make major emergency decisions based on incomplete but compelling information without having the luxury of waiting until incontrovertible evidence is available. This practice is performed daily by environmental health and protection personnel charged with managing such risks as food, water, air, radiation, toxics, noise, and unintentional injuries.

Most mathematical health risk assessment models have been developed to determine carcinogenic outcomes. Current models reflect single-agent exposure assessment. New models must be developed to assess effects of multiple incidents of exposures and multiple agents. Increasingly, researchers and practitioners are finding it necessary to develop knowledge and models to determine other types of health and ecological outcomes of various environmental exposures. Besides carcinogenicity, the health outcomes might include mutations, teratogenicity, altered reproductive function, mental health, neuro-behavioral toxicity and other specific organ systems.

Risk assessments generally follow the most conservative estimates that can be defended. The uncertainties in the degree of risk are frequently significant, and many issues in risk assessment can only be determined judgmentally. It has been shown that by taking nearly all relevant information about the test chemicals into consideration, a group of scientists correctly predicted the outcome at a higher success rate than computer-assisted models. Risk assessment remains as much an art as a science, and risk assessment models need significant improvement.

Personnel involved in risk assessment procedures rely on knowledge and skills from such fields as chemistry, epidemiology, toxicology, biology, engineering, geology, hydrology, statistics, meteorology, and physics. The practice of risk assessment is, therefore, multidisciplinary and interdisciplinary in nature. Risk assessment procedures are commonly practiced by a team of individuals representing a spectrum of required competencies.

Many individuals and agencies have recommended developing a uniform model for risk assessment. Others feel this would prevent needed improvements in the available models and would retard progress in risk assessment procedures and public acceptance.

While risk assessment modeling is practiced to some degree by all environmental health and protection agencies, many feel that formal risk assessment should be organizationally separate from risk management programs in order to reduce possible politicization of the process.

Interesting case studies iterating the politicization of several EPA standards and policies are detailed in the book *The Environmental Protection Agency: Asking the Wrong Questions*.

The U.S. Office of Management and Budget has noted "The need to keep risk assessment and risk management separate has long been the objective of responsible officials." The National Institute of Medicine (IOM) in its report *The Future of Public Health* recommends "there should be an institutional home in each state and at the federal level for development and dissemination of knowledge, including research and the provision of technical assistance to lower levels of government and to academic institutions and voluntary organizations." The U.S. Public Health Service Bureau of Health Professions publication *Educating Environmental Health Science and Protection Professionals* recommends that the foregoing "IOM and OMB recommendations could best be accomplished by providing start-up financial incentives for each state to organize and staff an Environmental Health Science and Protection Research and Service Institute within a university. By insuring good environmental epidemiology and risk assessment studies specific to each state, environmental health science and protection issues would be better defined and prioritized. In such a system, program funding could address science based recommendations rather than public hysteria. By basing such institutions in academic settings and separating them from operating agencies, emotionalism would be alleviated." The report of the Committee on the Future of Environmental Health recommends that "Environmental health and protection research institutes should be established in each state to ensure timely research that addresses local and regional issues."

Risk assessment is only one of the factors to be used to determine priorities. Other vital considerations include public health assessments, social factors, economic factors, political factors, technical feasibility, and community expectations.

Few jurisdictions have adequate multidisciplinary capacity to conduct and implement risk-based decision making and risk management. Increasingly, educational programs for environmental health and protection personnel are requiring formal risk assessment and risk communication course content. Programs accredited by the National Environmental Health Science and Protection Accreditation Council are required to include risk assessment and risk communication as educational competencies.

Training in risk assessment and risk communication procedures is available through various short courses and institutes sponsored by various universities, professional groups, EPA, and the U.S. Public Health Service.

··············

PUBLIC HEALTH ASSESSMENT

The Agency for Toxic Substances and Disease Registry has developed and emphasized the use of **public health assessments** in an effort to better measure public health problems and develop realistic solutions. Such public health assessments are increasingly being used to evaluate human health risk. They provide compelling additional information, as they provide direct measures of human exposures rather than the hypothetical and statistical findings of risk assessments. Public health assessments are based on the data from representative biologic samples and personal monitoring and, therefore, are targeted at actions directly related to the exposure. Public health assessments have enhanced interactions with individuals and communities, and have improved public health decisions and actions.

··············

RISK COMMUNICATION

Risk communication is the process of communicating risk with the public, including community groups, the private sector, the media, and public policy leaders. In the absence of timely and effective risk communication, risk assessment is merely academic. The utilization of risk assessment inherently requires effective risk communication if findings are to be utilized. Administrators must not confuse official pronouncements and the distribution of public information materials with the art of risk communication.

Environmental health and protection administrators must develop and demonstrate effective risk communication skills. Lack of such communication results in priorities and policies that differ considerably from those based on good environmental health and protection science. Effective risk communication requires complete openness throughout the planning and decision process, as well as embracing, including and involving appropriate groups. Failures in risk communication are frequently linked to the failure to involve the public early and openly discuss the needs, assumptions, alternatives, and data on which problems have been assessed and public health assessments conducted. Risk communication, like risk assessment, is multidisciplinary and interdisciplinary involving such disciplines as sociologists, political scientists, educators, and marketing professionals.

Effective risk communication requires a continuing relationship with the public even in the absence of risk communication crises. Risk communication on a single-issue crisis basis is doomed to be less than optimal.

• • • • • • • • • • • • • •

RISK MANAGEMENT

Risk management constitutes those measures designed to deal with risk that has been assessed. Most environmental managers and agencies routinely operate to manage risk, but may not use that terminology. Risk management is the process of integrating the results of risk assessment with economic, social, political and legal concerns to develop a course of action to prevent a problem, or solve an existing problem. Risk management methodologies include measures such as those listed on pages 304–305 of this chapter.

The issue of how risk is assessed, communicated, and managed is among the most critical environmental problems faced by society. Public perception drives the actions of elected officials.

However, public perception of environmental priorities and problems frequently differs from that of environmental scientists. We do not live in a zero-risk society, and it is essential that limited resources be utilized to address the higher-priority problems. The environment and the health of the public will be best served by prioritizing problems based on the best of risk and public health assessment measures and professional judgment coupled with effective risk communication and risk management.

• • • • • • • • • • • • • •

PRIORITIZATION

Globally, priority environmental health and protection issues include species extinction; wastes; desertification; deforestation; global warming and stratospheric ozone depletion; planetary toxification; and, most importantly, over-population.

Congress, as well as state and local legislative bodies, has authorized and funded our nation's various environmental health and protection programs with little regard for risk, relative risk, or priority. A December 1991 survey entitled "The Health Scientist Survey: Identifying Consensus on Assessing Human Health Risk," conducted by the Institute for Regulatory Policy of nearly 1,300 professionals in the fields of epidemiology, toxicology, medicine, and other health sciences, indicated that over 81% of the professionals surveyed believed that public health dollars for reduction of environmental health risk were improperly targeted. For many years, the U.S. Environmental Protection Agency (EPA) and many other federal, state, and local agencies have been attempting to request and allocate resources on the basis of relative risk, and EPA is now placing increased emphasis on ecological risk.

A Roper poll determined that, in terms of public perception, at least 20% of the U.S. public considered hazardous waste sites to be the most significant environmental issue. At the same time, the report of EPA's Science Advisory Board, *Reducing Risk: Setting Priorities and Strategies for Environmental Protection*, listed ambient air pollution, worker exposure to chemicals, indoor pollution, and drinking water pollutants as the major risks to human health. While not EPA programs, food protection, unintentional injuries, and childhood lead poisoning (in specified areas) should be added to this list by any reasonable public health priority.

As risks to the natural ecology and human welfare, *Reducing Risk* listed habitat alteration and destruction; species extinction and overall loss of biological diversity; stratospheric ozone depletion; global climate change; herbicides/pesticides; toxics, nutrients, biochemical oxygen demand and turbidity in surface waters; acid deposition; and airborne toxics. Among relatively low risks to the natural ecology and human welfare, the list also included oil spills, groundwater pollution, radio nuclides, acid runoff to surface waters, and thermal pollution.

Priorities at the local levels may vary considerably, but should be based on public health assessments, epidemiology, community risk assessment, cost-benefit analysis, and public demands, as well as legislative delegation of responsibilities.

· · · · · · · · · · · · · · ·

FEDERAL ORGANIZATIONS

In addition to the U.S. Environmental Protection Agency, other significant federal environmental health and protection agencies include the Occupational Safety and Health Administration of the U.S. Department of Labor, the U.S. Public Health Service (including the National Institute of Environmental Health Sciences, the Centers for Disease Control and Prevention, the Indian Health Service, the Food and Drug Administration, the Agency for Toxic Substances and Disease Registry, and the National Institute for Environmental Health and Safety), the U.S. Coast Guard, the Geological Survey, the National Oceanographic and Atmospheric Administration, the Nuclear Regulatory Commission, the Corps of Engineers, and the Departments of Transportation, Agriculture, and Housing and Urban Development.

· · · · · · · · · · · · · · ·

STATE ORGANIZATIONS

A study conducted by the Johns Hopkins School of Public Health, under contract with the USPHS Bureau of Health Professions, revealed that at least 85% of state-level environmental health and protection activities were being administered by environ-

mental health and protection agencies other than state health departments. Every state indicated that multiple agencies were involved in environmental health and protection activities. Data from the Hopkins study, coupled with data published by the Public Health Foundation, also suggest that states spend approximately as much on environmental health and protection as they do on all other public health activities combined. Another study conducted by the University of Texas School of Public Health leads to similar conclusions. It is clear that environmental health and protection is the largest single component of the field of public health. Regardless of titles, environmental health and protection agencies are components of the broad field of public health as their programs fall within any common definition (see page 305) of environmental health and protection and are based on achieving public health goals. Such agencies have various titles such as environment, environmental protection, ecology, labor, agriculture, environmental quality, natural resources, and pollution control.

In general, state environmental health and protection agencies are apt to have responsibility for administering water pollution control, air pollution control, solid waste management, public water supplies, meat inspection, occupational health and safety, pesticide regulation, and radiation protection.

· · · · · · · · · · · · · · ·

LOCAL ORGANIZATIONS

The majority of local environmental health and protection administration remains the responsibility of local health departments, but there is a trend to assign various responsibilities to local agencies other than health departments. Local activities tend to differ from those assigned state agencies, and focus on such programs as food protection, swimming pool inspection, lead in the environment, on-site liquid waste disposal, groundwater contamination, asbestos surveillance, water supplies, animal/vector control, radon testing, illegal dumping, hazardous materials spills, emergency response planning, health impact statements, and nuisance abatement. A few local jurisdictions administer comprehensive indoor and ambient air pollution control programs. Some local health departments indicate activities in water pollution control, solid waste management, radiation control, and hazardous waste management.

Most local governments have assigned certain environmental health and protection administration to agencies such as public works, housing, planning, councils of government, solid waste management, special purpose districts, and regional authorities.

....

FEDERAL, STATE, OR LOCAL?

Environmental health and protection services should be administered as close to the people as possible. Local agencies can do a better job of protecting the local environment than can a distant bureaucracy. There are, however, certain issues that have defined the responsible levels of government. These include the following:

- Problems of an interstate nature, such as interstate protection of food and food products, interstate solid and hazardous wastes transportation, interstate water pollution control, interstate pesticide regulation, and interstate air pollution resolution are administered by appropriate federal agencies.

- The federal government has retained partial or sole authority to administer many activities that have been federally mandated or funded including, but not limited to, certain aspects of radioactive waste management, water pollution control and facilities construction, air pollution control, meat inspection, occupational safety and health, and safe drinking water. State and local governments have frequently accepted primacy for administering some of these activities subject to adhering to federal requirements.

- State agencies or special districts may find it easier to administer certain issues on a problem-shed basis rather than on a limited local jurisdiction basis. Examples include water pollution control, air pollution control, solid waste management, and milk sanitation.

- In sparsely populated states as well as rural areas of some other states, the state agency may exercise direct administrative authority in all program areas.

- Many state agencies provide technical and consultative support to local environmental health and protection agencies.

- State agencies, as well as federal agencies, may develop criteria, standards, and model legislation for state and/or local adoption.

- State agencies administer state and federal grant-in-aid funds for local agencies.

- There may be a conflict of interest situation when local environmental health and protection agencies attempt to regulate local government proprietary functions such as public water supplies, solid waste disposal, and sewage treatment.

- Smaller local agencies may not have expertise in certain specialized areas such as epidemiology, toxicology, public health assessment, and risk assessment.

The trend to organizationally diversify environmental health and protection programs will continue in response to the priority of environmental health and protection, the demands of environmental advocates, and the trend for many health departments to become significantly involved in health care to the detriment of environmental health and protection and other public health priorities. It is unrealistic to develop programmatic relationships between water pollution control, for example, and any one of a number of health care (treatment and rehabilitation) programs. Increased health care responsibilities of federal, state, and local health departments may translate into inadequate understanding, leadership, and priority for environmental health and protection within health departments. Additionally, health departments find it difficult to deal with the ecological aspects of environmental health and protection.

Such organizational diversification does not mean that environmental health and protection programs are no longer basic components of the field of public health. While each community or state has only one health department, every community and state has several other public health agencies including numerous environmental health and protection agencies.

Academic institutions preparing students for environmental health and protection careers should orient students striving for leadership roles in the multitude of agencies involved. Public health leaders should help assure that the programs administered by such agencies are comprehensive in scope; based on sound epidemiology, toxicology, public health assessment, and risk assessment data; and help ensure that they have adequate legal, fiscal, laboratory, communications technology, epidemiological and other support resources to be effective.

PROGRAM DESIGN

An environmental health and protection program is a rational grouping of activities designed to solve one or more problems (see page 305).

Problems must be accurately defined as to cause, time of day or season, geographic area, nature, intensity, and public health and environmental effects prior to designing the program. Program design must stand the scrutiny of critical evaluation to ensure that the design will prevent or solve the problem(s) in an economical and societally acceptable manner.

The net health, environmental, social, and economic impacts of proposed requirements must be thoroughly evaluated prior to implementation. One seemingly desirable measure may result in undesirable problems of a more serious nature than the problem for which the program was intended.

Most environmental health and protection programs have been developed to address a single problem. This has led to unnecessary inefficiencies and ineffectiveness along with poor utilization of personnel and other resources. Properly designed, a program can address components of several environmental problems. This design practice is common in such programs as food protection, institutional environmental control, environmental control of recreational areas, and industrial hygiene and safety.

ADMINISTRATIVE SUPPORT

Administrative support elements as fiscal, audit, purchasing, budget, and personnel are required. A number of additional support functions are essential to the administration of environmental health and protection services.

LABORATORY

Comprehensive laboratory support must be available in quantity and quality for epidemiological investigations, public health assessment, risk assessment, determining environmental trends and needs, developing standards and regulations, regulation, public information, and program design. Such services may be available through public health laboratories, environmental laboratories, pollution control laboratories, agriculture laboratories, or in a few jurisdictions, comprehensive laboratories serving various governmental agencies. At the federal level, more specialized services may be requested from the Centers for Disease Control and Prevention, the Environmental Protection Agency, and the Food and Drug Administration.

EPIDEMIOLOGY

Environmental epidemiology is a specialized epidemiological function that deals with extrapolations and correlations as well as direct cause-and-effect investigations. Early day environmental health practice was geared primarily to communicable disease problems. Now, it also embraces the impacts of increasing amounts, types, and combinations of nonliving contaminants and other stresses. Such impacts are more subtle and long range in their effects. There is greater difficulty in measuring effects as well as in precisely isolating and understanding the cause(s).

Some state and local environmental health and protection agencies do not have in-house epidemiological support and must receive such services through another agency, usually a health department. Sound environmental surveillance data and epidemiology are essential to determine needs, trends, and priorities, and to design effective programs.

LEGAL

Environmental health and protection programs are authorized by legislative bodies at various levels of government, and provide for legal remedies when other efforts do not provide for compliance with specified requirements. When regulatory remedies are pursued, the advice, support, and involvement of legal counsel are desirable.

Many environmental health and protection agencies have specialized environmental law attorneys. Others may request assistance through a city or county attorney, a state attorney general, or the U.S. Department of Justice, depending on the nature of requirement(s). The involvement of a skilled legal draft person is also essential when legislation is being drafted.

PUBLIC INFORMATION AND EDUCATION

Environmental health and protection is the public's business, and will not be properly understood or supported in the absence of continuing public information and educational activities. While all environmental health and protection administrators should be involved in these activities, it may be desirable to utilize staff specifically skilled in assuring a free flow of information and the dissemination of new knowledge to the public, including the news media, citizen groups, professional groups, elected officials, and other agencies involved in the field of environmental health and protection.

RESEARCH

Environmental health and protection programs cannot be properly justified, prioritized, budgeted, designed, implemented, or administered without the benefits of peer-reviewed research. Research is essential to the development of new methodologies for preventing and controlling problems, environmental remediation, analyses, and public information.

Most official agencies and practitioners are not well equipped to conduct research, but should be active participants in the processes of identifying research needs and routinely communicating these needs to appropriate research institutions. The knowledge and skills of practitioners will be enhanced through continuing communication and coalitions with academic programs and individuals involved in environmental health and protection education and research.

DATA

Environmental health and protection surveillance and status data are currently inadequate. These data should include environmentally related morbidity and mortality, specified environmental contaminant and pollution levels, and other environmental/ecological conditions.

State-of-the art environmental health and protection information systems would enhance the level of informed administration at all levels of government and industry.

FISCAL SUPPORT

Environmental health and protection administrators are finding it necessary to be creative in funding services. Activities must be evaluated and prioritized to address the more significant priorities within the jurisdiction. Where additional general fund support is not available, administrators must consider reallocating budgets from lower-priority activities, or developing new sources of revenue such as fees for service and/or pollution taxes and other market-based incentives.

Prioritizing funding requests requires the best skills in administration, epidemiology, public health assessments, toxicology, and risk assessment. Developing creative funding mechanisms will require that administrators have basic knowledge and skills in public financing and environmental economics. Marketing such budget requests requires competencies in marketing, communication, and public policy development.

THE PRIMACY OF PREVENTION

EPA's Science Advisory Board publication *Reducing Risk* states:

> . . . end-of-pipe controls and waste disposal should be the last line of environmental defense, not the front line. Preventing pollution at its source—through the redesign of production processes, the substitution of less toxic production materials, the screening of new chemicals and technologies before they are

introduced into commerce, energy and water conservation, the development of less-polluting transportation systems and farming practices, etc.—is usually a far cheaper, more effective way to reduce environmental risk, especially over the long term . . .

Pollution prevention also minimizes environmental problems that are caused through a variety of exposures. For example, substituting a non-toxic for a toxic agent reduces exposures to workers producing and using the agent at the same time as it reduces exposures through surface water, groundwater, and the air.

Pollution prevention also is preferable to end-of-pipe controls that often cause environmental problems of their own. Air pollutants captured in industrial smokestacks and deposited in landfills can contribute to groundwater pollution; stripping toxic chemicals out of groundwater, and combusting solid and hazardous wastes, can contribute to air pollution. Pollution prevention techniques are especially promising because they do not move pollutants from one environmental medium to another, as is often the case with end-of-pipe controls. Rather, the pollutants are not generated in the first place.

PLANNING FOR ENVIRONMENTAL HEALTH AND PROTECTION

Environmental health and protection planning (as differed from program planning) is a fundamental prevention function. While environmental health and protection should be grounded on prevention, a preponderance of efforts and funds are currently devoted to remediation of contamination and pollution problems created as a result of earlier actions taken by other interests in the public and private sectors.

Environmental health and protection administrators must have the knowledge, skills, and authority to become effectively involved in prevention during the planning, design, and construction stages of energy development and production, land use, transportation methods and systems, facilities, resource development and utilization, and product design and development. Developing the capacity and authority to function effectively in environmental health and protection planning is necessary for environmental health and protection administra-

tors to strive to function in a primary prevention mode, rather than secondary prevention or treatment of the environment after the contamination or pollution has been produced and emitted.

BUILDING AND TRAVELING BRIDGES

Effective environmental health and protection administration depends on developing and utilizing constantly traveled communication bridges and network processes connecting a wide variety of groups and agencies involved in the struggle for a quality environment and enhanced public health. A few such interests include land use, energy production, transportation, resource development, the medical community, public works officials, agriculture, conservation, engineering, architecture, colleges and universities, economic development, chambers of commerce, environmental groups, trade and industry groups, and elected officials. Organizational policy, rather than being left to chance or personalities, should ensure these relationships.

PERSONNEL REQUIREMENTS

Environmental health and protection, like other components of public health, is not a profession or a discipline. It is a cause and a field engaged in by a wide array of personnel practicing within a broad and diverse spectrum of individuals, groups, and agencies.

The field of environmental health and protection requires the involvement of scores of disciplines as well as interdisciplinarily trained personnel. Personnel function in roles ranging from routine inspection and surveillance levels through administration, policy, education and research components. Depending on the type of agency and sophistication of programs, effective efforts demand an alliance of physical scientists, life scientists, social scientists, educators, physicians, environmental scientists, engineers, data specialists, planners, administrators, laboratory scientists, veterinarians, attorneys, economists, political scientists, and others in order to fully utilize the variety of environmental health and protection activities.

Environmental health and protection personnel may be grouped as environmental health and protection professionals, and professionals in environmental health and protection.

Environmental health and protection professionals are those who have been educated in the various environmental health and protection technical areas, as well as in epidemiology, biostatistics, toxicology, administration and public policy, risk assessment, communication, public health assessment, risk management, environmental law, and environmental finance. For the most part, such professionals are graduates of environmental health science and protection programs accredited by the National Environmental Health Science and Protection Accreditation Council, or of schools or programs accredited by the Council on Education for Public Health.

Professionals in environmental health and protection include other essential professionals and disciplines such as epidemiologists, biostatiticians, toxicologists, chemists, hydrologists, geologists, biologists, physicians, attorneys, administrators, economists, political scientists, educators, engineers, meteorologists, and social scientists.

The 1990 EPA Science Advisory Board publication, *Reducing Risk*, states that:

> The nation is facing a shortage of environmental scientists and engineers needed to cope with environmental problems today and in the future. Moreover, professionals today need continuing education and training to help them understand the complex control technologies and pollution prevention strategies needed to reduce environmental risks more effectively.
>
> .... Most environmental officials have been trained in a subset of environmental problems, such as air pollution, water pollution or waste disposal. But they have not been trained to assist and respond to environmental problems in an integrated and comprehensive way. Moreover, few have been taught to anticipate and prevent pollution from occurring or to utilize risk reduction tools beyond command-and-control regulations. This narrow focus is not very effective in the face of intermedia problems that have

emerged over the past two decades and that are projected for the future.

Competencies for environmental health and protection professionals as practitioners should include the following:

- Relevant environmental health and protection sciences such as biology, chemistry, physics, geology, ecology, and toxicology
- Environmental health and protection technical issues
- Epidemiology and biostatistics
- Etiology of environmentally induced diseases
- Risk assessment
- Public health assessment
- Risk communication
- Risk management
- Marketing
- Interest group interactions
- Personnel, financial, and program administration
- Organizational behavior
- Public policy development and implementation
- Planning for environmental health and protection
- Cultural issues
- Strategic planning
- Fiscal impacts of environmental health and protection
- Environmental health and protection law
- Organizational diversity
- Political processes

CONTINUING EDUCATION

Continuing education is an essential component of a career, not only to be effective, but personnel must learn more readily as they encounter specific needs. Such continuing environmental health and protection education should be budgeted, timely, relevant, economical, and convenient, as well as strongly supported by management.

THE FUTURE

Environmental health and protection administration will continue to assume a higher priority in our society, and the public will expect and demand greater levels of protection.

Demographic changes, resource development and consumption, product and materials manufacture and utilization, wastes, global environmental deterioration, technological development, changing patterns of land use, transportation methodologies, energy development and utilization, and continuing diversification of environmental health and protection efforts will create additional and unanticipated challenges. The competencies of properly prepared environmental health and protection administrators will be critical.

SUMMARY

Within the overall mission to administer services that will protect the health of the public and the quality of the environment, environmental health and protection planning emphasizes prevention over remediation. The goal is to ensure an environment that will provide optimal public health and safety, ecological well-being, and quality of life for this and future generations.

Environmental health and protection is the largest single component of the field of public health. At least 85% of state-level environmental health and protection activities are administered by agencies other than state health departments. The total process involves risk assessment, risk communication, risk management, and prioritization.

Environmental health and protection administration will continue to assume a higher priority in our society, and the public will expect and demand greater levels of protection. Population growth and shifts, resource development and consumption, product and materials manufacture and utilization, wastes, global environmental deterioration, technological development, changing patterns of land use, transportation methodologies, energy development

and utilization, and continuing diversification of environmental health and protection agencies will create additional and unanticipated challenges. The competency of properly prepared environmental health and protection administrators will be a critical component.

KEY TERMS

Environmental health and protection, p. 303

Risk assessment, p. 307

Public health assessment, p. 308

Risk communication, p. 308

Risk management, p. 309

REFERENCES

Abraham, John E., and Robert C. Williams. "Enhancing Risk Management and Public Health Decisions Through Exposure Investigations." Unpublished paper, Agency for Toxic Substances and Disease Registry, Atlanta, GA.

Browner, Carol. 1993. "Public Health—An EPA Imperative." *EPA Insight Policy Paper*. EPA-175-N-93-025. November.

Burke, Thomas A. 1996. "Meeting the Educational Needs of Risk Professionals and Professionals in Risk." *Risk Sciences and Public Policy Institute Newsletter* 4–7. Johns Hopkins University School of Hygiene and Public Health. Fall.

Burke, Thomas A., Nadia M. Shalauta, and Tran, Nga L. 1995. *The Environmental Web: Services, Structure, Funding*. U.S. Department of Health and Human Services, Health Resources and Services Administration, Bureau of Health Professions, Public Health Branch. Rockville, MD. January.

Center for Health Policy Studies. 1996. *The Professional Public Health Workforce in Texas*. University of Texas School of Public Health, Houston, TX.

Committee for the Study of the Future of Public Health, Division of Health Care Services, Institute of Medicine. 1998. *The Future of Public Health*. National Academy Press, Washington, DC.

Committee on the Future of Environmental Health, National Environmental Health Association. 1993. "The Future of Environmental Health, Part One." *Journal of Environmental Health* 55 (4):28–32.

———. 1993. "The Future of Environmental Health." *Journal of Environmental Health* 55(5):42–45.

———. 1993. "The Future of Environmental Health." *Journal of Environmental Health*, 55, nos. 4 and 5:28–32, 42–45. January/February and March.

Council on Education for Public Health. Council on Education for Public Health: *The Accrediting Agency for Graduate Public Health Education*. CEPH, Washington, DC.

Gordon, Larry J. 1990. "Who Will Manage the Environment?" *American Journal of Public Health*, August, 80:904–905.

———. 1993. "The Future of Environmental Health, and The Need For Public Health Leadership." *Journal of Environmental Health* 56(5):28–30.

———. 1994. "Public Health: A Blurred Vision*," Newsletter, Conference of Emeritus Members of the APHA*, 8, no. 2:2–8. Summer.

———. 1995. "Environmental Health and Protection: Century 21 Challenges," *Journal of Environmental Health*. 57, no. 6: 28–34. Jan/Feb.

———. 1995. "Risk Analysis." *McGraw-Hill Yearbook of Science and Technology, 1995*. McGraw-Hill, Inc.

Gordon, Larry J., and McFarlane, Deborah R. 1996. "Public Health Practitioner Incubation Plight: Following the Money Trail," *Journal of Public Health Policy*. 17, no.1:59–70.

Gordon, Larry J., and Stern, Barry. 2001. "Environmental Health and Protection: A Primer." Unpublished paper.

Health Resources and Services Administration, Public Health Service, U.S. Department of Health and Human Services. 1988. *Evaluating the Environmental Health Work Force*. Bureau of Health Professions, Rockville, MD.

———. 1991. *Educating the Environmental Health Science and Protection Work Force: Problems, Challenges, and Recommendations*. Bureau of Health Professions, Rockville, MD.

Hileman, Bette. 1993. "Expert Intuition Tops in Test of Carcinogenicity Prediction." *Chemical and Engineering News* 71(25):35–37.

Institute for Regulatory Policy. 1991. *The Health Scientist Survey: Identifying Consensus on Assessing Human Health Risk*. Institute for Regulatory Policy, Washington, DC.

Landy, Marc K., Marc J. Roberts, and Stephen R. Thomas. 1990. *The Environmental Protection Agency: Asking the Wrong Questions*. Oxford University Press.

National Association of County Health Officials. 1990. *National Profile of Local Health Departments*. National Association of County Health Officials, Washington, DC.

———. 1992. *Current Roles and Future Challenges of Local Health Departments in Environmental Health*. NACHO, Washington, DC.

National Environmental Health Science and Protection Accreditation Council. 1992. *Guidelines for Accreditation of Environmental Health Science and Protection Baccalaureate Programs*. Denver, CO.

———. 1993. *Guidelines for Accreditation of Environmental Health Science and Protection Master's Level Graduate Programs*. Denver, CO.

Public Health Foundation. 1991. *Public Health Agencies 1991: An Inventory of Programs and Block Grant Expenditures*. Public Health Foundation, Washington, DC. December.

Roper, William L., Edward L. Baker, William W. Dyal, and Ray M. Nicola. "Strengthening the Public Health System." *Public Health Reports* 107 (6):609–615.

Sorensen, A., and R. Bialek, eds. 1993. *The Public Health Faculty/Agency Forum: Final Report*. Florida University Press, Gainesville, FL.

U.S. Environmental Protection Agency, Science Advisory Board. 1990. *Reducing Risk: Setting Priorities and Strategies for Environmental Protection*. U.S. Environmental Protection Agency, Washington, DC.

U.S. Office of Management and Budget. 1990. *Regulatory Program of the United States Government*. Washington, DC.

SUMMARY OF ENVIRONMENTAL LAWS

NATIONAL ENVIRONMENTAL POLICY ACT

The National Environmental Policy Act, signed into law on January 1, 1970, established a framework for the government to assess the environmental effects of its major actions. It required federal agencies to prepare "environmental impact statements" assessing the environmental effects of proposed projects and requests for legislation. The act also created the Council on Environmental Quality (CEQ), a three-member presidential advisory group that is required to prepare an annual environmental quality report for Congress. The council also serves as mediator of disputes among federal agencies over environmental issues. As the administrator of federal pollution control programs, the EPA does not have to comply with the act, but it reviews environmental impact statements prepared by other agencies and makes comments and recommendations on the projects proposed. Environmental Impact Statements (EIS) must include the following:

1. The environmental impact of the proposed action.

2. Any adverse environmental effects that cannot be avoided if the proposal is implemented.

3. Alternatives to the proposed action.

4. The relationship between local short-term uses of the environment and maintenance and enhancement of long-term productivity.

5. Any irreversible and irretrievable commitments of resources that would be involved in the proposed action if it is implemented.

Prior to making any detailed statement, the responsible federal official must consult with and obtain the comments of any federal agency that has jurisdiction by law or special expertise with respect to any environmental impact involved. Copies of the statement and the comments and views of the appropriate federal, state, and local agencies, which are authorized to develop and enforce environmental standards, must be made available to the President, the Council on Environmental Quality, and the public.

CLEAN AIR ACT

The original Clean Air Act was passed in 1955, authorizing a research program in the Public Health Service and technical support for local agencies concerned with the abatement of air pollution. Amendments in 1960 directed the Surgeon General to study the problem of motor vehicle pollution. Amendments in 1963 directed research into fuel desulfurization and development of air quality criteria. Amendments in 1965 added the investigation of new sources of pollution.

In 1967 the Clean Air Act was replaced by the Air Quality Act of 1967, although the former name is still used. The 1967 act provided for the designation of air quality control regions, which originally were intended to include only areas with serious air pollution problems. When the Environmental Protection Agency was organized in 1970, it covered all areas of the United States.

The Clean Air Amendment of 1970 required the EPA to set ambient air quality standards to protect public health and welfare and environmental quality, to control emissions from stationary and mobile sources, to control emissions from new stationary sources, and to control hazardous air pollutants.

The 1977 amendments to the act adopted a standardized basis for rule-making regarding criteria for national ambient air quality standards, new source performance standards, hazardous air pollution standards, motor vehicle standards, fuel and fuel-additive provisions, and aircraft emission standards. The amendments established two programs to protect air quality in pristine areas such as national parks, where the air is required to be cleaner than in areas subject to the ambient standards. One program prevents significant degradation of air quality, and the other protects visibility.

······

CLEAN WATER ACT

The basic federal law authorizing regulation to prevent water pollution can be dated from the Federal Water Pollution Control Act of 1956, as amended in 1961, 1965, 1966, 1970, 1972, and 1977. The 1956 act was the beginning of the construction grants program and of the enforcement and research authorizations that form the key parts of the present program. The 1961 amendments increased the funding for construction grants and increased the research program set up under the act.

In 1965 the Water Quality Act created the Federal Water Pollution Control Administration within the Department of Health, Education and Welfare, but this was transferred to the Department of Interior in 1966 under a presidential reorganization plan.

The Water Restoration Act of 1966 authorized research to cover demonstration of industrial waste treatment methods, advanced waste treatment, and joint municipal and industrial treatment. The act required the states to establish standards for all interstate and coastal waters. Federal authority was moved from the Department of the Interior to the Environmental Protection Agency. If the EPA finds the state standards inadequate, it has the power to set the standards itself.

The Federal Water Pollution Control Act amendments of 1972 replaced the previous language of the Clean Water Act entirely. The act stated the goal of attaining zero discharge of pollutants by 1985, with an interim 1983 goal of attaining water quality to support fish and wildlife and to be suitable for recreation.

The National Pollutant Discharge Elimination System (NPDES) was set up to control pollution from point sources. Facilities are required to have an NPDES permit, negotiated with the EPA or the state water authority, to discharge pollutants into waters. Pretreatment standards for wastes discharged from industrial facilities to publicly owned sewage disposal plants also were provided for. The 1977 amendments strengthened and extended the regulation of toxic substances in water and extended some deadlines written into the 1972 law.

······

RESOURCE CONSERVATION AND RECOVERY ACT

The need to protect groundwater led Congress to enact the Resource Conservation and Recovery Act (RCRA) of 1976. Hazardous raw materials or products are not regulated under RCRA because they are regulated under the Toxic Substances Control Act or there are inherent economic incentives for their careful management. Instead, hazardous wastes have been targeted for regulation, because of their potential impact on groundwater supplies and the absence of an economic motive to ensure responsible management of spent and discarded materials. Shortly after the federal legislation was enacted, states enacted their own laws that greatly resembled RCRA.

Subtitle C of RCRA addresses five major elements for the management of hazardous waste:

1. Classifications of waste and hazardous waste.
2. Cradle-to-grave-manifest system, record-keeping and reporting requirements.
3. Standards to be followed by generators, transporters, and owners or operators of treatment, storage, or disposal facilities.
4. Enforcement of the standards through a permitting program and civil penalty policies.
5. Authorization of state programs to operate in lieu of the federal program.

The EPA took nearly 6 years to develop a near-complete set of regulations to implement the statute. This may explain in part the frequent complaint that the regulations are complicated and difficult to follow.

An entire section of the RCRA law is devoted to defining hazardous waste. This is the most challenging section of the regulations to understand. A waste is defined as "any material resulting from commercial or industrial operations which sometimes is discarded or is accumulated, stored, or treated prior to such abandonment." Recent amendments to RCRA also have included most materials that are recycled or reclaimed in the definition of waste.

Once something has been established to be a waste, the next step is to determine whether it meets the narrower category of hazardous waste. Hazardous waste is defined as any waste that is not excluded from the regulations, and that is either listed or exhibits one or more of the characteristics of hazardous waste.

If the waste is not one of the several hundred ones listed, laboratory analyses must be performed to determine whether it qualifies as hazardous waste by possessing at least one of the four characteristics of hazardous waste: ignitability, corrosivity, reactivity, and EP toxicity. The regulations describe parameters for determining whether a waste qualifies as being characteristically hazardous. *Reactivity* refers to chemical instability or the tendency to release a toxic substance into the air. A flashpoint threshold (less than 140°F) is specified for the *ignitability* characteristic. Specific pH values (greater than 12.5 or less than 2.0) and a steel corrosion rate define the *corrosivity* characteristic. EP *toxicity* involves testing the waste for concentrations of certain soluble heavy metals or pesticides. These wastes are hazardous if extract concentrations are more than 100 times the primary drinking water standards. An array of contaminants may indicate EP toxicity, and wastes exhibiting this characteristic often are denoted for the specific constituent.

Even though they exhibit a characteristic of hazardous waste, several wastes are excluded from full regulation as hazardous wastes. Examples include wastes generated from the processing of ores and minerals, residues remaining in empty containers, certain small quantities of hazardous waste

(small quantity generators generate between 100 and 1000 kg/mo), samples, etc.

Generator Standards

A generator is a person, or site, whose act or process produces a hazardous waste, or whose act first causes a hazardous waste to become subject to regulation. Even though generating hazardous waste is not unlawful, a generator must certify that an effort is being made to reduce the quantity of hazardous waste generated. Once a hazardous waste is generated, the generator must notify the EPA (or an authorized state) of that waste. No permit is required to generate hazardous waste, and generators are allowed to store their hazardous waste on site for no more than 90 days without a permit, provided they comply with certain conditions. These conditions include: storing the hazardous waste in either tanks or containers, making or labeling containers or tanks, training personnel, conducting at least weekly inspections, and developing and maintaining a contingency plan for accidents.

When the generator ships the hazardous waste off-site, a hazardous waste manifest must be completed properly. The generator must identify on the manifest the type and quantity of hazardous waste being shipped, the transporters to be used, and the designated treatment, storage, or disposal facility (TSDF). The generator also must ensure that the designated facility received the hazardous wastes shipped. If the manifest is not returned to the generator within 45 days of the date the waste was accepted by the initial transporter, the generator must submit an exception report to EPA or an authorized state. Periodically, generators must submit a summary (annual or biannual report) of the hazardous waste shipped off-site.

Transporter Standards

A transporter's responsibility is summarized best as ensuring that the hazardous waste accepted is received by either the next designated transporter or the designated TSDF. In the event of a hazardous waste discharge during transportation, the transporter must take appropriate and immediate action to protect the public health and the environment. The transporter also has limited responsibility for cleaning up the contaminated area.

TSDF Standards

The owner or operator of every TSDF that receives a regulated hazardous waste for TSD must obtain a permit under RCRA, unless the activity is excluded specifically from the permitting requirements. The permit for TSDF is the key mechanism for reinforcing control of hazardous waste management facilities. The permitting process is structured to allow the EPA or an authorized state to write facility-specific permits. The owner or operator has the opportunity to write facility-specific plans and procedures that are added to the permit as attachments.

Permitting Process

The first major step of the permitting process is the submission by the applicant. After detailed technical review, the EPA or an authorized state determines that the application is complete or makes a tentative decision to either grant or deny the permit. A public notice then is published regarding the tentative decision, allowing the affected community and the owner and operator 45 days to comment. A public hearing may be held if it is requested and warranted. The EPA or an authorized state will respond to comments received and make the final permit decision. This final decision can be appealed.

Authorization of State Programs

From the inception of RCRA, Congress intended to grant states the authority to administer the hazardous waste program, rather than having the EPA implement and manage RCRA on a national scale. A significant amount of federal grant money is appropriated to states each year to facilitate the development and administration of state-run hazardous waste regulatory programs. A state seeking federal authorization is subject to probation under EPA for a period of time, and full delegation is conferred when the state becomes trained and experienced in administering the program. Although a state is never fully autonomous from the EPA, decisions can be made and acted on by an authorized state without lengthy overview by the federal agency.

· · · · · · · · · · · · · · · ·

COMPREHENSIVE ENVIRONMENTAL RESPONSE, COMPENSATION, AND LIABILITY ACT OF 1980

The Comprehensive Environmental Response, Compensation, and Liability Act (CERCLA) of 1980, commonly known as the Superfund Act, was passed by Congress in response to a growing national concern about the release of hazardous substances to the environment primarily at inactive sites but also from actively managed facilities and vessels that are not subject to the Resource Conservation and Recovery Act (RCRA). The key purpose of CERCLA is to establish a mechanism of response for the immediate cleanup of hazardous waste contamination from accidental spills or from abandoned hazardous waste disposal sites that may result in long-term environmental damage.

In general, if a release to the environment is considered a "federally permitted release," it is not subject to CERCLA reporting requirements. A federally permitted release is any discharge that is in compliance with a permit issued under other environmental laws. This exemption applies whether the permit is issued by a federal, state, or local authority. The intent of CERCLA is to provide for response to and cleanup of environmental problems that are not covered adequately by other environmental statutes.

Three basic types of responses may be taken under CERCLA: removals, remedial actions, and enforcement actions. All three actions may be taken at any site. Enforcement actions, either administrative or judicial, always are initiated at the time a site is discovered. The goal of CERCLA is to compel those parties responsible for a non-permitted release to pay for the cleanup of that release. If a potentially responsible party cannot be identified quickly enough to address an imminent and substantial endangerment, the federal government will respond.

The National Priorities List (NPL) is a list of sites that present the greatest danger to public health or welfare or the environment. The list is promulgated by the EPA. The sites on the NPL are prioritized according to the Hazard Ranking System (HRS). Cleanup of the sites must conform to the EPA's National Contingency Plan (NCP).

The NCP specifies the planning, coordination, and communication networks. The NCP requires that each federal region prepare regional contingency plans similar to the NCP. Each EPA region is to have its own regional team and coordinators to oversee responses for removal of oil and hazardous substances, as well as remedial project managers to oversee remedial activities involving hazardous substances. Releases of oils, PCBs, or hazardous substances in excess of reportable quantities must be reported to the National Response Center.

CERCLA has been amended four times. The most recent amendment, the Superfund Amendments and Reauthorization Act of 1986 (SARA), was signed on October 17, 1986. SARA is the first major revision of CERCLA since it was enacted. Some of the major issues addressed by SARA include:

- Cleanup standards—Adopted to discourage moving waste from one location to another without reducing the long-term threat.

- Fund replenishment—Provides for an $8.6 billion, 5-year replenishment of the Superfund.

- Settlement provisions—Deal with provisions that facilitate voluntary settlements by offering a variety of techniques for carrying out such actions.

- Liability—Defines four categories of people as liable for response costs incurred as a result of the release or threat of release of hazardous substances:

  1. The current owner or operator of a vessel or a facility.

  2. The owner or operator at the time of disposal.

  3. Any person who by contract, agreement, or other arrangement is responsible for the disposal or treatment of hazardous substances at, or transported to, a facility from which a release has occurred.

4. Transporters who selected the disposal facility. SARA also provides a new defense for innocent landowners who acquire property without knowledge that it was used previously for waste disposal.

- State participation—Requires states to provide assurances to the EPA that they have sufficient treatment and disposal facilities complying with RCRA that are adequate to meet the state's needs for 20 years.

- Public participation—Gives the public an opportunity to comment both on a proposed remedial action and on the consent order settling a case. The EPA must respond to these comments. Furthermore, a citizen suit provision is established. Private persons may petition the EPA to have risk assessments performed on any site, and technical assistance grants to Superfund site community groups may be made.

- Health-related authorities—Greatly expands the expertise in health risk assessment to be utilized at Superfund sites. Responsibility for implementing many of these requirements rests with the Agency for Toxic Substances and Disease Registry (ATSDR) in consultation with the EPA. The ATSDR is required to perform health assessments at all NPL sites. Upon request of a state or the EPA, these assessments must be conducted at other sites. Citizens also are allowed to petition directly to ATSDR for health assessments.

- Federal facilities cleanup program—Makes each department, agency, and instrumentality of the United States subject to CERCLA in the same manner as any nongovernmental entity.

- Radon Gas and Indoor Air Quality Research Act—Emphasizes coordination of efforts and gathering of data.

- Underground storage tank (LUST) trust fund—Establishes a comprehensive corrective action program for releases of petroleum from underground storage tanks. The fund is financed at $600 million from a new tax on fuel.

TOXIC SUBSTANCES CONTROL ACT

Passage of the Toxic Substances Control Act (TSCA) in 1976 culminated 5 years of intensive effort by Congress to provide a regulatory framework for dealing comprehensively with risks posed by the manufacture and use of chemical substances. Prior to passage of TSCA, these substances were largely unregulated. TSCA was enacted in large part because of the discovery of widespread contamination by polychlorinated biphenyls (PCBs) and the EPA's lack of regulatory tools to control PCB material. TSCA authorizes the EPA to:

- Obtain data from industry regarding the production, use, and health effects of chemical substances and mixtures.

- Regulate the manufacture, processing, and distribution in commerce, as well as use and disposal, of a chemical substance or mixture.

Premanufacture Notification (PMN)

In May 1977, the EPA published its initial inventory of chemical substances. Any chemicals not listed were considered new chemicals subject to premanufacture review as of July 1, 1979. As new chemicals complete premanufacture review and begin to be manufactured, they are added to the inventory.

If a chemical is not listed already on the inventory, a premature notification (PMN) must be submitted. This notification, among other things, must identify the chemical, provide information on use, method of dispersal, production levels, worker exposure, and potential byproducts or impurities. In addition, the manufacturer must provide data on health and environmental effects of the product and a description of known or reasonably ascertainable data. After submittal of the PMN, the EPA has 90 days to complete the review and either approve production of the chemical or act to ban or otherwise restrict manufacture or use. The EPA may extend the review period for an additional 90 days. If additional time is needed, the EPA and the manufacturer may interrupt the 180-day review to develop additional data.

Testing Requirements

If the EPA determines that data are insufficient to evaluate whether a chemical poses unreasonable risk to health or the environment, it can require testing of the material. Some studies that may be required include: carcinogenicity, mutagenicity, teratogenicity, behavioral modification, synergisms, and various types of toxicity. An Interagency Testing Committee composed of representatives from eight federal agencies select chemicals for testing. Once selected, these chemicals or groups of chemicals are placed on a priority list for testing that may never contain more than 50 chemicals or chemical groups.

Data Gathering

For the EPA to perform an adequate risk assessment of a chemical substance, the agency must have access to all available data regarding the substance. TSCA authorizes the EPA to require industries to provide these data. The agency requires four types of reporting under this section.

1. General data collection: Data must be submitted on chemical substances as they are added to the list.

2. Health and safety studies: Manufacturers test their chemicals routinely for efficiency and safety. Health and safety studies allow the EPA to require a manufacturer to provide copies of these studies. In addition, if the company has copies of, knows of, or reasonably could determine that other reports or studies exist, regardless of their origin, it also must provide copies or lists of these reports.

3. Notification of substantial risk: Industry is required to notify EPA if any evidence of substantial risk is identified.

4. Significant adverse reactions: Industry is required to maintain records of significant adverse reactions alleged to have been caused by a chemical because they "may indicate a tendency of a chemical substance or mixture to cause longlasting or irreversible damage to health or the environment." Records relating

to possible health reactions of employees must be kept for 30 years. All other allegations must be kept for 5 years.

The EPA may move to ban the manufacturing and distribution in commerce, limit the use, require labeling, or place similar restrictions on specific chemicals. It also may issue public warnings, require situational notification, record-keeping, reporting, or other measures as the agency deems appropriate.

PCB Regulation

Regulation of PCBs (polychlorinated biphenyls) represents the full extent of powers granted to the EPA under TSCA. Nowhere else in environmental statutes is a substance banned by name. Further, what started out to be a rather simple ban on manufacturing and use has developed into a complex set of regulations restricting PCB use, requiring inspections, reporting, and record-keeping; establishing labeling and marking requirements, and outlining disposal criteria.

....

HAZARD COMMUNICATION STANDARD (RIGHT-TO-KNOW LAW)

Numerous state and municipal governments' worker right-to-know laws resulted in the promulgation of a federal right-to-know law entitled the Hazard Communication Standard. The objective of this law is to communicate to the worker the presence and effects of hazardous chemicals in the workplace that are known to be present in such a manner that employees may be exposed under normal conditions of use or in a potential emergency. With a few exceptions (labeling on pesticides, foods, distilled spirits and consumer products, and total exemptions on regulated hazardous wastes, tobacco, wood and foods, drugs and cosmetics intended for personal use), all workers must be informed. Training for worker identification evaluation and protection was required to be in place by May 25, 1986.

To accomplish this training, each employer must establish a hazardous chemical list. This list is defined in a written hazard determination program developed by each employer. The chemical list required of each employer is composed of two parts:

1. A list of hazardous chemicals as determined from the Material Safety Data Sheet (MSDS) from chemical manufacturers, distributors, and importers, in the "hazardous ingredients" section.
2. A list of in-house reaction products such as welding fumes, carbon monoxide from lift trucks, wood dust, and chemical intermediates.

A MSDS should be requested from suppliers for all incoming materials used and developed and evaluated for reaction products by a qualified person such as a chemist or industrial hygienist. Physical hazards of chemicals, as well as health hazards, must be addressed.

Employee recall is perhaps the most effective measurement of communication. The required information must be in simple and understandable language, as used by the worker. The MSDS probably cannot be used directly as the medium of communication because the language often is too technical. The information must be simplified, summarized, and communicated. In some parts of the country, 20% of the workforce cannot read or write effectively. Written information transfer is not the preferred method. Supervisor-to-worker communication is essential, using visual aids and dialogue.

The basic areas of the employee knowledge are: purpose, what, where, effect on body, detection, protection, and written program and MSDS.

Employers are not only responsible for preparing a written plan for determining whether chemicals they use or store are hazardous (which must be shown and explained to the worker), but they also must develop a written program of the plan they will use to effect the hazard communication program. This plan should designate a person in charge of the various responsibilities and generally explain how they will be carried out. These responsibilities are: provision and maintenance of MSDS, preparation and maintenance of labels, execution and sources for a good training program, production of a hazardous chemical list, description of the methods the employer will use to inform employees of the hazards of non-routine tasks, and description of the methods the employer will use to inform any contractor employees working in the employer's workplace of the hazardous chemicals they may be exposed to while performing their work, and any suggestions for appropriate protective measures.

SAFE DRINKING WATER ACT

The Safe Drinking Water Act was passed in 1975 (and amended in 1986) to protect groundwater and drinking water sources. The law requires the EPA to establish recommended maximum contaminant goals (RMCG) for each contaminant that may have an adverse effect on the health of an individual. Two types of drinking water standards were established to limit the amount of contamination that may be in drinking water:

1. Primary standards with a maximum contaminant level (MCL) to protect human health;
2. Secondary standards that involve the color, taste, smell, and other physical characteristics of drinking water sources.

The Safe Drinking Water Act stipulated 83 contaminants for which regulations were required to be developed by 1989. These include:

14 volatile organic compounds

29 synthetic organic compounds

13 inorganic chemicals

4 microbiological contaminants

2 radiological contaminants

A second major provision of the Safe Water Drinking Act for the purpose of protecting groundwater is the regulation of underground injection of toxic chemicals. Injection of liquid wastes into underground wells is used as a means of disposal. Controls were needed to assure that this means of disposal did not damage the quality of aquifers. The act established five classes of underground injection wells. Class IV wells, where hazardous wastes are injected into or above a formation within one-quarter mile of an underground source of drinking water, were to be phased out. Under the 1986 amendments, states must adopt a program for protecting wellheads. The pro-

gram must include the surface and subsurface surrounding a well or well field through which contaminants are reasonably likely to move toward a well.

COASTAL ZONE MANAGEMENT ACT OF 1972

In 1972, Congress declared that it is national policy to preserve, protect, develop and, where possible, restore or enhance the resources of the nation's coastal zone. The Coastal Zone Management Act declared that it is public policy to:

- Encourage and assist the states to exercise effectively their responsibilities in the coastal zone through the development and implementation of management programs that will achieve wise use of the land and water resources of the coastal zone, giving full consideration to ecological, cultural, historic, and aesthetic values, as well as needs for economic development.

- Encourage the preparation of special area management plans that provide for increased specificity in protecting significant natural resources, reasonable coastal-dependent economic growth, improved protection of life and property in hazardous areas, and improved predictability in governmental decision making.

- Encourage participation and cooperation of the public, state and local governments, and interstate and other regional agencies, as well as the federal agencies having programs affecting the coastal zone.

The management program for each coastal state must include each of the following requirements:

- Identification of the boundaries of the coastal zone subject to the management program.

- A definition of what constitutes permissible land uses and water uses within the coastal zone that have a direct and significant impact on the coastal waters.

- An inventory and designation of areas of particular concern within the coastal zone.

- Identification of the means by which the state proposes to exert control over land uses and water uses, including a listing of relevant constitutional provisions, laws, regulations, and judicial decisions.

- Broad guidelines on priorities of uses in specific areas, including specifically those of lowest priority.

- A description of the organizational structure proposed to implement a management program, including the responsibilities and interrelationships of local, areawide, state, regional, and interstate agencies in the management process.

- A definition of the term "beach" and a planning process for the protection of, and access to, public beaches and other public coastal areas of environmental, recreational, historical, aesthetic, ecological, or cultural value.

- A planning process for energy facilities likely to be located in, or that may significantly affect, the coastal zone, including, but not limited to, a process for anticipating and managing the impacts from such facilities.

- A planning process for assessing the effects of shoreline erosion and studying and evaluating ways to control, or lessen the impact of, such erosion, and to restore areas affected adversely by such erosion.

· · · · · · · · · · · · · ·

OCCUPATIONAL SAFETY AND HEALTH ACT OF 1970

The Occupational Safety and Health Act (OSHAct) was enacted in 1970 "to provide for the general welfare to assure so far as possible every working man and woman in the nation safe and healthful working conditions and to preserve our human resources." The act grants the Secretary of Labor the authority to promulgate, modify, and revoke safety and health standards; to conduct inspections and investigations and to issue citations, including proposed penalties; to require employees to keep records of safety and health data; to petition the courts to restrain imminent danger situations; and to approve or reject state plans for programs under the act. The Secretary's authority includes right of access to the records of other federal agencies, and a shared responsibility with other federal agency heads for the adequacy of programs in the organizations reporting to them.

The act authorizes the Secretary to have the Department of Labor conduct short-term training of personnel involved in performance of duties related to their responsibilities under the act, and in consultation with the Department of Health, Education and Welfare, and to provide training and education to employers and employees. The Secretary and his or her designees are authorized to consult with employers, employees, and organizations regarding prevention of injuries and illnesses. The Secretary, after consultation with the Secretary of Health, Education and Welfare, may grant funds to the states for identification of program needs and plan development, experiments, demonstrations, administration, and operation of programs. In conjunction with the Secretary of Health and Human Services, the Secretary of Labor is charged with developing and maintaining a statistics program for occupational safety and health.

The OSHAct sets out two duties for employers and one for employees. The general duty provisions are:

1. Furnish to each employee a place for employment that is free from recognized hazards that are causing, or are likely to cause, death or serious physical harm to employees.

2. Comply with occupational safety and health standards under the act.

3. Each employee shall comply with occupational safety and health standards and all rules, regulations, and orders issued pursuant to the act that are applicable to the employee's own actions and conduct.

Health standards are promulgated under the OSHAct by the Labor Department with technical advice from the National Institute for Occupational Safety and Health (NIOSH) in the Department of Health, Education and Welfare. NIOSH provides information and data in the area of health hazards, but the final authority for promulgation of the standards remains with the Secretary of Labor.

Consumer Product Safety Act

The Consumer Product Safety Act of 1972 created the Consumer Product Safety Commission (CPSC), whose mission was to reduce product-related injuries to consumers by regulation of product design, labeling, and use instructions. The CPSC is a five-member independent commission with authority to set safety standards for consumer products and to ban those providing an unreasonable risk of injury. The commission also has authority to recall products. The only consumer products not covered were those governed by other regulatory agencies, such as aircraft, automobiles, food, drugs, and pesticides. The CPSC has been provided with a substantial budget to undertake its legal and administrative processes, test products, gather medical statistics pertaining to product-related injuries, and disseminate information to consumers.

Congress included a provision that requires manufacturers and sellers of covered consumer products to report to the CPSC the existence of any substantial product hazards. Rulemaking, rather than administrative adjudication, was to be the principal means by which the CPSC would ensure rapid decision making. Stiff penalties imposed upon violators of the standards set forth in the rules were intended to ensure effective compliance.

Establishment of safety standards was to involve an "offeror process" under which the commission was required to solicit draft standards from outside parties.

In 1981, the act was amended to abolish the offeror process. The CPSC was directed to rely on voluntary rather than mandatory safety standards wherever voluntary standards would "adequately" reduce risk—a potentially major curtailment of its authority.

SELECTED ENVIRONMENTAL ORGANIZATIONS

American Public Health Association

An association for the enhancement of public health.

800 I Street, NW
Washington, DC 20001
(202) 777–2742
www.apha.org

Centers for Disease Control and Prevention

The national focus for developing and applying disease prevention and control, environmental health, health promotion and education activities designed to improve the health of individuals.

1600 Clifton Rd.
Atlanta, GA 30333
(888) 232–6789
www.cdc.gov/nceh

Congress Watch Lobbying

Consumer health and safety, pesticides.

1600 20th Street, NW
Washington, DC 20009
(202) 588–1000
www.citizen.org

Environmental Defense Fund

Research, litigation, and lobbying: cosmetics safety, drinking water, energy, transportation, pesticides, wildlife, air pollution, cancer prevention, radiation.

257 Park Avenue South
New York, NY 10010
(212) 505–2100
www.environmentaldefense.org

League of Conservation Voters

Political arm of the environmental community. Works to elect candidates to U.S. House and Senate who will vote to protect the nation's environment, and holds them accountable by publishing the National Environmental Scorecard *each year, which can be ordered for $6 and is free to students.*

1920 L Street, NW
Suite 800
Washington, DC 20036
(202) 785–8683
www.lcv.org

National Environmental Health Association

Professional organization for environmental health professionals, and offers registration services for environmental health specialists.

720 S. Colorado Blvd.
Suite 970-S
Denver, CO 80246
(303) 756–9090
www.neha.org

Planned Parenthood Federation of America

Education service, and research: fertility control, family planning.

810 7th Ave.
New York, NY 10019
(212) 245–1845
www.plannedparenthood.org

Population Reference Bureau, Inc.

Engaged in collection and dissemination of objective population information. Excellent publications.

1875 Connecticut Ave., N.W.
Suite 520
Washington, DC 20009
(202) 483–1100
www.prb.org

U.S. Environmental Protection Agency, Public Information Center

Provides general information about environmental topics.

401 M Street, S.W.
Washington, DC 20460
(202) 260–7751
www.epa.gov

World Watch Institute

Research and education: energy, food, population, health, women's issues, technology, the environment.

1776 Massachusetts Ave., N.W.
Washington, DC 20036
(202) 452–1999
www.worldwatch.org

GLOSSARY

Activated sludge   Sewage sediment that contains a heavy growth of microorganisms, resulting from vigorous aeration.

Acute   Having a sudden onset and rapid recovery.

Acute toxicity   A response to a chemical that occurs within minutes, hours, or days of exposure.

Aeration   Introducing oxygen (in air) to water to encourage bacterial growth and decomposition of organic material.

Aeration tank digestion   The tank in which aeration takes place.

Aerobic   Requiring free oxygen.

Aerosol   Liquid droplets or solid particles that remain dispersed in the air a prolonged time.

Anaerobic   Living in environments void of free oxygen.

Anthropogenic   Refers to air pollutants that may adversely impact human health.

Aquifer   A porous stratum that stores water underground.

Arachnids   A class of Arthropods in which the head, thorax, and abdomen are unified in one body region.

Arthropods   Animals belonging to the phylum Arthropoda, meaning "jointed foot."

Asbestos   The mineral chrysotile, used for making incombustible or fireproof articles.

Ashes   Combusted materials that have been burned to total breakdown.

Avalanche   A sliding mass of ice and snow.

Backsiphonage   The backflow of used, contaminated, or polluted water from a plumbing fixture or vessel or other source into a potable (or clean swimming) water supply as a result of negative pressure in the pipe/system.

Bar screen   Device that strains out large materials that may damage a wastewater treatment plant.

Biochemical oxygen demand (BOD)   Amount of oxygen microorganisms require while stabilizing decomposable organic matter under aerobic conditions.

Biohazards   Living organisms that are infectious agents and represent a potential risk to human or animal health.

Biosphere   Air, water, and land.

Bored well   A well in which a mechanical device bores into the ground to reach water; limited by underlying consolidated bedrock or impervious strata.

Box and can   A self-contained, above-ground chamber to collect urine and feces that can later be disposed of properly; sometimes termed "port-a-john" or "portable toilet."

Canning   Process of sealing a metal container of food with the microorganism potentially in it and heating the can to kill the organism.

Carbon monoxide   Colorless, odorless, poisonous gas, CO, which burns with a pale blue flame, produced when carbon burns with insufficient air.

Carrier   A person who harbors and spreads disease without necessarily showing symptoms of the disease.

Catalytic converter   Device installed in automobiles to control volatile hydrocarbons and carbon monoxide exhaust.

Causative agent   That agent which causes disease.

CERCLA   Comprehensive Environmental Response, Compensation and Liability Act, known as Superfund, passed in 1980 by the U.S. Congress to clean up and monitor hazardous waste.

Channel of infection   Portal of entry of a causative agent of disease.

Chemical oxygen demand (COD)   Test that allows measurement of waste in terms of total quantity of oxygen required for oxidation to carbon dioxide and water.

Chronic   Refers to diseases that linger and often become worse over time.

Chronic toxicity   A response to a chemical that occurs after years or nearly a lifetime of exposure.

Cistern   A tank for storing rainwater from a catchment area or for storing water hauled in from some outside source.

Coliform group   Microorganisms whose presence indicates that contamination is entering a water supply.

Communicable   Infectious, contagious.

Comminuter   A unit that grind up the large solids to prepare them for digestion by microorganisms in a wastewater treatment plant.

Composting   Taking biodegradable materials and, through natural processes, producing humus.

Conduction   The transfer of heat between the human body and surrounding substances or objects by direct contact.

Convection   Transfer of heat from one place to another by moving fluid (gas or liquid). Natural convection results from differences in temperature. As related to hypothermia and frostbite, the difference in heat in the fluid is caused by fluid in contact with the (human) body gaining heat from the body.

Corrosive   Having a pH below 2 or above 12.5; capable of eating away living tissues or nonliving materials through chemical reaction.

Cyclo-propagative   Refers to a condition in which the disease agent undergoes a change in form and increase in number within the vector.

DNA   The genetic instructions for cell survival and reproduction.

Decibels (dB)   A unit of measure of sound.

Deep wells   Wells dug deep into the earth where hazardous waste is injected as a means of disposal.

Deforestation   Permanent decline in trees in an area to less than 10% of its original extent; usually denotes human activity.

Dermatitis   A skin condition caused by the mite called chiggers, or redbugs.

Desiccation   *See* drying.

Digester   A large sealed unit in a wastewater treatment plant where anaerobic decomposition takes place.

Disease   Deviation from the normal physiological state of the host.

Dissolved oxygen (DO)   Factor in liquid wastes that determines whether biological changes are brought about by aerobic or by anaerobic organisms.

Dose-response relationship   The percentage of subjects exhibiting a response to a chemical as the dose increases.

Doubling time   Time required for a population to double its size.

Drilled well   Well that is drilled mechanically through rock and compacted areas; not limited to depth of rock. Water is less subject to reduced flows in times of drought and less subject to biological contamination.

Driven well   Well created by driving a pipe with a special screened point into the ground until reaching water; limited to areas where soil particles are large and coastal regions with shallow water tables.

Drying   Process that removes the moisture from a product to kill the bacteria; also termed *desiccation*.

Dug well   Well constructed by digging straight down into the earth manually until reaching water; limited by the depth of the dense bedrock.

Dust   Solid particles produced by crushing, grinding, drilling, and otherwise handling materials.

Ecological system   A natural association of populations of plants and animals that persists over time.

Electrostatic precipitator   Air pollution control device in which particles are electrically charged, then collected on metal plates that are oppositely charged.

Endemic   Refers to diseases with the expected number of cases for a specific human population at a specific time.

Environmental health and protection   The art and science of protecting against environmental factors that may adversely impact human health or the ecological balances essential to long-term human health and environmental quality. Includes, but not limited to, air, food and water contaminants; radiation; toxic chemicals; wastes; disease vectors; safety hazards; and habitat alterations.

Environmental health practice   Study of the relationship between environment and health.

Epidemic   Refers to diseases with a greater than normal rate of disease in a population.

Epidemiology   Study of the distribution and determinants of diseases and death in specified populations.

Epidermis   Outer layer of skin.

Evapotranspiration   Plants' drawing water from soil by capillary action, where it evaporates into the air.

Evaporation   Physical transformation of a liquid to a gaseous state at any temperature below its boiling point.

Facultative   Having the ability to exist either aerobically or anaerobically, depending on the surrounding environment.

Fermentation   Action of specialized bacteria or yeast to produce alcohol or acid by-products that prevent the growth of flora.

Fomites   Any inanimate objects that provide a "resting place" for causative agents of disease.

Frostbite   Damage to or destruction of bodily tissue as a result of exposure to extremely cold air or objects.

Fumes   Solid particles created by condensation of a substance from a gaseous state.

Garbage   Organic putrescible matter resulting wherever people live, work, travel, and recreate.

Gases   Fluids that take the shape of whatever container is available to them.

Greenhouse effect   The effect produced by certain gases, such as carbon dioxide, on a planet's atmosphere by raising the temperature of the surface of the planet, thus preventing the outward transmission of long-wave radiation from the surface but permitting the inward transmission of short-wave radiation from the sun to the surface.

Grinder   *See* Comminuter.

Grit chamber   A basin that slows the water entering a wastewater treatment plant just enough to allow time for heavy particles to settle out.

Growth rate   Difference between live birth rate and death rate in a given population.

Half-life   The time required for half of the atoms of a particular radionuclide to decay.

Humidity   Humid condition; dampness.

Hypertonic environment   A condition in which the environment surrounding the cell contains a greater saline concentration than that within the cell.

Hypochlorous acid   (H_oC_l) An unstable acid with excellent bactericidal and algicidal properties.

Hypothermia   Abnormal, potentially dangerous, low body temperature (= or > 95°F). Most commonly caused by loss of body heat as a result of contact with cold air or objects.

Hypotonic environment   A condition in which the saline content within the cell is greater than that of the surrounding environment; allows moisture to enter cell by osmosis.

Industrial hygienist   Person assesses and recommends methodology for controlling environmental hazards and toxic substances for a company.

Industrial health educator   Person who educates workers in the prevention of occupational diseases/ injuries; counsels workers; and conducts health and safety surveys.

Industrial toxicologist   A toxicologist who practices toxicology in an industrial setting.

Ignitable   Refers to liquids having a flashpoint below 60°C or nonliquids liable to cause fires via friction, moisture absorption, or spontaneous chemical change.

Immunity   The quality or state of being immune to a disease.

Incineration   Burning waste at high temperatures.

Incubation period   The time that elapses between the organism entering the body and appearance of the first symptoms.

Injury   Physical damage to the body that results when energy is transferred to the body in amounts greater than it can withstand

Ionizing radiation   Radiation that interacts with matter to produce charged particles.

Isotonic environment   A condition in which the saline solution surrounding a cell has the same salt concentration as that within the cell and provides optimum growth potential.

Joules   Gram in any specified material.

Lead (Pb)   A heavy, comparatively soft, malleable, bluish-gray metal, sometimes found in its natural state but usually combined as a sulfide.

Loose-snow avalanche   An avalanche that starts at the point or side of a slope when unattached snow crystals slide downward, growing in size, and the quantity of snow involved, as it descends. Loose snow moves as a formless mass with little internal cohesion.

Maggot   The larva form of the housefly.

Mass gathering   Precise legal definition varies by state and may be determined on basis of a minimum number of persons in attendance, time duration of the activity, its sponsorship, or its location. In general, an assembly of people requiring planning in aspects such as sanitation, emergency preparation, and environmental health precautions to ensure a safe and recreational experience for those in attendance.

Maximum contaminants levels (MCLs)   The concentration of water pollutants that may have adverse effects on human health, according to EPA standards.

Mesophilic   Refers to organisms that grow in a medium range of temperatures, from about 69°F to 113°F.

Metamorphosis   Life cycle of arthropod from egg to adult with various stages.

Minimum separation distance   The distance that the health department allows between drinking water wells and pollution sources.

Mist   Composed of liquid droplets suspended in air and formed by condensation from a gas to a liquid or by dispersing liquid into tiny particles.

Mode of action   The interaction between the chemical and a specific cell structure that results in a response.

Myiasis   Invasion of the flesh of the host animal by the larva of the fly.

NPDES   National Pollutant Discharge Eliminations System, established to control wastewater discharges.

National Electronic Injury Surveillance System (NEISS)   An electronic system that monitors admissions to selected hospital emergency rooms daily for injuries involving consumer products.

Nitrogen oxides   Compounds formed by the fixation of nitrogen at high temperatures, as in furnaces and internal combustion engines. Primary product is nitric oxide (NO), which slowly oxidizes in air to nitrogen dioxide (NO_2)

Noise   Unwanted sound.

Objective   Something toward which effort is directed.

Occupational health nurse   A nurse responsible for the care of illnesses and injuries occurring at the workplace.

Occupational physician   A medical doctor who typically performs pre-employment physicals, treats work-related injuries and illnesses, supervises drug screening, and determines the presence and extent of workers' disability.

Ootheca   The egg-containing pouch carried from the abdomen by the German cockroach.

Ozone   A form of oxygen (O_3) produced by a reaction of photochemical smog and in electrical discharges; a powerful oxidizing agent, toxic to plants and animals at relatively low concentrations.

Ozone layer   That portion of the stratosphere surrounding the earth that shields the earth's surface from the sun's harmful ultraviolet rays.

Pandemic   Refers to diseases with a greater than normal rate of disease in the human population covering several countries, maybe worldwide.

Particulate air pollution   Small particles suspended in the atmosphere, such as smoke from industrial processes.

Pasteurization   Time-temperature process that destroys the pathogenic organism.

Pediculosis   Infestation with lice.

Phagocytosis   The ingestion and destruction of particlelike matter by cells, especially of infectious microorganisms in man.

Pharmacology   The study of drugs and their actions.

Photochemical smog   Air pollution derived mainly from emissions from automobiles and other sources interacting in the atmosphere in the presence of sunlight to create ozone and other oxidants.

Physiological needs   Physical needs of humans such as light, space, favorable temperature and ventilation.

Pit privy   Underground area where urine and feces can be deposited and retained in a sanitary manner.

Planning   Advanced thinking as a basis for doing.

Planning premises   Assumptions forming the basis for planning and implementation that will take place in the future.

Plasmolysis   Shrinking of *bacterium cytoplasm* as a result of loss of water.

Plasmoptysis   The bursting of protoplasm from a cell, resulting from the rupture of the cell wall because of high osmotic pressure within the cell.

Playground   A recreational area encompassing program activities, play apparatus, and an open-space area designed to focus on the physical and social development of children.

Potable   Describes water of good taste, odor, and microbiological quality.

Primary clarifier   A device, also called a settling basin, through which water moves slowly, allowing a large amount of suspended solids to accumulate on the bottom, producing sludge.

Primary irritants   Material that exerts little systemic toxic action.

Priority setting   Determining the relative importance of various problems under consideration.

Proboscis   Collective mouthparts of the insect.

Proventriculus   Gizzard in some insects, where food is ground into smaller particles.

Psychrophilic   "Cold-loving"; organisms that grow in a range from 19°F to 68°F.

Public health assessment   A process by which human exposure to environmental agents determined through environmental sampling at the point of exposure, and through human biologic testing, personal monitoring, and reviewing existing medical information.

RAD   The dose of any form of ionizing radiation that produces energy absorption of 1×10^{-5}.

REM   Major unit of exposure to radiation based on dose equivalency in the U.S. customary set of units.

Radiation   The emission through space, or through a medium such as air, of energy, as related to human body temperature, specifically heat energy.

Radioactivity   Characteristic of an isotope such that it emits radiation.

Radon   A dense gas that is radioactive and may enter buildings from the earth.

Reactive   Capable of exploding and generating toxic gases when combined with air or water.

Refuse   Waste material composed of garbage, rubbish, and ashes.

Resistance to disease   Ability to ward off disease such as by immunity.

Risk analysis   A qualitative and quantitative process used to evaluate hazardous conditions and to characterize the resulting risk.

Risk assessment   The process by which the form, dimension, and characteristics of risk are estimated.

Risk communication   A process whereby individuals, groups, or the public are informed and involved concerning the existence, nature, form, severity, and/or acceptability of risks.

Risk management   The process of integrating the results of risk assessment with economic, social, political, and legal concerns to develop a course of action to prevent or solve a problem.

Rubbish   Combustible and noncombustible solid waste generated from people's activities; includes paper, beverage cans, yardwork trimmings, and many other materials.

Safety engineer   Person who has the responsibility of developing complex systems for the analysis and control of occupational hazards.

Sanitary landfill   Site where solid waste is buried systematically in sections and covered with soil.

Scabies   A mite infestation by *Sarcoptes scabiei*.

Secure landfill   Site for hazardous waste disposal consisting of ground excavation and some sort of insulation to prevent waste from escaping into air, water, and land.

Settling basin   *See* Primary clarifier.

Sick building syndrome   Term used for buildings that spread the causative agent of disease.

Slab avalanche   An avalanche that starts when a solid area of snow breaks away at once, leaving a well-defined fracture line where the moving snow has broken away from the stable snow. Slab avalanches are characterized by the tendency of snow crystals to stick together and may contain angular blocks and/or chunks of snow.

Sludge   Suspended solids that accumulate in a wastewater treatment plant.

Smog   Combination of the words *smoke* and *fog* to describe polluted air.

Smoke   Incomplete combustion of organic materials such as wood, coal, and petroleum products.

Snowmobile   A self-propelled vehicle steered by skis, runners, or caterpillar treads, and designed to be used principally on snow or ice.

Sporadic diseases   Those diseases that occur in scattered cases, such as rabies.

Spring   A surface water supply arising from a groundwater source.

Storm sewer   Wastewater system that collects surface runoff only from rainwater.

Sulfur oxides   Products of the oxidation of fuels containing sulfur; include both sulfur dioxide (SO_2) and sulfur trioxide (SO_3) and the acids formed by their combination with water. Sulfuric acid (H_2SO_4) is of principal interest.

Superfund   *See* CERCLA.

Synanthropic   Refers to the close association of the fly with humans.

Threshold limit values (TLVs)   Guidelines in the control of occupational exposures.

Thermal inversion   A layer of the atmosphere in which the temperature increases with height; may prevent air pollutants from dispersing, leading to high concentrations of pollutants, which may impact human health.

Thermophilic   "Heat-loving"; microbes that grow in the range of around 113°F to 167°F.

Toxic   Potentially poisonous to humans.

Toxic effect   Any noxious effect or undesirable disturbance of the body's physiologic function whether reversible or irreversible.

Toxicology   The study of poisons.

Transovarian transmission   Transmission of pathogenic organisms from one stage to the next stage in the life cycle of the arthropod.

Transstadial transmission   Transmission of pathogenic organisms from one stage to the next stage in the life cycle of the arthropod.

Tumbler   Pupa form of the mosquito.

Turbidity   Cloudy looking water resulting from particles suspended in the water.

Undertow   A current resulting from waves breaking upon a beach, then receding toward the lake or ocean. If the waves are large enough and the beach has a slope, the undertow will have a force great enough to pull a person into the water.

Vapor   Gaseous forms of substances that exist normally as liquids or solids at room temperature and pressure.

Vector   An organism that transmits a pathogen.

Vehicle of infection   Mode of transport from one individual or group to another; water, food, insects, and inanimate objects.

Venturi meter   A device for measuring the rate of flow through a wastewater treatment plant.

Volatile organic compounds (VOCs)   Organic matter capable of being vaporized or evaporated quickly.

Waste to energy (WTE)   Burning solid waste and generating energy or steam or electricity.

Wastewater stabilization pond   Water body engineered to utilize biological decomposition as a means of wastewater disposal.

Wetland   An area that is partially or completely saturated or occasionally inundated with water. Examples are swamps, marshes, bogs, fens, estuaries, intertidal mud flats, and river deltas.

Winter white-out   Condition existing when an overcast sky or snow precludes shadows, causing the horizon to be indistinguishable from the terrain.

Wriggler   Larvae form of mosquito.

Years of potential life lost (YPLL)   A measure of the impact of premature death on a population, calculated as the sum of the differences between some predetermined minimum or desired life span and the age of death for individuals who died earlier than that predetermined age.

Zoonoses   Diseases of animals that are transmitted to people.

ZPG   Zero population growth; no overall growth or decline in the total population.

ABOUT THE AUTHOR

Monroe T. Morgan, Dr.P.H., M.S.P.H, R.S.

Dr. Monroe T. Morgan, Sr., grew up on a farm near Mars Hill, North Carolina. After graduating from Mars Hill Junior College, he earned a B.A. degree from East Tennessee State University, and later an M.S.P.H. from the University of North Carolina and a Doctor of Public Health from Tulane University School of Public Health and Tropical Medicine. He worked as an environmentalist in Fairfax County, Virginia, and later as Training Officer for the state of Virginia. He developed and chaired for 22 years, the first academic department of environmental health in the world to offer B.S.E.H. and M.S.E.H. degrees, which became the first two such programs to become professionally accredited.

Dr. Morgan has served as a consultant to the National Institutes of Heath, the Carter Center, the World Health Organization, and the National Academy of Science to study the U.S. Environmental Protection Agency. He served as president of the National Environmental Health Association (NEHA) in the mid-1970s. He has received many awards and honors, including the National Environmental Health Association's highest honor, the Walter S. Mangold Award, in 1979, and the NEHA Outstanding Award for Leadership to the Environmental Health Profession. Dr. Morgan has 36 years of teaching experience, teaching students from the 50 states, including those from most American Indian tribes, and students from 56 countries. He chaired the first Earth Day Forum at ETSU on April 14, 1970.

Five of the contributing authors are his former students.

ABOUT THE CONTRIBUTING AUTHORS

Darryl B. Barnett, Dr.P.H., M.P.H., R.S.

Dr. Barnett is currently the chair of the Clinical Laboratory Science/Environmental Health Science Department at Eastern Kentucky University, Richmond, Kentucky. A native of Johnson City, Tennessee, he earned a B.S. in Environmental Health (1970) at East Tennessee State University, and an M.P.H. (1977) and Dr. P.H. (1993) at Oklahoma University Health Sciences Center in Oklahoma City, Oklahoma. He retired from the Commissioned Corps of the U.S. Public Health Service in 1991 where he served in various positions specializing in Institutional Environmental Health. Between 1991 and 1998 he served as an Associate Professor at EKU in Environmental Health Science and from 1998 to 2001 he served as Kerr chair and chair of the Environmental Health Science Department at East Central University, Ada, Oklahoma. Dr. Barnett also serves as the chair of the NEHA Technical Research Section and as member of the NEHA REHS/RS Credentialing Committee.

Joe E. Beck, D.A.A.S., R.S.

Professor Beck is a tenured associate professor of Environmental Health Science at Eastern Kentucky University in Richmond, Kentucky. He has over 30 years of experience in the field of environmental health of which a great deal has been spent in the area of institutional and shelter environments. He holds undergraduate degrees in the life and physical sciences; a graduate degree in Public Administration and Academy status with the American Academy of Sanitarians. He is past chair of a number of national organizations, including the American Academy of Sanitarians, the National Council for Accreditation of Graduate and Undergraduate Environmental Health Curricula, and as the chair of the Institutional Section of the National Environmental Health Association. Professor Beck developed the CDC home study course Environmental Health Sciences, 3010, currently in use. Past positions include: member of the faculty of the Business School, Washington State University; Senior Staff Scientist, Pacific Northwest laboratory, Battelle Memorial Foundation; associate professor and academic unit chair of Environmental Head Sciences, Western Carolina University. He began his teaching career at Illinois State University in the Environmental Health Sciences Department.

Franklin B. Carver, Ph.D., M.S.E.H., R.S.

Dr. Franklin B. Carver, a native of Fayetteville, North Carolina, is currently the vice chancellor for University Programs and a tenured professor in the environmental science program at North Carolina Central University, located in Durham, North Carolina. He also holds the rank of Commander in the U.S. Navy Reserves as an Environmental Health Officer.

With over 25 years of experience in the environmental health science field, Dr. Carver holds a B.S. degree in Health Education from Fayetteville State University (N.C.), a Master of Science in Environmental Health from East Tennessee State University, along with a Doctorate Degree from Ohio University. Dr. Carver has worked in industry for over three years as an Occupational Health and Safety Director, and in Liberia, West Africa, for more than four years in environmental health.

He has taught and directed environmental health science programs at the University of Liberia, Mississippi Valley State University, Western Carolina University, and Ohio University. His most recent position before going to North Carolina Central University was director of the School of Health Sciences at Ohio University in Athens, Ohio, where he was employed for over ten years.

Dr. Carver is an active member of the National Environmental Health Association, the National Association of Environmental Professionals, the American Public Health Association, and many other national and state professional organizations. He has served as a councilman on the National Environmental Health Accreditation Council for colleges and universities for more than six years and served as the editor of the *Journal of Environmental Health*, which is distributed throughout the world. Dr. Carver also serves on the Environmental and Public Health Council for Underwriters Laboratories, Incorporated, and is on the Board of Directors for a North Carolina Long-Term Care Foundation.

His areas of research include: (1) Minority Concerns In Environmental Health; (2) Environmental Health Issues In Developing Countries and Rural America; and (3) Curriculum Development and Manpower Needs In Environmental Health.

Trenton G. Davis, Dr.P.H., M.P.H.

Dr. Davis is a professor in the Department of Environmental Health Sciences and Safety, East Carolina University. He received a B.S. degree from East Tennessee State University, an M.P.H. degree from Tulane University, and a doctorate in Public Health from the University of Oklahoma. During his 37 years in public health and academics, he has held a number of positions including Sanitarian; assistant professor of Environmental Health, East

Tennessee State University; associate vice chancellor for Academic Support, East Carolina University; interim dean, School of Industry and Technology, East Carolina University; associate dean, School of Allied Health Sciences, East Carolina University; and chair, Department of Environmental Health, East Carolina University.

Dr. Davis is the recipient of numerous awards including the Walter Mangold Award (National Environmental Health Association), the Walter Snyder Award (National Sanitation Foundation/National Environmental Health Association), the William Broadway Award (North Carolina Public Health Association), and the Trenton G. Davis Award (Eastern District, North Carolina Public Health Association). On the national level, he has served as President of the National Environmental Health Association and as technical editor of the *Journal of Environmental Health*. He has written papers for publication in the *Journal of Environmental Health,* the *North Carolina Medical Journal,* the *Oklahoma Medical Journal,* the *North Carolina Public Health Forum*, the *Journal of Public Health Policy,* and other journals.

L. Fleming Fallon, Jr., M.D., M.B.A., Dr.P.H.

Dr. Fallon received his M.D. degree from St. Georges University School of Medicine in 1984. He completed his residency in Occupational and Environmental Medicine and also earned a Dr.P.H. from the Columbia University School of Public Health. He is currently a faculty member at Bowling Green State University in Bowling Green, Ohio, where he also directs a Master of Public Health degree program. He also teaches for St. Joseph's College in Maine and holds a faculty position at the Columbia University School of Public Health. He has formerly taught at Slippery Rock University. Dr. Fallon is a reviewer for the *American Journal of Occupational and Environmental Medicine* and the *Journal of Rural Health*. He has received three awards for teaching and the President's Award from the National Association of Local Boards of Health. Dr. Fallon is a licensed Health Officer (NJ). He has written a weekly newspaper column entitled *Health Thoughts* since 1995.

Frank C. Gomez, Dr.P.H., M.P.H.

Frank C. Gomez earned his Doctorate in Public Health from UCLA's School of Public Health. Previous to this he graduated from California State University Los Angeles with a B.S. in Environmental Health Science and completed his M.P.H. in Environmental Health from UCLA's School of Public Health a year later. He worked for 29 years with Environmental Health, Department of Health Services, County of Los Angeles. He headed the Department's Environmental Impact Unit for nine years and served as Environmental Health Training Coordinator for over 18 years. He served as an appointed member on the state of California's Registered Environmental Health Specialists Committee for nine years. He has served as a subject matter expert for several national certification examinations. Dr. Gomez has also taught at various universities, including CSULA, UCLA SPH, and CSUDH, for over 22 years. Presently, he is a professor at Touro University International.

Larry Gordon, M.S., M.P.H.

Mr. Gordon has been an adjunct professor at the University of New Mexico since 1988. Previously he was the New Mexico Cabinet Secretary for Health and Environment; Deputy Secretary for Health and Environment; State Health Officer; New Mexico Scientific Laboratory System Director; Albuquerque-Bernalillo County Environmental Health Department Director; and a Commissioned Officer in the U.S. Public Health Service.

He has served as president of the American Public Health Association; chair of the National Conference of Local Environmental Health Administrators; and president of the New Mexico Public Health Association. He was a founding member of the Council on Education for Public Health and has been a member of the National Environmental Health Science and Protection Accreditation Council.

A few of the numerous honors and awards he has received are: Sedgwich Award, from American Public Health Association, 1987; Wagner Award, from American Academy of Sanitarians, 1984; Snyder Award, from National Environmental Health Association, 1978; and Mangold Award, from National Environmental Health Association, 1961.

Gordon planned and gained legislative authorization to create the Albuquerque-Bernalillo County Environmental Health Department (the nation's *first* local environmental health department), the New Mexico Scientific Laboratory System, the New Mexico Scientific Laboratory System, and the New Mexico State Health Agency. He also has contributed to enactment of numerous state and local environmental health and protection laws. He earned an M.S. at University of New Mexico, and an M.P.H. at the University of Michigan School of Public Health. He has written more than 225 publications.

Carolyn Hester Harvey, Ph.D., C.H.M.M.

Dr. Harvey is currently an associate professor of Environmental/Occupational Health at Eastern Kentucky University, Richmond, Kentucky. A native of Harriman, Tennessee, she earned her B.S. in Microbiology at East Tennessee State University, a Master of Science in Environmental Management from University of Houston/Clear Lake, and her Ph.D. in Occupational/Environmental Health from University of Texas School of Public Health, Houston, Texas. Before becoming a college professor at East Tennessee State University, Dr. Harvey worked in the environmental/occupational health field for over 29 years. She has been a college professor since 1996. At present she serves as the president-elect of the Association of Environmental Health Academic Programs.

Albert F. Iglar, Ph.D., M.P.H.

Dr. Iglar holds a B.S. degree in Chemical Engineering and is a Registered Professional Engineer. After undergraduate study, he was employed in water-related programs by the Pennsylvania Department of Health. He obtained M.P.H. and Ph.D. degrees from the University of Minnesota, where he also was a research fellow. Beginning in 1970, he was a professor at East Tennessee State University, but now is retired. His academic efforts included the direction of many M.S.E.H. theses. Among diverse professional contributions he has focused on radiological health and hazardous waste management.

Maurice Knuckles, Ph.D., M.S.P.H.

Dr. Maurice Knuckles received his B.S.E.H. degree from East Tennessee State University, his M.S.P.H. from UNC Chapel Hill, and his Ph.D. from the University of Alabama, Birmingham. After receiving his B.S.E.H. degree he worked as an environmentalist in the newly developed Soul City, North Carolina. After receiving his Ph.D. he taught toxicology at Meharry Medical College in Nashville, Tennessee. Recently he was employed in the Washington, D.C., Department of Public Health.

R. Steven Konkel, Ph.D., AICP

Dr. Konkel was born in Denver, Colorado. After graduating from the University of Colorado, Boulder, in 1972, he earned a master's degree in City Planning from Harvard University's Graduate School of Design. He then worked in Portland, Maine, on projects to clean up Maine's lakes and ponds and to evaluate proposals for electricity generation, including environmental impact assessments on the Dickey-Lincoln School hydroelectric project and a proposed Sears Island nuclear power plant. Later he moved to Tennessee, where he was hired as a Cost-Benefit Analyst in the Energy Division at Oak Ridge National Laboratory. From 1980 to 1984 he served in the Office of the Governor, state of Alaska and had oversight responsibilities involving rural energy conservation programs and renewable energy R&D programs— including wind generators.

In 1985 Steve began his doctoral work, culminating in the award of a Ph.D. in Urban and Environmental Planning & Policy by the Massachusetts Institute of Technology.

In 1998 Dr. Konkel was hired in a tenure-track position as an assistant professor in Environmental Health Science at Eastern Kentucky University in Richmond, Kentucky, on to program coordinator of the Master of Public Health—Option in Environmental Health. He has over 25 years of experience in the field of environmental health planning, environmental regulation and policy, and decision making. He is a certified mediator and member of the American Institute of Certified Planners (AICP) of the American Planning Association and editor of the *Chronicle of the Association of Environmental Health Academic Programs* (AEHAP). He has published several recent articles in the *Occupational Health and Safety Magazine* and he has co-authored many articles with Professor Joe Beck.

David McSwane, H.S.D., M.P.H.

Dr. David McSwane is an associate professor in the School of Public and Environmental Affairs at Indiana University—Purdue University at Indianapolis. Dr. McSwane has published numerous articles in peer-reviewed journals in the fields of environmental health, food protection, and public health. He is co-author of *Essentials of Food Safety and Sanitation.* Dr. McSwane also created a drinking water handbook for the public officials. Prior to joining the faculty and Indiana University, Dr. McSwane was a Public Health Sanitarian and Administrator of the Monroe County Health Department in Bloomington Indiana. Since joining the public health profession in 1970, Dr. McSwane has served as president of the Indiana Environmental Health Association and the Indiana Public Health Association. Dr. McSwane is a Registered Environmental Health Specialist, a Certified Food Safety Professional, and a Diplomate of the American Academy of Sanitarians. Dr. McSwane's professional achievements have been recognized through such honors as the Walter S. Mangold Award presented by the National Environmental Health Association, the W. George Pinnel Award, the Tony and Mary Hulman George Achievement Award, and the American Cancer Society's St. George Medal.

Burton R. Ogle, Ph.D., M.S.E.H., C.I.H., C.S.P.

Dr. Ogle is an Assistant Professor in the Department of Environmental Health Sciences, Western Carolina University. He received a B.S. degree from the University of Tennessee, an M.S.E.H. degree from East Tennessee State University, and a Ph.D. from Virginia Commonwealth University. Over the past 19 years, he has been involved with occupational health and safety as a manager, industrial hygienist, and teacher. He has held a number of positions including OSHA inspector and OSHA consultant for the Virginia Occupational Safety and Health program; Environmental Health Specialist for the Fairfax County school system, Fairfax Virginia; institutional biohazard officer and chemical hygiene officer for Virginia Commonwealth University; and a variety of industrial hygiene consultation experiences.

Dr. Ogle served as a member of the Richmond Emergency Planning Commission and other regional committees for emergency preparedness. He provided on-call assistance for the Medical College of Virginia Hospitals chemical emergency response program. He has been an active member of the American Industrial Hygiene Association, serving on committees for toxicology and confined space entry.

Welford C. Roberts, Ph.D., M.S., D.A.A.S., R.S., R.E.H.S.

Dr. Welford C. Roberts is a native of Philadelphia, Pennsylvania. At Hampton University (Virginia) he obtained Bachelor and Master of Science degrees in Biology. He holds a Ph.D. in Environmental Health, with an emphasis in Occupational Health and Industrial Toxicology, from the University of South Carolina Norman J. Arnold School of Public Health. Dr. Roberts currently is an assistant professor in the Division of Environmental and Occupational Health, Department of Preventative Medicine and Biometrics, at the Uniformed Services University of the Health Sciences (USUHS) and the F. Edward Hebert School of Medicine, Bethesda, Maryland. He serves as an Environmental Health and Toxicology Consultant and Research Investigator for the Environmental and Occupation Health Center, USUHSs Centers for Preventive Medicine. He is a co-director and lecturer for graduate courses in Environmental Health Sciences for Master (M.P.H., M.S.P.H.) and Doctoral (Dr.P.H., Ph.D.) level degree programs, and a co-director of the Environmental Health Postgraduate Training Program.

Dr. Roberts served as an Environment Science Officer with the U.S. Army where he was awarded the U.S. Army Surgeon General's highest professional designation for the specialty and other awards including the Defense Meritorious Service Medal, two Meritorious Service Medals, three Army Commendation Medals, the Army Achievement Medal, the Army Service Ribbon, the Overseas Service Ribbon and numerous certificates of achievement.

Dr. Roberts is the technical section chairman for Emerging Diseases, Vector Control, and Zoonotic Diseases for the National Environmental Health Association. He also is the chairman of the National Environmental Health Association and Underwriters Laboratory Indoor Air Quality Committee. He has authored or co-authored more than 75 professional environmental health publications, and co-edited two books.

About the Authors

INDEX

Swimming pools (*continued*)
   drownings and, 240
   fill and draw, 84
   filtration systems for, 86–88
   flow-through, 84–85
   parts of, 89–90
   pH of, 85
   recirculatory, 85
   skimmers for, 86
Sylvatic rodents, 142–143
Synanthropic flies, 145–146

Tattoo facilities, environmental health in, 227
Technology, health and, 14
Temperature
   extremes in, as physical hazard, 278
   recommended levels for, 211
   requirements for microorganisms, 16
Temperature pressure relief (TPR) valve, 210
Tenement Housing Act of 1867, 204–205
Tenement Housing Act of 1901, 205–206
Termite shields, 209
Therapeutic pools, 91. *See also* Pools
   chlorine and chlorination of, 91
Thermal energy, 232
Thermal inversion, 249
Thermal Plasma technology, 130–131
Thermodynamic and equilibrium modeling, 157
Thermophilic microbes, 16
Thrackrah, Charles, 264
33/50 program, EPA, 296–297
Threshold dose, 154
Threshold limit values (TLVs), 279–280
Ticks, 42–44, 142, 148–149
Toxic effects, 279
Toxic materials, 17
Toxicology
   defined, 151–152
   industrial, 278–280
   resources for, 158–159
Toxic Substances Control Act (TSCA) of 1976, 324
Toxin-mediated infections, 175–176
Toxins, food-borne diseases and, 190–192
Train, Russell, 29
Trampolines, 202
Transovarian transmission, 148
Transportation safety, 242–245
Transstadial transmission, 148
Travel sanitation, 15
Trihalomenthanes (THMs), 66
Tuberculosis, 5, 34
Tumbler, 143
Turbidity, 62
Turbine well pumps, 59
Typhoid fever, 5, 30–31
Typhus, 5, 149
Typhus fever, 40

Ultraviolet light (UV), 200–201
Ultraviolet radiation, 19, 30
Undertow, 84
Undulant fever (brucellosis), 37–38
Unintentional injuries, 232
Unitary materials, for playgrounds, 95
United Nations Environment Program, 259
United Nations Fund for Population Activities, 7
United Stated Public Health Service (USPHS), 264, 269
U.S. Consumer Product Safety Commission (CPSC), 93, 95
United States Council for Automotive Research (USCAR), 119
U.S. Department of Agriculture, 269–270
Universal precautions, 225–226
Unknown, as disease agent, 19–20
Urbanization, 7, 8
Urban planning, 290
U traps. *See* P traps

Vapors, 273
Vectors, 137
Veiller, Lawrence, 205
Ventilation, 211–212
   indoor carbon monoxide levels and, 218
Venturi meter, 109
Vibrio cholerae, 181
Vibrio parahaemolyticus, 181–182
Vibrio vulnificus, 182–183
Viruses, 18–19
   Black Creek Canal, 142
   of food-borne diseases, 185–187
   Hepatitis A virus, 185–186
   Norwalk, 186–187
   occupational diseases and, 270
   rabies, 5, 30, 36–37
Vitamin K, 141–142
Volatile organic compounds (VOCs), 219–220
Voluntary Protection Program (VPP), 293

Wading pools, 91. *See also* Pools
   chlorine and chlorination of, 91
   pH of, 91
Warfarin, 141
Waste. *See also* Hazardous waste; Solid waste
   human, 100–101
   industrial, 99
   radioactive, 170
Waste-to-energy (WTE) technology, 123
Wastewater. *See also* Water
   municipal treatment systems for, 108–113
   non-water-carried systems for, 101–102
   stabilization ponds for, 112–113
   treatment of, 100–101
   water-carried systems for, 102–107

Water, 51. *See also* Wastewater
   chemicals in, 62
   conservation of, 73
   consumption of, 72–73
   distribution, 62–64
   ground, 53–54
   hardness, 62
   hazardous chemicals in, 61
   microorganisms in, 51
   municipal distribution systems, 64–66
   national primary regulations for, 67–71
   national secondary regulations for, 66, 72
   natural bathing, 84
   physical parameters of, 62
   potable, 52
   protecting supplies of, 60–61
   recreation, 83–92
   surface, 53
   surface supplies of, 54–56
   treatment process for, 65
   world population and, 73–74
Waterborne diseases, 51–53
Water-carried wastewater systems, 102–107
Water heaters, 210
Water pollution, 99
Water pollution control, 15
Water quality management, 14
Water tables, 57
Weiel's disease (leptospirosis), 39
Wells. *See also* Groundwater
   bored, 59
   community water systems and, 72
   contamination and, 57
   drilled, 59–60
   driven, 59
   dug, 58–59
   testing water quality of, 661
West Nile Fever, 49, 145
Wetlands, preservation of, 78
Whooping cough, 35
Wiesel, Elie, 24
Winter recreation, 79–82
Winter white-outs, 81
World Health Organization, 73
World Meteorological Organization, 259
Worms, parasitic, 188–190
Wriggler, 143

Xenobiotics, 151
X-rays, 15, 163–164

Years of potential life lost (YPLL), 232
Yellow fever, 2, 5, 41

Zero population growth, 7
Zoning regulations, 207–208, 290
Zoonoses, 36–40

Photo Credits

Chapter 2
p. 21, © PhotoDisc

Chapter 3
p. 29, © Digital Vision
p. 32, © Digital Vision

Chapter 5
p. 82, © PhotoDisc
p. 83, Joanne Saliger
p. 93, © PhotoDisc

Chapter 6
p. 100, photo courtesy of East Tennessee State University
p. 101, photo courtesy of East Tennessee State University

Chapter 7
p. 117, Dr. Monroe T. Morgan

Chapter 12
p. 200, Joe Beck
p. 214, Dr. Monroe T. Morgan
p. 218, John Crawley

Chapter 14
p. 260, both photos by Fred Milenovich